Residential Facilities for the Mentally Retarded

Modern Applications of Psychology
under the editorship of
Joseph D. Matarazzo
UNIVERSITY OF OREGON MEDICAL SCHOOL

Residential Facilities for the Mentally Retarded

ALFRED A. BAUMEISTER

University of Alabama

and

EARL BUTTERFIELD

University of Kansas Medical Center

ALDINE PUBLISHING COMPANY

Chicago

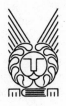

This book is dedicated to the
memory of our colleague
Harvey F. Dingman
1925–1969

First published 1970 by
Aldine Publishing Company
529 South Wabash Avenue
Chicago, Illinois 60605

Library of Congress Catalog Card Number 72–91724
SBN 202–26016–x
Printed in the United States of America

Preface

During the little more than a century of its fitful being the American residential institution has become our society's primary solution to the problem of mental retardation. Since its tentative beginning as a small "experimental" school, it has grown into a vast and perplexing complex that critically affects the lives of thousands upon thousands of people.

Originally the institution for the retarded was lauded as inspired. More recently it has been maligned as a living hell. In the larger picture, it is neither. Like any social institution, it can only be construed as "good" or "bad" in relation to society's values. Values change and, consequently, so do our definitions of problems and approaches to managing them. If the retarded have at various times been regarded as sinful or sick, repugnant or pitiful, menacing or mindless, indeed they were. What is today just and good institutional practice may tomorrow be evil and bad.

A new set of attitudes toward the mentally retarded is in the making. Perhaps the most fundamental manifestation of the emerging view is the belief that the retarded person is a genuine member of our society with a valid and equal claim to all its privileges, resources, and, indeed, even its adversities. The residential institution is now damned by some because it has not kept pace with the public spirit. But it will change in response to that spirit.

In this book we interpret the institution as a part of the culture which it serves. We have tried to avoid the emotional responses that have characterized much of the recent discussion concerning institutions. We do suggest changes for conditions we find deplorable. Indeed, the purpose of this book is to stimulate meaningful alterations in the fabric of the institution and in its interaction with the community. But we have tried to ground our suggestions in the sciences and technologies that contribute to our understanding of mental retardation and to recognize that institutional administrators, even more than society in general, wish to serve the retarded in the best possible way.

We examine, in detail, all of the institution's major facets—its history, its organization, its programs, its goals, and its prospects. We have tried to produce a comprehensive picture of the institution: what it is and what it might reasonably be. Each author was encouraged to couch his views within their major historical perspectives. The reader will note that many of the views expressed within this book derive from the same antecedents. In this manner we hope that we have reliably identified the most significant historical and conceptual developments that have shaped and continue to affect the course of the residential facility.

We have tried to produce a "handbook" of residential institutions for workers and students in the field of mental retardation. It is written from the perspective of many disciplines and reflects a wide array of conceptions, special interests, problems, and objectives that make up the very complex character of institutions. Inevitably, certain areas of interest have been emphasized more than others, but we hope that there are no critical omissions. We have endeavored to deal with all areas that seem relevant to the welfare of the residents of institutions.

Contents

Preface   v

1   The American Residential Institution: Its History and Character, *Alfred A. Baumeister*   1

2   Evolutionary Changes of the Residential Facility, *Philip Roos*   29

3   Planning a Residential Facility for the Mentally Retarded, *James D. Clements*   59

4   Statistics in Institutions for the Mentally Retarded, *Harvey F. Dingman and Richard K. Eyman*   117

5   Dimensions of Institutional Life: Social Organization, Possessions, Time and Space, *Charles C. Cleland and Harvey F. Dingman*   138

6   Institutional Programming and Research: A Vital Partnership in Action, *Michael Klaber*   163

7   Behavior Modification of Residents and Personnel in Institutions for the Mentally Retarded, *Luke S. Watson, Jr.*   199

8   Functions and Problems of Social Workers in Institutions for the Mentally Retarded, *James E. Payne*   246

9   Education of the Mentally Retarded in Residential Settings, *C. Milton Blue*   272

10   Medical Services in Institutions for the Mentally Retarded, *James D. Clements*   315

11   Residential Speech and Hearing Services, *C. Milton Blue and F. G. Sumner*   326

12   Adjunctive Therapy in Residential Institutions for the Mentally Retarded, *Neland C. Hibbett*   357

13   Psychological Services in the Institution, *R. L. Forehand, T. Mulhern, and D. A. Gordon*   373

Index   397

Contributors

Alfred A. Baumeister
Professor of Psychology and Director of the Center for Developmental
  and Learning Disorders
University of Alabama

C. Milton Blue
Professor of Special Education
Division of Exceptional Children
University of Georgia

Earl Butterfield
Research Associate and Associate Professor
The University of Kansas Medical Center

Charles C. Cleland
Professor of Educational Psychology and Special Education
The University of Texas

James D. Clements
Director, Georgia Retardation Center

Harvey F. Dingman
Associate Professor of Educational Psychology
University of Texas

Richard K. Eyman
Chief of Research
Pacific State Hospital
Assistant Research Psychologist and Research Associate
University of California at Los Angeles

Rex Lloyd Forehand
Department of Psychology
University of Alabama

Donald A. Gordon
Department of Psychology
University of Alabama

Neland C. Hibbett, Jr.
Director of Adjunctive Therapy
Clover Bottom Hospital and School

M. Michael Klaber
Professor of Educational Psychology
University of Hartford

Tom Mulhern
Department of Psychology
University of Alabama

James E. Payne
Assistant Professor
Graduate School of Social Work
University of Texas

Philip Roos
Executive Director
National Association for Retarded Children

F. G. Sumner
Department of Speech Pathology
University of Georgia

Luke S. Watson, Jr.
Columbus State Institute

The American Residential Institution: Its History and Character

The institution for the mentally retarded is an invention of modern times. So too, for that matter, is mental retardation.

Deviance, of course, has existed since the beginning of human history. Variability is inherent in nature, human or otherwise. There must always have been some people who were noticeably less adequate than others. The Greeks called them *idiots,* and the Romans labeled them *morons.* However, very little seems to have been said by early writers about mental retardation as a behavioral concept. Rather, references were made to a variety of neurologic and emotional disorders, some of which were accompanied by gross behavioral impairment.

References to mental deficiency appeared first in literary or religious contexts rather than in scientific works. Substantial and systematic discussion of retardation has appeared only comparatively recently in the scientific literature. Viewed from today's perspective, the treatment accorded mentally defective individuals has had, in spite of a few occasional bright spots, a generally sordid history. Even today we emphasize how the retarded are different, not how they are similar. Deprived of ordinary rights and privileges, misunderstood and scorned, they were more often than not treated inhumanely. In ancient Rome, for example, the wealthy often kept "fools" for amusement. This practice apparently continued for many centuries, reaching its greatest respectability in the courts of medieval nobility (Horsfield,

1

1940). Generally these jesters were mental defectives with unusual physical anomalies, and they fared poorly, though a few achieved fame and distinction.

Although religious teachings usually have advocated compassion for the unfortunate, the period of Protestant Reformation in Europe lent, for a time, a peculiar religious significance to deviant behavior. People who behaved oddly were, according to the teaching of Luther and Calvin, possessed by the Devil, "a mass of flesh . . . with no soul." Lacking souls, the odd were often treated harshly. Paradoxically, during this period it was the churches that provided a sanctuary for many handicapped persons, including mental defectives.

In more recent times societies have had to make special provisions for dealing with the retarded. With the rapid and dynamic growth of highly technological cultures, there have been increasing numbers of individuals who cannot adapt sufficiently to their environment. Thus while retardation as a concept must be as old as man himself, as a problem of major social and economic dimensions it is largely a product of the modern world.

Beginnings of Institutional Care in Europe

Credit for the first successfully established training school for mental defectives is usually accorded to Edward Seguin, who began his private school in Paris in 1837. The school was expressly established to put into practice the techniques of "physiological education" first developed by Itard and later extended and elaborated by Seguin in his book, *Theory and Practice of the Education of Idiots,* published in 1842. A subsequent work, *The Moral Treatment, Hygiene, and Education of Idiots and other Backward Children* (1848), became a classic landmark in the field of mental deficiency. These, together with a third book (1866), provided the scientific, philosophical, and social rationale that guided the establishment of institutions in the United States for about fifty years.

Actually, the significance of Seguin's work lies not so much in the fact that he probably founded the first permanent school for the retarded, but rather that in the field of mental retardation his work was a practical culmination of sensationalist philosophy, nineteenth-century humanitarianism, and the scientific method. The influence of these converging trends on the initial development of institutions in this country, and, indeed, upon our conceptions of mental retardation, would be difficult to exaggerate.

Seguin had a faith in the pliability of human behavior. He did not regard feeblemindedness as an irremedial defect, but rather as a product of a weakened nervous system that "removed the organs and faculties of the child from the will." The child, thus cut off from the moral world, could act only on instinct. The objective of Seguin's training regimen was to establish contact with the environment, first by systematically training the senses and muscles. Then he worked the child through an orderly progression from simple to complex activities, from concrete to abstract notions, and from instinctual to moral control. The theory was that the nervous system, awakened and developed, would bring behavior under control of the will and, consequently, of the moral world.

In practice the physiological method was an elaborate system of sensory-motor activities that varied from exceedingly simple and rudimentary muscular activities to complex vocational and social skills. The underlying principle of the physiological method derived from the natural law of action and repose—that is, each function is called into action and then to rest. Imitation was the major teaching technique. Reflecting the prevailing sensationalist philosophy, Seguin placed great stress on the development of the basic sensory modalities, particularly touch.

The physiological method was widely hailed a century ago. In 1844 the Paris Academy of Science officially declared that Seguin had solved the problem of idiot education. Seguin's techniques provided the impetus to the organization of training programs in numerous countries, including the United States. Most of the first institutions in this country were founded expressly to "treat" mental deficiency by the application of Seguin's methods. The techniques are still employed by institutions, particularly in the form of sensory training. But, by and large, the system of education envisioned by Seguin has little direct effect on current practice. His system is significant because it provided the technical rationale for the founding of institutions for the feebleminded. Unfortunately, these early residential facilities, founded on such a positive and optimistic basis, were to result in disillusionment and despair.

Another aspect of Seguin's views markedly affected prevailing attitudes in this country during the latter portion of the nineteenth century. As Kraft has observed (1961), Seguin's theories regarding *moral treatment* may ultimately be more influential than his contribution to the physical aspects of therapeutic education. To be sure, the time was right for humanitarian concern. Pinel, for instance, as early as 1880 had removed the inmates of Bicetre from their chains. Morel, too, had advocated (1842) psychotherapy in the place of extreme and harsh methods of treatment. But it was Seguin who translated the concept of moral treatment into a practical concept.

By "moral" education, Seguin meant that the mental defective, regardless of the reasons for his backwardness, was entitled to be treated with dignity, warmth, and kindness and with the best skills and resources available. The basic element in this concept was reliance on a spirit of love and on the exercise of the will of the teacher. As Seguin indicated, the goal of his system was to make "the child feel that he is loved, and to make him eager to love in his turn." It should be stressed that Seguin was talking about children who are not very lovable. In this prescription for the education of idiots, it is obvious that the institution would require services of a patient, dedicated, and skilled staff. Apparently this influence was keenly felt by those men who were responsible for the institutional movement in this country. If one may take statements made by the first superintendents at face value, their institutions were indeed founded and operated in a larger spirit of benevolence, enthusiasm, patience, and democracy than most of those which were to follow.

In addition to his influential books, Seguin contributed to the development of American institutions by actively advising in their organization. When political events became unbearable to him in France following the Revolution of 1848, he emigrated to the United States (1850). At the request of Samuel Howe, Seguin spent his first months in this country assisting in the organization of the Massachusetts School for the Feebleminded. He also actively assisted in organizing schools in New York, Ohio, Connecticut, and Pennsylvania. For a time he was head of a public institution in Philadelphia and later founded a private school in New York City in 1880, the year of his death. In addition to his involvement in institutional work in this country, Seguin published his widely read book (1866) *Idiocy and its Treatment by the Physiological Method* and served as the first President of the Association of Medical Officers of American Institutions for Idiotic and Feebleminded Persons (1876).

Early Provisions in the United States

During the Colonial Period, the first public provisions for the feebleminded came in the form of statutes designed to allow officials to take certain necessary actions to deal with individual cases that came to attention. Maryland, in 1650, apparently was the first colony to pass a law authorizing the appointment of special guardians of feebleminded children. By the time of the Revolution, a number of colonies had made funds available to certain individuals in the community who would care for feebleminded children. In some cases, the feebleminded, along with paupers and other deviants, were auctioned to the highest bidder who was allowed to use them for manual labor in return for caring for them (Deutsch, 1949). Apparently, the first state to make a general provision of this type was Kentucky, where in 1793 a "pauper idiot law" was enacted which allowed a subsidy to families with feeble-minded individuals (Best, 1965).

However, few systematic approaches to the problem of feeblemindedness were attempted before 1850. For the most part, the feebleminded were a neglected lot. To the extent that any form of public residential provision was made, the feebleminded were found in alms houses, incarcerated in jails, and confined to insane asylums. In no instance does there seem to have been attention given to remediation or rehabilitation.

Actually, it appears that the mentally deficient were among the last of the deviant individuals to arouse constructive public interest in this country. Provisions had already been organized for the blind, deaf, and insane. If services for these individuals were not widespread before 1850, at least they were well established in principle. Possibly, what was needed was some sort of evidence that something positive and constructive could be done for the mentally defective. Thus, the much heralded work of Seguin in France and Guggenbuhl in Austria, stressing the treatment of mental deficiency, created an impression that constructive educational programs could be devised for the feebleminded.

It was not long after the establishment of permanent residential schools in Europe that the first such facility was founded in the United States. By 1850, a number of Americans had suggested that special schools be created to care for, protect, and treat the feebleminded. In 1845 the superintendents of the institutions for the insane in the states of Massachusetts and New York had indicated that special schools were needed for the feebleminded (Best, 1965). Apparently, the first formal effort to seek public provisions for the mentally defective was made by Dr. F. F. Backus who, on March 25, 1846, introduced a bill in the state legislature of New York for the establishment of an asylum for idiots. The bill survived the Senate but was defeated in the House. In spite of considerable public and personal pressures and strong encouragement from the governor, the Legislature refused to pass a bill for the establishment of a state institution. It was not until 1851 that New York provided money for its first public institution for defectives.

Credit for the enactment of the first legislation making provision for a public facility for defectives goes to the state of Massachusetts. In April of 1846 the general court of the commonwealth of Massachusetts passed into a law a bill requiring the governor to appoint a commission "to inquire into the condition of the idiots of the commonwealth, to ascertain their number, and whether anything could be done for their relief." Dr. Samuel G. Howe, director of the Perkins Institute and Massachusetts School for the Blind, was chosen to head the commission.

Howe's capacity for becoming involved in various social causes seems to have been limitless. Among his various causes were the blind, the deaf, the slaves, and the politically oppressed of various nations of Europe, as well as the mental defective. Howe was familiar with the developments in Europe, having visited Guggenbuhl's Abendberg and probably with Seguin in France. It is certain that he was an admirer of Seguin and had a great deal to do with Seguin's eventual emigration to this country.

The commission submitted its report, written mostly by Howe, to the Massachusetts legislature in 1848. This report is remarkable not only because of its thoroughness in its analysis of the extent and causes of mental deficiency, but also in its eloquent appeal for compassion, understanding, and action. He asked of Massachusetts ". . . Will she longer neglect the poor idiots—the most wretched of all who are born to her—those who are usually abandoned by their fellows—who can never, of themselves, step upon the platform of humanity—will she leave them to their dreadful fate, to a life of brutishness, without an effort in their behalf?" About the defective he said, " . . . there is not one of any age who may not be made more of a man and less of a brute by patience and kindness directed by energy and skill." It is indeed unfortunate that the movement inspired by this visionary report was soon to produce "hospitals" and "schools" whose effects were quite often the opposite of the goals set forth by Howe.

The Massachusetts legislature cautiously responded to this appeal by providing $2,500 per annum to establish an "experimental" school. On October 1, 1848, the first permanent institution in the United States was opened. Ten feebleminded children were placed together in a wing of Perkins Institute under the guidance of James J. Richards, a teacher.

Three years later, having decided that its experiment was successful, the Massachusetts legislature passed a law which incorporated Howe's school, giving it the name of Massachusetts' School for Idiotic and Feebleminded Youth. In 1855 the school was moved to a new site in south Boston and in 1887 was finally moved to its present location in Waltham. At that time it was renamed the Walter E. Fernald State School, in honor of its influential superintendent.

A number of the first public institutions apparently began as private schools. James Richards, after working with Howe for a period, opened a private institution at Philadelphia in 1852, the Elwyn Training School, which became one of the most well known and influential private institutions in the United States. His school attracted considerable attention and sympathy throughout Pennsylvania. Following the efforts of several prominent individuals, the state appropriated $10,000 to assist in maintaining the school. It has remained a private institution but is subsidized by the state.

The first institution in Connecticut (1858) also began as a private enterprise, but with state aid. This institution was taken over by the state in 1861. A source of a number of innovations, this school existed until 1917 when Connecticut opened the Mansfield Training School.

The founders of the first residential institutions set forth as their purpose the treatment of mental deficiency with a view toward returning them to the community—a community, to be sure, less complex than today's. The early literature is replete with statements reflecting an uncritical and overriding faith in the efficacy of the physiological method. Mental deficiency was regarded basically as a lag of the development of intelligence. With proper diligence and skill, the mind could be trained. Indeed, Seguin even noted that the effects of education demonstrated an enlargement of the cranium. Seguin, reflecting on his long experience, said, "Idiots have been improved, educated, and even cured. Not one in a thousand has been entirely refractory to treatment." However, in fairness, it should also be stated that some of these men were aware that even hope has its rational limits. Wilbur, for example, wrote: "We do not propose to create or supply faculties absolutely wanting . . ."

Writing in his first report as superintendent of the institution at Syracuse, Wilbur represented the views of most superintendents of his day: "At the basis of all our efforts lies the principle that the human attributes of intelligence, sensitivity, and will, are not absolutely wanting in an idiot, but dormant and undeveloped." Howe pleaded that the new schools be regarded as educational institutions rather than asylums. The term *asylum* was in particular disfavor, for it carried the implication of a custodial function. In fact, most of these schools made no provision for permanent custody. A concerted effort was made to impress upon the public that these new institutions were *schools* charged with the same responsibilities as other schools in the community—a link in the chain of the common school system.

Moreover, there were many favorable (and probably exaggerated) reports of the wonders that the early institutions worked upon their students. The "experimental school" in Massachusetts declared that it was entirely successful and that the "popular air that idiocy is a positive incurable malady had been disproved. . . . " In one report after another, in state after state, the conviction was expressed, often in glowing language, that access had been found to the idiotic brain. One report, representative in sentiment, waxed so eloquently that it is worth citing: "Some of our little ones imprisoned in the gloom of imbecility have been liberated from darkness and sorrow to possess a share of light and gladness, such as they have never known before."

Lest one condemn these writers for being carried away with their enthusiasm and even euphoria, it should be recalled that sometimes they had to convince a skeptical citizenry and often recalcitrant legislature that their work was worthy of public support. Furthermore, as Best (1965) has observed, this was, in many ways, an age of professional altruism in America. Not only the feebleminded, but all classes of defective individuals, became the object of concern and sympathy, at least among the professionals. Best describes the prevailing attitude in this way: "Probably the world has never known, before or since, such a pouring out of sympathy for the afflicted of society, a more zealous resolve to speed to their relief, nor a more ornate faith in the possibilities of education." (p. 185). Altruism may have been the mother of excess—for their claims were indeed excessive. Clearly, the statistics show that, even by today's standards, much was accomplished in behalf of the retardate. But the accomplishment could not match the hope. For this, and for other reasons, the pendulum was in its back swing by the turn of the century and the institution moved into a much darker and forlorn era from which we are only now beginning to emerge. Within fifty years after the founding of the first institution in New England, opinion on the role of the institution in American society had almost reversed. Whereas formerly the concern was with helping the defective, the goal soon became to protect society.

Acceptance of the institutions by the general public was something short of overwhelming. Indeed, growth of the institutional concept often proceeded in the face of considerable skepticism, if not outright opposition both from the general public and from state legislatures. Many people were convinced that not much, if anything, could be done to benefit the feebleminded. Consequently, the large expenditures of funds might well be put to more constructive purposes. In 1857 the governor of Massachusetts justified his veto of a bill for increases for state allocations for Howe's institution by reasoning that it was a "reversal of the law of survival of the fittest, to attempt the education of the feebleminded, an asylum being best for them." He went on to express the sentiment that would certainly find its modern advocates: "When the state shall have sufficiently educated every bright child within its borders, it will be time enough to undertake the education of idiots and feebleminded children." An official summation of public opinion concerning mental defectives in Connecticut in 1856 reported that most people considered idiots so utterly hopeless that it was a waste of time even to try to collect statistics regarding them (Best, 1965). This attitude was widespread and was encountered without exception by those who championed the educational institution. Even after the institutions had been established in many states, efforts were made to close them, succeeding briefly in Kentucky.

Feelings of aversion and revulsion and fear were and still are often conjured up in relation to the mental defective. (Curiously, when these feelings are given to expression they are often couched in an even more degrading form of pity.) If many people were suspicious that feeblemindedness was connected to criminality, pauperism, perversion, and degeneracy, their worst fears were confirmed by the early eugenists. It is no accident that so many institutions were located in the countryside out of sight.

In spite of the abounding faith and enthusiasm diplayed by many of the earlier workers in this field, the construction of residential institutions did not proceed at a "break-neck" pace. Indeed, these facilities were built at a much faster rate when they were regarded as custodial rather than educational.

The first institutions, by modern standards, were quite modest enterprises. They had relatively few students and tended to accept only those who offered a reasonable prognosis of response to treatment. These schools were frankly regarded as educational institutions (see Chapter 9). It is clear that certain types of severe retardates were regarded as completely intractible and that educational efforts should be directed toward those with the prospect of being cured or, at the very least, who showed promise of considerable improvement. From the very beginning, Howe himself warned that these schools should not be made into "asylums for incurables." More than one institution followed the policy of admitting only the higher grade cases. Howe, for example, excluded epileptic, insane, and hydrocephalic children. Staff-patient ratios were usually quite high and each child was made the object of an all-out intensive treatment effort in the spirit of Seguin's physiological method. A generally enthusiastic, optimistic tone pervaded discussion of this new movement. And some professionals even complained that, in view of the demonstrated success of such schools, the public was too slow in responding with support.

However, by the 1880's, evidence was beginning to accumulate to show that many, if not most, of the early claims of success were ill-founded. The physiological method had not produced the remarkable changes in behavior that would have permitted these defectives to make a satisfactory adjustment upon return to the community. Although the early institutions were not established as permanent custodial facilities, a number of authorities were beginning to express regret that they had to return some of their students to the community unfit and unprepared. More and more frequently, mention was made of the "hopeless ones."

Out of this concern came the distinction between trainables and untrainables. But this distinction did not alter the fact that very few of the feebleminded were being "cured." The dream of the institution as an educational program began to evaporate. Those in charge of institutions came to believe that their function must be extended beyond relatively short-term training to include comprehensive care for the individual for long periods of time—even a lifetime.

In reading statements concerning the aims and goals of institutions only twenty-five years after Massachusetts organized its first school, one can readily discern a cooling of attitude concerning what might be accomplished in behalf of the feebleminded. By 1875 a trend began toward construction of more and larger institutions whose role was more frankly conceived as custodial. Part of this reaction to the mental defective can be linked to a more general aversion to all forms of deviancy. This attitude was most marked during the first quarter of the 20th century.

Leaders in the field began to press for long-term custodial care of the retarded. Barr, writing in the *Journal of Psycho-Asthenics* in 1899, expressed the new sentiment by noting that experience and indeed every consideration for the individual and society, points to the absolute necessity of permanent segregation. A year later in the same journal Johnson wrote that " . . . the proportion of feebleminded who are fit to go out from our schools to take . . . a place in the great world, with all that implies, is so small that it may be safely disregarded in adopting a policy." Johnson was so disappointed in the prospects of any meaningful outcome from education programs for defectives that he was moved to declare, somewhat melodramatically, that "They must be kept quietly, safely, away from the world, living like the angels in Heaven, neither marrying nor given in marriage." Literally dozens of such expressions can be found in the literature after 1875. It is remarkable what a pronounced change in attitude the first quarter of a century of institutional experience produced.

By 1875 a number of states began to plan and build custodial institutions. In 1878 New York opened a facility at Newark for custodial care for deficient women. (Female defectives were often feared more than males.) Even the names of the new institutions reflected the change in philosophy. For example, in 1894 New York constructed the Rome State Custodial Asylum for low-grade and delinquent individuals.

With the abandonment of the concept of cure, the nature of the institution, both in service and in its physical plant, began to change. By the end of the 19th century the now familiar large isolated residential institution, with well diversified buildings, with a highly organized custodial staff, with its own social structure began to emerge. As someone recently observed to the effect: "Institutions were built to last forever, and, unfortunately, they did." "Villages of the simple," Kerlin called them. Only the last decade has witnessed a significant general change in the public and professional conceptions of institutional residence. And, this chapter in history is far from finished.

By and large, institutional programs originally had been motivated by the desire to protect and benefit the intellectually disadvantaged and allow them to live happily with their "own kind." At least this was the rationale usually given. However, by 1900 the emphasis began to shift from the feebleminded to society. The change in institutional philosophy accompanied a widespread concern that maybe society needed to be protected from the feeble-minded. This concern arose largely from the eugenics scare that began early in this century and is still reflected in some current practices and research studies. Attitudes toward the mental defective were also greatly affected by intelligence tests. Not only did these tests provide a rapid and systematic means of measuring intellectual capabilities, but they also revealed how extensive stupidity really was. Goddard's discovery of the "moron" was a shock from which we have yet to recover. The eugenics movement and intelligence testing together exerted a tremendous effect on the concept of institutionalization for mental defectives in this country.

The Eugenics Movement

The eugenics movement owes its original impetus to Sir Francis Galton who, if he did not invent the concept (Plato advocated a similar notion), was more articulate in advancing eugenics as a social concept than any other individual. The eugenics movement, concerned primarily with the nature and ability of man, played an important role in shaping American attitudes about the solution of social problems, and particularly the problem of mental deficiency. Eugenics is still a live issue.

Charles Davenport, one of the first American proponents of eugenics described it as " . . . the science of the improvement of the human race by better breeding (1911)." The fundamental idea is an appealingly simple one: to create a better breed of people, those with desirable traits must be encouraged to propagate. Those with undesirable traits should not propagate. Because the mental defective possesses undesirable traits he should not reproduce.

Many years before the appearance of the eugenics movement heredity had been implicated as an etiological factor in mental deficiency. Seguin, for example, had observed "the circumstances which favored the production of idiocy are endemic, hereditary, parental, or accidental." But, by and large, during these early years there was a tendency to discount heredity as a major cause. For example, the report of the Massachusetts commission prepared in 1848 found inheritance of feeblemindedness as a prime factor in only 22 per cent of the cases included in its survey. Little was understood of the mechanisms of heredity and besides, Howe, Seguin, and the others were inclined to be highly optimistic about the effects of intervention, an attitude hardly reinforced by the notion of an inborn disposition to be defective.

However, studies were not long in coming that would not only reveal the major influence of heredity in relation to mental deficiency, but would show the close connection between feeblemindedness and various forms of degeneracy. Moreover, the development of intelligence tests revealed how numerous the defectives really were. Butler's view was representative (1915): "When we view the number of the feebleminded, their fecundity, their lack of control, the menace they are, the degradation they cause, the degeneracy they perpetuate, the suffering and misery and crime they spread—these are the burden we must bear." Fernald called this burden "disgusting," and Goddard (1915) did the retardate little good by saying of the moron " . . . he is a burden to society and civilization . . . he is responsible to a large degree for many, if not all, of our social problems." That was quite an indictment—which Goddard apparently lived to regret. Goddard was not alone, for literally dozens of similar expressions appeared in the literature during this period. The studies of Dugdale, Goddard, and McCullough are too well known to be documented in detail here. These studies had a tremendous impact both on public and professional opinion. Whereas earlier little concern was given to inheritance of feeblemindedness, by 1915 the root of the problem was seen to be in defective germ plasma. Goddard (1912) stated "There is not the slighest evidence that . . . any environmental condition can produce feeblemindedness."

The "eugenics scare" of the early 20th century led to a number of measures to halt the menace of the defective to society. These measures included larger and more durable institutions designed to segregate the defective from society. A rash of sterilization laws were passed in many states, beginning with Indiana in 1907. Sterilization became closely identified with the concept of institutionalization, for the failure of eugenics measures had a great deal to do with the course of institutional development. Moreover, the great majority of such operations have been performed in institutions. In addition to the protection that sterilization presumably afforded society there were other benefits to be derived from such operations. Frequently it was observed that patients became more manageable following such an operation. Barr even cited, as one of the benefits of castration, the fact that some nice male soprano voices could be obtained for the institutional choir.

By 1926 sterilization statutes had been passed in 23 states. Many of these laws were obviously motivated by therapeutic and punitive considerations. However, sterilization practices were actually quite variable and in some states only a comparatively few operations were performed.

The courts have generally held that sterilization is unconstitutional if employed as a punitive measure, as it clearly was in some of the early statutes. However, a U.S. Supreme Court decision in 1927 upheld the Virginia sterilization law which was founded on the principle that heredity is an important etiological factor in mental pathology including feeblemindedness. Justice Holmes summed up the genesis of eugenics in his famous opinion: "Three generations of imbeciles are enough." The Virginia law subsequently was used as a model for sterilization statutes in a number of states.

The whole concept of eugenics and the accompanying issue of sterilization has undergone considerable criticism on moral, legal, and scientific grounds. What value there may have been to the family studies by Goddard and others was obscured by some of their technical and methodological naiveté and often outright absurdity. It was frequently pointed out that sterilization programs would be ineffective in reducing the incidence of mental retardation. The observation was repeatedly made that the vast proportion of inheritable mental deficiency is transmitted by individuals who are not themselves retarded and confined to institutions. If there was any justification for sterilization it had to be on grounds other than inheritance of undesirable traits. This is probably still the most prevalent view regarding sterilization. The issue, however, is far from being settled.

By far the most thorough and sophisticated longitudinal family study has been reported recently by Reed and Reed (1965). These workers, starting with the families of 289 probands who were institutionalized at the Faribault State School and Hospital during the years 1911 to 1918, obtained IQ data on over 80,000 persons. This is the largest investigation ever conducted on the effects of genetic variation on intelligence. The conclusions reached by Reed and Reed are strikingly similar to those made by earlier investigators. Some which are relevant to the issue of eugenics are presented here:

(1) The most obvious implication of these studies is that the greatest predisposing factor for the appearance of mental retardation is the presence of retardation in one or more relatives of the person concerned. (p. 72).

(2) One of the important humanitarian implications of our demonstration of the importance of the transmission of mental retardation is that a better legal basis must be provided for the voluntary sterilization of the higher grade retardates in the community. (p. 77).

(3) Few people have emphasized that where the transmission of a trait is frequently from parent to offspring, sterilization will be effective and it is irrelevant whether the basis for the trait is genetic or environmental. (p. 77).

(4) When voluntary sterilization for the retarded becomes a part of the culture of the United States, we should expect a decrease of about 50 per cent generation in the number of persons as a result of all methods combined to reduce mental retardation. (p. 78).

A final conclusion is almost straight from the eugenics handbook.

(5) . . . the intelligence of the population is increasing slowly, and that greater protection of the retarded from reproduction will augment the rate of gain. The elevation of the average intelligence is essential for the comprehension of our increasingly complicated world. (p. 79).

In spite of the heat generated by the issue of sterilization, or asexualation as it was frequently called, as a means of dealing with mental deficiency it has yet to gain widespread acceptance. While sterilization was typically rationalized on eugenics grounds, even those who were the most alarmed about the menace of the feebleminded still opposed this procedure on other bases, usually moral. In fact, some of the most effective critics of sterilization were to be found among the eugenists.

Actually, a number of recommendations have been suggested as possibly effective for controlling defective strains in the race. In 1911 the Research

Committee of the Eugenics Section of the American Breeders' Association listed nine alternatives in addition to sterilization (Davies, 1930):

1. Segregation
2. Restricted marriage laws
3. Eugenics education of the public
4. Systems of matings purporting to remove defective traits
5. General environment improvement
6. Polygamy
7. Euthanasia
8. Neo-Malthusianism
9. Laissez-faire

The Committee recommended sterilization and segregation as the most efficacious, at least immediately. Sterilization has not proven to be either very popular or very effective.

Segregation

Segregation as a means of controlling the defective in the population was widely adopted as policy for many years and had a considerable impact on the institutional movement in this country. The apparent failure of education and the ineffectiveness of eugenic recommendations left rigid segregation as the only practical way of meeting the dangers presented to society by the defective. Most leading professionals of the age raised the cry for more and larger institutions. Representative of this view is the impassioned plea by Martin Barr, one of the most highly regarded professionals of his age. As usual Barr was a few years ahead of his time when in 1902 he wrote: "I think we need to write it very large, in characters that he who runs may read, to convince the world that by permanent separation only is the imbecile to be safe-guarded from certain deterioration and society from depredation and contamination . . . " From these sentiments came the legacy with which we deal today.

In the first half of the present century:

1. The number of institutions increased.
2. Institutions grew larger.
3. Institutions became custodial rather than educational.
4. The medical model was widely adopted, with most institutions organized in terms of a "hospital" hierarchy. In fact, the trend was to label most institutions *hospitals*. At the same time, the notion that mental deficiency was incurable became the prevalent view. What was never there, could not be restored.

5. Institutions became self-sustaining and managed as economically as possible.
6. New institutions were constructed in rural areas to provide farming opportunities and to remove the defective as far as possible from the populace. (Apparently, the rule-of-thumb was one acre of land per inmate.)
7. Inmates were completely segregated by sex, age, and ability level (and, in some states, by color).
8. Institutional architecture became very distinctive, with the emphasis on highly specialized and sturdy buildings. Large dormitories were the rule, constructed with the intention of economically housing as many residents as possible.
9. The number of professionals employed became generally inadequate to carry on meaningful treatment and rehabilitation programs. Moreover, quality of professional services was typically very poor relative to other types of exceptionality. As Cleland and Peck (1967) have observed the employees also became "institutionalized."
10. Increasing emphasis was placed on the legal aspects of commitment and release.
11. The residents were dehumanized, deprived of many legal rights, frequently subjected to physical and psychological abuse and personal indignity, and their welfare generally neglected.

In effect institutions became the antithesis of what the original founders had hoped. Indeed, the very rationale had changed. Only since World War II, and particularly in the past decade, have the professional community and the public begun to question the traditional institutional model. To be sure, there were those who earlier expressed doubt about and even repudiated the direction in which the American institution headed. But they were few and their voices unheeded. By 1925, the concept of permanent segregation for all defectives was widely questioned, but there seemed to be no practical alternative. Deprived of a rationalization and caught in the economic squeeze of the depression and the War, the institution simply stagnated for a quarter of a century. Today the emphasis seems to be shifting to another of the ten remedies suggested over a half-century ago by the American Breeders' Association—namely, general environment betterment.

Community Provision

Although historically, segregation of the mental defective from the rest of society was the approach generally advocated by professionals, the emphasis has shifted in recent years to making provisions within the community for as many retarded individuals as possible. As this trend continues, it will have a profound effect upon the character of residential institutions. The most obvious and immediate consequence will be a decrease in gross ability level of the resident that will result from selective admission.

There are several reasons for the growing interest in providing public school classes for the retarded. It is less expensive to keep an individual in the community where he may achieve some degree of self-sufficiency. The effects of institutionalization are widely thought to be debilitating in themselves. The well known studies by Skeels and others have convinced many workers in the field that individuals should be kept out of institutions whenever possible. The dominant educational philosophy seems to be that the public schools should provide a wide area of experiences and services to the community to include more than solely academic preparation. The public schools have gradually become more responsive to the broad spectrum of needs within the community.

Special classes for the mentally retarded were first established in Germany around 1870. The purpose of these classes, "Hilfschule," was to prepare their pupils for return to their regular classes. France and England were not long in providing special educational programs in the public schools. Like their institutional counterparts, the special class programs were based largely upon Seguin's physiological method.

The first public school class in the United States was established in 1896 in Rhode Island (Wallin, 1966). By 1967 special classes for the mildly retarded were included in the programs of approximately half of U.S. school districts, enrolling about 590,000 pupils. Programs differ markedly in terms of organization, content, and numbers of children enrolled. Some current estimates place the number at 2,000,000 children who could benefit from some type of special class placement. Recently, more attention has been directed toward the moderately or trainable retarded with a number of states making formal distinctions for purposes of special class placement. During the 1967 school year about 90,000 children were enrolled in special classes for the trainable. Other developments within the community affecting the residential institution include day care centers, diagnostic and evaluation clinics, sheltered work-shops, vocational training centers, and an assortment of federal programs.

Population Growth of the American Institution

By 1890 approximately 20 residential schools had been established in 15 states. This represented almost every geographical area in the country. Following is a list of the first institutions by state, date of founding, and number of residents (Haskel, 1944).

Table 1–1. Institutions for the Feebleminded, 1888

State	Name	Founded	Pupils
1. Massachusetts	School for the Feebleminded	1848	230
2. New York	State Asylum for Idiots	1851	492
3. Pennsylvania	Training-School for Feebleminded Children	1853	654
4. Ohio	Institution for Feebleminded Youth	1857	824
5. Connecticut	School for Imbeciles	1858	127
6. Kentucky	Institute for the Education and Training of Feebleminded Children	1860	166
7. Illinois	Asylum for Feebleminded Children	1865	409
8. Iowa	Institution for Feebleminded Children	1877	370
9. New York	State Custodial Asylum for Feebleminded Women	1878	194
10. Indiana	School for Feebleminded Youth	1879	240
11. Minnesota	School for Feebleminded	1879	191
12. Kansas	State Asylum for Idiotic and Imbecile Youth	1881	116
13. California	Home for the Care and Training of Feebleminded Children	1885	92
14. Nebraska	Institution for Feebleminded Youth	1887	81
15. New Jersey	Home for the Education and Care of Feebleminded Children	1888	30

There followed a period of fairly rapid growth, both in terms of numbers of institutions and patients that (except during World War II) has continued until the present day.

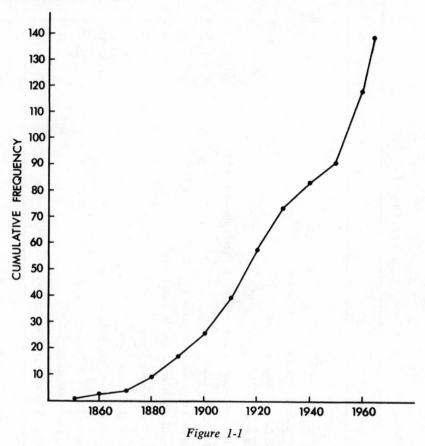

Figure 1-1

Figure 1–1 graphically displays the cumulative growth curve of public institutions. This graph indicates that the period of most rapid growth occurred in the post World War II years.

Of course, it is possible to evaluate the increase in number of institutions only in relation to the growth to the general population. Furthermore, many states, rather than building new institutions as the need arose, chose to expand existing plants. In view of these considerations, the most valid data concerning the growth of institutionalization are to be found in relative population figures. Figure 1–2 shows the increase in residential population from a few thousand in 1880 to the present level of approximately 200,000 persons.

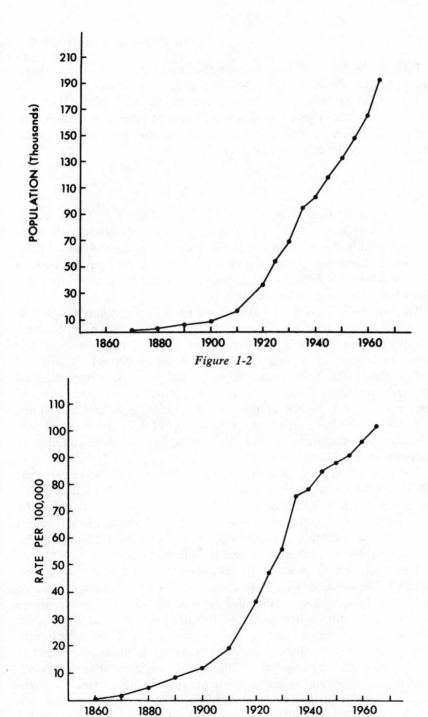

Figure 1-2

Figure 1-3

Perhaps the most revealing data are shown in Figure 1–3 which reports rate of institutionalization per 100,000 of general population.

From this last figure it can be seen that the period between 1915 and 1935 was associated with a relatively high rate of institutionalization. The two factors related to this trend were the widespread application of intelligence tests and the eugenics movement.

Current Status

According to the most recent survey (1968) conducted by the American Association on Mental Deficiency there are 167 public facilities for the mentally retarded in the 50 states and the District of Columbia. A few of these are new and had not, at the time of the survey, accepted any patients. In some instances, the facilities for the retarded were part of larger units that housed other types of patients as well.

Most of the 167 residential institutions in this country are designed as large multi-purpose facilities to serve all types and levels of patients over a long period of time. This is the traditional model which lately has been subjected to increasing criticism (President's Panel on Mental Retardation, 1962). Some institutions, particularly in recent years, have been designed for more specialized functions, to serve a relatively homogenous group of residents. This may become a trend. A few facilities have been established to provide short-term care. Although the concept of short-term care has only recently been rediscovered in the United States, one can discern an increasing emphasis on this type of facility.

There is a tendency, as noted in an earlier survey (Scheerenberger, 1965), for the newer institutions to be somewhat smaller. More than half of the new institutions have a rated capacity of fewer than 500 residents. Of course, it should be noted that almost all of the older institutions began as relatively small facilities, and have added more buildings. Undoubtedly this will be true of some of the more recent institutions as well.

The rated capacity of all public institutions included in the survey was 191,587. The actual resident population was 199,694. These data indicate that, even by traditional standards, there is considerable overcrowding. Actually, this estimate is conservative because the "rated capacity" figure included some institutions that had not yet opened. In addition, most institutions have long waiting lists, including as many applicants as 25 per cent of their actual residential population. The waiting period for admission is two years in most states and as long as five or six years in other states. There are at least 31,000 individuals on waiting lists, while only 9,000 patients are released annually and another 3,000 die. Thus there are 2.5 persons waiting for every bed that becomes available.

Most of the residents are housed in large rooms. The average number of residential units per institution is 14. Approximately 40 per cent of the population is housed in rooms holding 30 or more residents. There is a tendency for the institutions constructed since 1960 to have smaller cottages with fewer residents per room. Roughly three-fourths of the institutional population live in buildings that are over 50 years old.

The native white population in the United States accounted for approximately 83 per cent of the general population according to the 1960 census. This group represents about 91 per cent of the total in public institutions. Although these figures suggest a racial bias in admissions of persons to public institutions, it should be noted that there are generally fewer institutional provisions in those areas of the country where the Negro population is the greatest.

CHARACTERISTICS OF RESIDENTS

Approximately half of the 200,000 residents in state institutions in 1968 were adults. Fifty-five per cent were males. The distribution by ages was as follows:

Under 5 years	—	3 per cent
5–9	—	11 per cent
10–14	—	18 per cent
15–19	—	19 per cent
20–24	—	12 per cent
25–29	—	9 per cent
Over 30 years	—	28 per cent

Many institutions have minimum age requirements for admission. Moreover, there is a definite difference in the ages of residents between older and newer institutions. The tendency seems to be to admit younger patients in new institutions. Approximately 80 per cent of first admissions to institutions are under 20 years of age. These data represent a slight shift toward younger admissions compared even with the 1965 survey conducted by AAMD. The vast majority of those institutions that limit admissions to minors were established since 1950. Many individuals who are now adults have spent most of their lives in an institution. Obviously, these individuals are more likely to be found in the older institutions.

BEHAVIOR CLASSIFICATION

More than half of all the institutionalized retarded are classified as profoundly or severely retarded. The distribution of IQs, by level of retardation, is:

Profound (IQ < 20)   29 per cent
Severe (IQ 20–35)   28 per cent
Moderate (IQ 36–50)   24 per cent
Mild (IQ 51–67)   14 per cent
Borderline (IQ 68–83)   6 per cent

There seems to be a definite trend toward admitting less intelligent individuals. Community resources for the mildly and moderately retarded have improved markedly within the past decade. At the same time, many institutions have placed their higher level residents in the community. This trend has many implications for institutional functioning and objectives. There is considerable variability from state to state with respect to the type of patient served. This stems in part from differences in resources, but it can also be related to philosophical and policy distinctions. The better the community facilities and programs, the lower the level of institutional retardates.

ETIOLOGY

The etiological factors responsible for the defects of about 75 per cent of the institutional population are largely unknown. There is a tendency for younger patients, particularly in newer institutions, to have more definite diagnoses. Table 1–2 provides an approximate summary of the percentages in the major medical classifications as outlined by the American Association on Mental Deficiency (Adapted from Best, 1965).

PROGRAMS

Virtually all institutions operate programs for the "educable" and "trainable" residents. Most also have vocational training programs. The relevance of these vocational training activities to the needs of modern society and to the individual resident is often difficult to appreciate. About 60 per cent of the institutions also have some type of adult educational program. Table 1–3 indicates the numbers of residents participating in the various programs.

MAINTENANCE COSTS

Maintaining residential institutions is expensive. In fact, more public money is spent on the five per cent of mental retardates who are institutionalized than upon the 95 per cent who are not. Data taken from the U.S. Census Reports indicate that mean per capita expenditures have risen gradually over the years, with the exception of a decline during the depression period. Per capita maintenance costs for five year intervals beginning in 1930 are presented in Table 1–4.

Table 1–2

Classification	Per cent	Number of Residents
Infection	6.7	13,400
Intoxication	.6	1,200
Trauma or Physical Agent	8.5	17,000
Disorder of Metabolism, Growth, or Nutrition	1.2	2,400
New Growths	.3	600
Unknown Prenatal Influence	36.6	73,200
Unknown or Uncertain with Structural reaction manifest	1.7	3,400
Uncertain or presumed Psychologic, with functional reaction alone manifest	32.0	64,000
Unclassified	9.7	19,400
Without Mental Retardation	2.7	5,400
Total	100	200,000

Of course, these data are somewhat misleading in that the dollar has undergone considerable inflation over this period. Even allowing for this consideration, however, it is clear that expenditures per patient have increased several times over the last 40 years. Currently, over one-half billion dollars are spent in maintaining public institutions.

There is considerable variability from state to state in the amount spent to operate institutions. For example, in 1966, five states spent less than $4 a day as compared with over $10 a day spent by five other states. Moreover, per capita expenditures are dependent upon the size of the institutions and the type of patient served. Southern states generally allocate the least money per patient. In general, the small institutions have higher per capital costs. In 1967 the average national per capita cost was $6.71. This figure is much

Table 1–3

Education	15875
EMR	15875
TMR	28172
Adult	5953
Vocational Rehab.	26613
Non Residents	2100
Summer Camp	19641

Table 1–4

Year	Per Capita Expenditures
1930	$265
1935	252
1940	291
1945	386
1950	746
1955	1093
1960	1660
1965	2375

lower than per patient costs for other types of facilities. It is interesting to note that some zoos spend more than this for the care and feeding of animals of human size (Blatt, 1968).

PERSONNEL

Approximately 94,000 persons are employed full time in public residential institutions. Another 3,000, mostly professionals, are employed on a part-time basis. Of the total, about half are attendants. The overall ratio of attendants to patients is 1:4. Ratios of staff to patients have increased in every state within the past decade. During this period, the total number of persons employed in institutions has doubled. The relative increase in professional personnel has been particularly marked. Figure 1–4 presents a break-down by category of the numbers, percentages, and ratios of various occupational groups as of 1968.

The "Other" category includes maintenance, clerical, secretarial, and like personnel not directly involved in patient care. There is one other large group of individuals, not indicated among employee statistics, who nevertheless contribute substantially to the operation of the institution. These are the patients themselves. Without working patients many institutions simply could not operate. Estimates of the contribution of the patients to the maintenance and operation of the institution are difficult to obtain, but in many instances patients may constitute 25 per cent or more of the maintenance staff. Some institutions have experienced staffing crises when large groups of high level working residents have been moved into the community. It should go without saying that a decision to keep a particular patient in a working position is deplorable when some other course of rehabilitation would be more meaningful.

Although there is not a great deal of information available regarding the qualifications of professional workers in institutions, it is probably true that, as a group, they are not highly qualified. Many institutional physicians are not even licensed for private practice. A survey by Baumeister (1967) indicated that over 10 per cent of those individuals designated as psychologists do not possess a masters degree. Only 29 per cent have the doctorate. Most

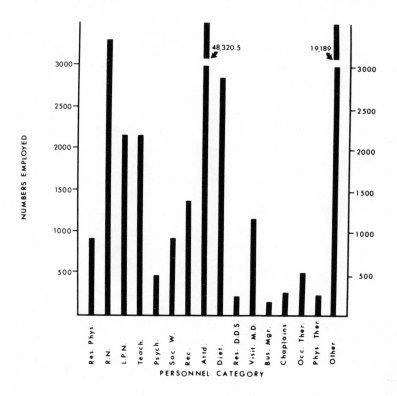

Figure 1-4

institutional social workers do not hold the masters degree and are not certified. This is not to criticize those professionals who are employed in institutions, but rather to indicate that professional staffs generally do not meet the qualification levels that are standard for their respective fields.

No one among the institutional staff is so vital to the program as the attendants. They are responsible for the day-to-day care, management, and rehabilitation of the residents. For better or worse, the welfare of the patient is in the direct hands of the attendant personnel. The attendants perform a fantastic array of responsibilities, many of which they are not trained to carry out (Butterfield, 1967). Why institutional administrations typically have difficulty recruiting and retaining a highly motivated and competent staff is no great mystery. Inadequate pay and low social status account for the high turnover and low ability level. Salaries are generally below the average in the surrounding community. Most attendants probably earn less than $350 monthly, particularly in the South. Too, they hold a low position in the institution "pecking order." Typically they are the last to be consulted in policy decisions affecting patients and the first to be blamed when something goes awry.

About the only formal training that many attendants receive is a brief "orientation" when they first arrive. The most significant training is usually the result of their personal interactions with "veterans" on the ward. What is learned under these conditions may not always serve the best interests of the patients.

Most institutions have introduced some type of in-service training programs. A special federal program provides some financial assistance for this effort. There is considerable variability in content, duration, and numbers of employees involved in in-service training. This is partly due to differences in resources but it is also related to the fact that nobody seems to be entirely sure what the attendant ought to be trained to do. The relevant criterion measures of effectiveness have escaped precise measurement. For a detailed consideration of the role and characteristics of attendant personnel the reader is invited to examine a review by Butterfield (1967).

Prospect

Social institutions are not changed easily. A functional autonomy sustains them, even when it is clear that their contribution to society no longer warrants their being. Nevertheless, the character of the residential institution is slowly changing. One must, of course, evaluate such changes in terms of what is actually accomplished in institutions, rather than in terms of what those responsible say is done. There is some discrepancy between verbalization and practice.

One may separate the residential institution from the concepts that gave birth to it and which nurture it. Our society will continue to segregate certain groups of individuals and put them into institutions. In fact, there is reason to believe that more, rather than less, institutionalization is the prospect for the immediate future. But, it is clear that the basic rationalizations justifying this practice are being modified. Perhaps the most fundamental trend lies in the conceptualization of retarded behavior in scientific rather than moral issues. There will be a time when people react to the retarded not out of fear, nor pity, nor even a misguided sense of humanitarianism, but with the simple realization that whatever produces a better behavioral adjustment for the individual also benefits society.

The development of the public residential institution is dependent upon the vicissitudes of public sentiment. The professionals may provide the models, but it is the "Great Public" who supply the wherewithal. Current support, by all levels of government and in the private sector, while not extravagant is at an all-time high. Moreover, antipoverty programs and other welfare legislation will have an impact on the field of mental retardation.

Several trends are discernible that will produce significant changes in the traditional role of the institution:

The resident population is generally becoming younger and more severely retarded. Due to a lowered mortality rate, an increasing proportion have secondary handicaps.

Institutions will be increasingly integrated into a continuum of public services with greater flexibility for movement within the entire system. More emphasis will be placed on short-term care with a view toward utilizing other services available within the community. The days of the monolith, separated from the mainstream of society and unresponsive to the needs of the individual and society, are numbered.

More institutions will be constructed, but they will be smaller and more strategically located. They will be designed to more closely parallel "normal" society with greater stress on normal living patterns.

More concern will be directed toward programming environments for individual residents at all levels of functioning.

Professional resources, both in quantity and quality, will improve. Institutions will accept broader training responsibilities, particularly in conjunction with universities.

Research, clinical as well as basic, will also become a recognized responsibility of institutions. Well equipped and competently staffed research units will be a common feature of institutions.

The millennium is a long way off. But, the institution has entered a new period in its development, a turn in the right direction.

References

Barr, M. W. The how, the why, and the wherefore of the training of feeble-minded children. *Journal of Psycho-Asthenics,* 1899, 4, 204–212.

————. The imperative call of our present to our future. *Journal of Psycho-Asthenics,* 1902, 7, 5–14.

————. *Mental defectives: Their history, treatment, and training.* Philadelphia: P. Blakiston's Son & Co., 1913.

Baumeister, A. A. A survey of the role of psychologists in public institutions for the retarded. *Mental Retardation,* 1967, 5, 2–5.

Best, H. *Public provision for the mentally retarded in the United States.* Worcester: Hefferman Press, 1965.

Blatt, B. Non-progress and non-change. *President's Committee on Mental Retardation Message,* 1968, 11, 3.

Butler, A. W. The feeble-minded: The need of research. *Proceedings of the National Conference of Charities and Correction,* 1915, 356–361.

Butterfield, E. C. The characteristics, selection and training of institutional personnel. In A. A. Baumeister (Ed.), *Mental Retardation: Appraisal, education and rehabilitation.* Chicago: Aldine Publishing Co., 1967. Pp. 305–328.

Cleland, C. C. and R. F. Peck. Intra-institutional administrative problems: A paradigm for employee stimulation. *Mental Retardation,* 1967, 5, 2–8.

Davenport, C. B. *Heredity in relation to eugenics.* New York: Henry Holt & Co., 1911.

Davies, S. P. *Social control of the mentally deficient.* New York: Thomas Y. Crowell Co., 1930.

Deutsch, A. *The mentally ill in America: A history of their care and treatment from colonial times.* New York: Columbia University Press, 1949.

Goddard, H. H. *The Kallikak family.* New York: Macmillan Co., 1912.

————. The possibilities of research as applied to the prevention of feeble-mindedness. *Proceedings National Conference of Charities and Correction,* 1915, 307–312.

Haller, M. H. *Eugenics: Hereditarian attitudes in American thought.* New Brunswick, N.J.: Rutgers University Press, 1963.

Haskell, R. H. Mental deficiency over a hundred years. *American Journal of Psychiatry,* 1944, 100, 107–118.

Horsfield, E. Mental defectives at the court of Philip IV of Spain as portrayed by the great court painter Velasquez. *American Journal of Mental Deficiency,* 1940, 45, 152–157.

Howe, S. G. *Report made to the legislature of Massachusetts upon idiocy,* 1848.

Johnson, A. Discussion on care of the feebleminded. *Proceedings National Conference of Charities and Correction,* 1889, 318–319.

————. The self-supporting imbecile. *Journal of Psycho-Asthenics,* 1900, 4, 91–100.

Kraft, I. Edouard Seguin and the 19th century moral treatment of idiots. *Bulletin of the History of Medicine,* 1961, 35, 393–418.

President's Panel on Mental Retardation. *A proposed program for national action to combat mental retardation.* Washington, D. C.: Superintendent of Documents, U.S. Government Printing Office, 1962.

Reed, E. W. and S. C. Reed. *Mental retardation: A family study.* Philadelphia: W. B. Saunders, 1965.

Scheerenberger, R. C. A current census of state institutions for the mentally retarded. *Mental Retardation,* 1965, 3, 4–6.

Vail, D. J. *Dehumanization and the institutional career.* Springfield: Charles C. Thomas, 1967.

Wallin, J. E. W. Training of the severely retarded, viewed in historical perspective. *Journal of General Psychology,* 1966, 107–127.

Evolutionary Changes of
the Residential Facility

Darwin's conclusion that the survival of organisms is a function of their adaptability to environmental change is, no doubt, equally valid for social agencies and institutions. The large, traditional residential facilities for the retarded are in danger of emulating the dinosaur and becoming extinct unless they undergo adaptive modifications in response to the rapid changes occurring in the field of mental retardation.

The Changing Environment

The pall of pessimism which enveloped the field of mental retardation during the early decades of the 20th century is being replaced by growing optimism. This swing in the pendulum from skepticism to enthusiasm reflects encouraging scientific advances in a number of fields. Probably of considerable importance is the modification of the concept of the "constancy of the I. Q." The traditional concept of irreversibility and of ingrained genetic limitations is being replaced by a much more flexible model, reflecting the empirical evidence which emphasizes the potency of the environment in modifying intellectual functioning (Skodak & Skeels, 1949; McCandless, 1964). Mental retardation no longer needs to be considered an "irreversible condition," but may be approached as a potentially modifiable syndrome.

Significant advances in prevention of specific forms of mental retardation through medical intervention have raised new hopes regarding possible treatment and prophylaxis. Although effective discoveries have been limited to only a small fraction of the retarded population, these "breakthroughs" tend to be interpreted as precursors of more extensive advances. Success in cases of phenylketonuria and galactosemia, and in hydrocephalus and craniosynestosis, emphasizes that early intervention *can* prevent severe intellectual impairment. Discoveries of the possible effects of prenatal maternal infections and malnutrition and of obstetrical difficulties further underline the growing emphasis on prevention.

Recent applications of principles derived from the behavioral sciences to training the retarded are demonstrating that significant progress can be made, even with the profoundly retarded (Ellis, 1963; Dayan, 1964; Roos, 1965; Watson, 1967). Derivatives of operant conditioning and classical conditioning procedures are proving effective in changing types of behavior considered for many years to be unmodifiable. As one result of these advances, the term *subtrainable* is being abandoned, and workers in the field of mental retardation are being challenged to train retardates of all levels.

Increasing recognition of the potentially damaging effects of early deprivation (Goldfarb, 1945; Spitz, 1945, 1949; Rosenzweig, 1960; Provence & Lipton, 1962; Shotwell & Shipe, 1964; Stedman & Eichorn, 1964; Harlow, 1964, 1965) has led to energetic attempts to stimulate and train the retarded—or potentially retarded—as early in life as possible. Encouraging—though as yet not adequately validated—results have been reported through exposure to "autotelic responsive environments" (Moore, 1963) and to a regimented program of "patterning" and sensory-motor procedures (Institutes for the Achievement of Human Potential, 1963; Doman, 1967). Strategies aimed at prevention of culturally derived retardation are being mounted as part of massive anti-poverty programs.

A potent factor in the institutional environment was highlighted by the establishment of the National Association for Retarded Children in 1950. From a modest beginning, this organization claimed 1,200 affiliated units in 1968, including professionals, civic leaders, and parents. Because it is estimated that roughly one-tenth of our population is directly affected by mental retardation, it is not surprising that parent groups have exerted considerable influence and that their efforts have brought about encouraging changes, both in state and federal programs. The basic concern of these groups has been to improve services to the retarded. They have demanded that training and habilitation replace custodial maintenance. Increased pressures can be anticipated from these interested groups both as a function of growing awareness of new treatment and training techniques and as a function of social change.

Increased popular concern with the problem of the retarded was reflected by the massive state-wide planning efforts recently completed in each of the 50 states. Stimulated by a federal grant program (P.L. 88–156), these efforts were aimed at developing comprehensive planning for the retarded in each state, based on detailed analysis of current needs and available services. Literally thousands of citizens, often including leading legislators, were participants in every state. In general, these studies not only uncovered areas of unmet needs, but they stimulated considerable interest and concern in the lay public, professionals, and legislators.

Yet another factor exerting pressure on the institution is the recent project sponsored by the American Association on Mental Deficiency to evaluate institutions systematically. Participating institutions were requested to complete a self-evaluation before evaluation by an outside team of expert consultants. The detailed standards against which institutions were compared were derived from the AAMD's Standards for State Residential Institutions for the Mentally Retarded (American Association for Mental Deficiency, 1964). Through this evaluation process, shortcomings and needs have become obvious, not only to residential administrators and their staffs but also to state and federal agencies and legislatures. The President's Committee on Mental Retardation reported in 1967, for example, that staffs in state residential facilities were barely more than half of what is considered minimal by the AAMD (President's Committee on Mental Retardation, 1967).

The numerous federal grant programs which have become available to residential centers are likewise exerting considerable pressure toward change. Motivated by the need for additional funds, residential administrators have been willing to modify existing philosophies or policies to qualify for the federal programs. Facilities participating in these programs have often been better able to innovate and expand programs than non-participating facilities, while becoming more vulnerable to outside regimentation. Introduction of federal programs within facilities is also likely to disturb the internal homeostasis, precipitating somewhat chaotic changes.

Another factor exerting pressure toward institutional change entails shifts within the composition of the institution's resident population. There has been a general increase in the proportion of severely and profoundly retarded institutionalized cases. At least three variables have been operating to foster this trend: a decrease in birth and infant mortality; an increase in the lifespan of the profoundly and severely retarded; and increased availability of community services for the mildly and moderately retarded. Within the mildly retarded segment of the residential population, an increase in the proportion of the emotionally disturbed and the socially adjusted mildly retarded individual is increasingly able to remain in the community, whereas the mildly retarded whose behavior is socially unacceptable is selectively being referred for residential placement.

As a corollary to these changes in admissions, a corresponding decrease is being noted in that segment of the resident population which has been relied upon to help operate the facility. The decrease in resident helpers is being reflected by greater demands on the time of the paid staff. The over-all effect of this gradual change in resident population is that the residential facility is being required to handle cases necessitating more intense management with a decreased manpower supply.

These changes in the environment of the residential facility are translated into demands that the institution meet the changing needs. These demands are sometimes unrealistic in view of the facilities' limited resources, but of greater concern to the residential center are those situations where it is subjected to incompatible and conflicting demands. The following are examples of typical situations of this type:

"Waiting lists should be abolished by expediting admissions, while conditions of overcrowding and understaffing should be remedied by reducing the number of residents." Both of these demands are certainly legitimate, but—unless increased appropriations for staff and construction are available —they cannot be met simultaneously. Administrators often become quite sensitive to this particular "double bind" situation, because it offers concrete ammunition for criticism by legislators, news media, and community representatives.

"Buildings unsuited to implement modern concepts of training the retarded should be replaced (preferably by 'cottage-type' construction), while minimizing budget requests and instituting 'economic means of operation'." Frequently the situation is further complicated by the need for new construction to accommodate expanding waiting lists. Older residential facilities are in a particularly difficult position because costs of programming and maintenance are typically higher, and cost of replacement may be higher than cost of new construction. Furthermore, building new facilities tends to have greater political appeal and is more in keeping with the trend toward small, easily accessible facilities.

"Residential programs should aim at maximal habilitation of residents through fostering community-oriented activities and freedom of residents while protecting communities from exposure to residents." As the mildly retarded residential population becomes increasingly composed of rejects from community programs, community concern with socially unacceptable behavior of residents is likely to increase. While the institution may be justly criticized for "locked doors," "detention units," regimentation, and other policies tending toward institutionalization of its residents, it is also open to criticisms stemming from allowing residents to "escape," failing to prevent damage to property or minor theft, inadequately monitoring sexual behavior, or failing to "protect" families from unwanted visits by offspring. Often community agencies are eager to institutionalize "trouble makers" for habilitation (even though the presence of mental retardation may be questionable), only to become highly resistive to reaccepting the "habilitated" subjects at a later time.

"Residential facilities should specialize so as to maximally serve the needs of specific sub-populations, while remaining in close proximity to the families of the residents being served." While it may be true that specialized facilities can deliver a higher quality of service, the geography of many states makes such institutions relatively inaccessible to major numbers of parents. Most of these states are unable—or unwilling—to appropriate the funds which would be required to develop enough specialized facilities to maintain proximity to the communities being served.

"Residential facilities should remain small (often the figure of 500 residents is mentioned as the maximum desirable size), while grouping all residents homogeneously in living units, developing adequate programs for atypical populations (e.g., blind, deaf, emotionally disturbed), and operating at maximum economy." If, in addition, the facility is required to offer a multi-purpose program serving all levels of retardation to offer proximity to families, the task becomes extremely difficult. The complexity of the problem becomes apparent when planning for a multi-purpose facility is considered. Assuming that residents are to be grouped in terms of four levels of retardation (profound, severe, moderate, and mild), four age levels (below six, six to twelve, teens, and adults), two sexes, and three catagories of gross motor handicap (ambulatory, semi-ambulatory, bed-fast), it becomes apparent that *96 buildings* would be required to house the population in relatively homogeneous living units. If the number of residents per unit is limited to 32 (and smaller units are frequently rejected by budget agencies as inordinately expensive to build or staff), the facility's population would be *3,072*. If such a facility were, in addition, to include an infirmary unit for acute illness and surgery and units for atypical cases (e.g., blind, deaf, cerebral palsied, emotionally disturbed), it would need to be even larger.

"Residential facilities should meet the minimum standards established by the AAMD, while instituting economic strategies aimed at reducing budget requests." It is estimated that the 94,000 persons employed in 1968 throughout the nation in publicly operated residential facilities for the retarded are barely more than half the number required to meet the AAMD minimum standards (President's Committee, 1967). Inadequacies of physical plants have already been documented. Upgrading these institutions would obviously be an extremely expensive proposition, and in most states a sizable portion of state appropriations are being directed into the construction and staffing of new facilities (to absorb waiting lists) and into emerging community programs.

"Residential facilities should insist on highest quality staff to implement their increasingly sophisticated programs, while minimizing costs of operation by maintaining moderate salary levels and relying primarily on untrained labor in recognition of professional manpower shortages." Competition for scarce professionals appears to be rapidly increasing as the result of burgeoning and expanding programs throughout the nation. In general, residential programs for the retarded rate low in attractiveness to professionals, who seem to prefer university, clinic, community or industrial settings. Residential administrators are faced with problems of recruitment and retention which are all too often aggravated by noncompetitive salaries.

"Residential facilities should develop into regional centers serving communities within their catchment area, while not competing for limited funds with community-sponsored mental retardation centers." Because most facilities' budgets do not allow adequate services to their own residents, expansion into regional services is dependent on additional funds. Such funds are often actively sought by community-sponsored centers or agencies. In the resulting competition for funds—and later for staff—residential centers are usually at a serious disadvantage.

New Trends in Residential Philosophy

Institutional goals are increasingly emphasizing prevention of institutionalization and reduction of the length of institutional placements. Whereas until recently parents were usually advised to institutionalize obviously retarded offspring (e.g., Mongoloids) as early as possible, such advice is currently judged to be unsound. This shift in philosophy, in many cases, reflects increasing drains on state fiscal resources for operation of residential institutions. A more fundamental reason for this reversal in institutional philosophy stems from studies interpreted to demonstrate that institutionalization or separation from parents has detrimental effects on young children (Goldfarb, 1943, 1945; Spitz, 1945, 1949; Rosenzweig, 1960; Provence & Lipton, 1962; Shotwell & Shipe, 1964; Stedman & Eichorn, 1964; Harlow, 1964, 1965). Recent investigations, however, have begun to explore differences among institutions (Butterfield & Zigler, 1966; Klaber & Butterfield, 1968) and to suggest that institutional effects may not be uniformly detrimental (Zigler & Williams, 1963; Butterfield & Zigler, 1966; Cleland, Patton & Dickerson, 1968). In spite of these indications that institutional placement may be beneficial for some retardates in some institutions, the current trend is overwhelmingly to discourage placement except for the most severely handicapped.

In an attempt to fulfill this goal, institutions are placing increasing stress on pre-admission services, including evaluation, parent counseling, and referral. These services may be implemented by the institution itself, by separate state-operated centers, or by community-operated centers. In general, emphasis is placed on screening applications to the institutions and referring applicants to alternate services. The success of this strategy is dependent, of course, on the availability of these alternatives. In most states, alternatives are still grossly inadequate.

To minimize the length of institutional placement, habilitation programs are being developed to return residents to the community. Socialization programs for the mildly retarded, often incorporating behavior shaping techniques (e.g., Roos, 1968), are yielding encouraging results. Success of such programs is dependent upon reversing the "institutionalization syndrome," developing residents' behavior to make it acceptable to the subculture to which they are to be returned, and providing post-discharge services. Only few programs currently effectively combine these three components. All too often the behavior reinforced by institutional programs is aimed to equip the resident for institutional life which results in the institutionalization syndrome of passivity, submissiveness, ingratiation, inertia, and related behaviors. Or he is supposedly prepared for life in the prevailing middle-class subculture, but the discharged resident is not equipped for life as he is liable to find it, leading to frustration and disillusionment.

Recognizing that many institutionalized residents are unable to achieve full community independence, an array of sheltered living arrangements are being evolved. Probably the most widely used facility is the half-way house, typically considered a transitional service, from which residents are discharged to independent (or semi-independent) living after having acquired the necessary social and vocational skills. The half-way house is a specialized habilitation service, and hence part, or all, of the program cost is often borne by the state Division of Vocational Rehabilitation.

A similar facility located on the institution grounds and providing greater supervision is usually referred to as a quarter-way house. Frequently, residents living in such a facility work in the community, while participating in an active socialization program. Typically, residents are referred from the quarter-way to the half-way house as they develop the needed social skills.

Terminal sheltered living arrangements away from the institution are being developed in some states as an alternative to life-long institutionalization. So-called *colonies,* operated by the state residential institutions, have housed mildly retarded adults in New York State for years. Some of these facilities are currently being replaced by *hostels,* consisting of small living units (10 to 20 residents) located in urban areas and operated by community agencies. New York State assumes acquisition or construction costs and a significant proportion of operational costs. This program is planned to handle hundreds of mildly and moderately retarded adults who are able to be employed in community jobs or in sheltered workshops.

Other states have developed variations on this program. Oklahoma, for example, has developed an extensive program whereby private nursing home operators are paid by the state for housing retarded adults. Some of these facilities house more than 100 moderately and mildly retarded residents. Attempts are made to furnish activity programs and to include residents in community recreation. Other states are exploring use of private nursing homes for housing geriatric or bedfast residents (e.g., Texas, Kansas, Indiana).

A different form of sheltered living alternative to institutional placement is placement in a private home referred to as *foster care* or *family care*. Typically, the state monitors the program and pays the family a fixed rate for each retarded person placed in the home. Several states have transferred hundreds of institution residents to such family situations (e.g., California, New York). In many cases the placement is considered a transition from institutional to independent status, and residents participate in local special education classes, sheltered workshop programs, or work in the community.

The increasing emphasis on habilitation programs aimed at discharging residents from institutions is gradually being paralleled by increasing concern that all institutionalized residents achieve maximum level of functioning. Energetic programs are being tried in many states to eliminate the "back wards" and to expand intensive training programs to all levels of retardation and handicap. The term *sub-trainable* is being abandoned as programs of behavior shaping are proving their effectiveness in developing self-help skills, social skills, and communication skills in even the profoundly retarded (e.g., Ellis, 1963; Dayan, 1964; Roos, 1965; Watson, 1967). Institutions are attempting to expand programs in education, language, physical therapy, pre-vocational training, and related modalities to include the profoundly retarded.

The changes taking place in the residential institution are beginning to modify its long-standing image as a custodial "warehousing" operation. Increasingly, institutions are describing themselves as active training, educational, and socialization centers. Re-definition of institutions in these terms promises changing relationships with community agencies, parents, educational facilities, and professionals.

Strategies for Implementing Goals

Modification of institutional programs to implement changes in philosophy is an extremely complex and difficult process. Wide variations in the degree to which the new philosophy is being met are evident among the states, and among institutions within the states. In spite of these variations, some consistency can be noted in strategic methods to implement change. The following approaches appear to be among the most successful and are widely used today:

1. Recognizing that the new programs require upgrading of staff, most institutions have expanded in-service training programs. The primary emphasis has been on caretaker personnel, as exemplified by the Southern Re-

gion Education Board's Attendant Training Project (Bensberg, Barnett & Hurder, 1964). The Inservice Training Program funded by the Department of Health, Education, and Welfare has been a potent catalyst in upgrading attendant training programs throughout the country. Although studies suggest these types of programs have been successful in increasing attendants' fund of information, there is a dearth of data indicating significant changes in attitude or behavior (Thorne, 1968).

Part of the problem in modifying attitudes and behavior of attendants stems from the potency of the attendant sub-culture within the institution. Frequently, the in-service training program is undermined by a small core of attendants and supervisors who control staff behavior in the wards or dormitories. Failure to include these powerful ward staff and supervisory personnel often contributes to the inefficacy of the in-service training program. Furthermore, the fact that training programs are usually conducted in a didactic manner in classrooms removed from wards has tended to isolate the experience and to minimize generalization to the ward situation.

In-service training programs have not been limited to attendant staff. Some institutions have established specialized training for supervisory and administrative staff, for volunteers, and for resident helpers. Preemployment training programs have been instituted by some states (e.g., Texas).

Training strategies have become increasingly sophisticated. Some institutions are pioneering the use of role-playing, management seminars, sensitivity training, programmed instruction, audio-visual aids, closed circuit television, and video-taping (Schein & Bennis, 1965; Robins & Burns, 1968). The use of specialized training wards where on-the-job training is conducted seems particularly promising.

2. In an effort to maximize the impact on resident services of limited manpower, institutions are redeploying their staff. Traditionally, most institutional programs have organized professional services along departmental, discipline-based dimensions, so that each department has tended to evolve its own programs frequently uncoordinated with other programs. As a result of this type of organization, departments have competed with each other, and many residents have "fallen in the cracks" and remained neglected. A related problem stems from the relative isolation of professionals from ward activities. As a result, professionally proposed programs are frequently not implemented in the residents' daily life, and detailed evaluation and program plans remain relatively meaningless. A number of institutions have attempted to improve this situation by institutional reorganization.

Institutions have been evolving techniques for maximizing staff-resident interactions. Because the personnel-to-resident ratio is usually far below that recommended by the AAMD project on technical planning (Scheerenberger, 1965), institutions have increased their budget requests in attempts to increase staff size. Typically, some form of unitization has replaced the departmental organization, so that multi-disciplinary teams are assigned to specific sub-groups of residents. Usually, these sub-groups are given responsibility for residents grouped homogeneously according to age, level of retardation, and—occasionally—special handicaps such as "emotional problems" or ambulation difficulties. Each team is responsible for full programming for all residents in its assigned group, including admission, evaluation, and post-discharge services. This form of organization reduces fragmentation of services and involves the professional staff in more direct contact with daily ward activities.

In spite of encouraging changes in deployment of professional resources, available evidence suggests that the current rate of training professionals for the field of mental retardation will not satisfy the growing need (President's Panel on Mental Retardation, 1962). It is becoming increasingly apparent that professionals are unable—and probably will continue to be unable—to give direct service to the majority of the institutionalized retarded. As a result, there has been a gradual abandonment of the one-to-one therapeutic model as being neither practical nor particularly effective. Professionals are beginning to function primarily as consultants, teachers, trainers, and supervisors.

The responsibility for program implementation through clinical interaction with residents is increasingly being delegated to relatively untrained personnel, such as ward attendants, teacher aides, and recreation assistants. Efforts are also being directed at the development of new kinds of staff having formal training at the Associate of Arts or Bachelor of Arts level. Community colleges are developing curricula which would prepare their Associate of Arts graduates for positions in institutions referred to as *Child Care Workers, Human Development Specialists,* etc. These graduates would be assigned to direct resident services, with primary responsibility for implementation of such specialized techniques as operant conditioning, language development, physical therapy, and recreation. Technician level personnel are also being developed in many of the professions, and they are increasingly being delegated routine technical duties under professional supervision. Several states are developing "career ladders" whereby relatively untrained persons may proceed through a sequence of work and educational experiences from untrained staff to technical specialists and, finally, to full professional status (e.g., Illinois, New York, Colorado).

Many institutions are expanding the use of non-staff resources for program implementation. The value of non-ward personnel on wards has recently been experimentally demonstrated (Klaber, 1968), but workers in the field have long emphasized the importance of interpersonal warmth and friendship. Volunteers are increasingly being involved in direct training and treatment programs. A recent research project at Austin State School has demonstrated the effectiveness of volunteers as members of treatment teams implementing technical procedures under professional guidance (Hinojosa, 1966, 1968).

The recent development of the TARS (Teens Aid the Retarded) program under the auspices of the National Association for Retarded Children has already demonstrated the immense value of bringing normal young people into regular contact with institutionalized retardates. The federally funded Foster Grand Parent program is likewise proving the effectiveness of using older persons as surrogate "grandparents" in residential institutions. Even residents' parents are finally being recognized as important members of the treatment team by a number of institutions, and they are increasingly included in program planning and implementation.

3. Because most institutions are still seriously impaired by insufficient funds in development of training and treatment programs, they have tended to develop specialized demonstration projects. The availability of federal funds for beginning such projects has acted as a strong catalyst (e.g., Hospital Improvement Program, Elementary and Secondary Education Title I and Title III). Institution administrators have tended to use demonstration projects to evaluate the effectiveness of special procedures, to demonstrate the value of new approaches to the institution staff, and to use the results as a justification for requesting additional state funds to expand the projects.

Some administrators have supported demonstration programs in a highly visible manner, capitalizing on the "Hawthorne" and "ripple" effects to maximize impact on their staff (Roos, 1968). Manifestation of "sibling" rivalry among institution sub-units has been channeled into constructive competitiveness for program excellence.

4. Frustrated by the serious limitations of knowledge in the area of mental retardation, institutions are placing increasing emphasis on programs of research. It is now evident that many significant research questions can be answered most meaningfully within the institutional setting. Previous artificial barriers between applied and basic research are gradually disappearing. In spite of the contention by budget agencies of a number of states that research should be confined to specialized research institutes, a number of institutions have succeeded in developing sophisticated full-time research staffs (e.g., Parsons State Hospital, Kansas; Pacific State Hospital, California). The development of more sophisticated budgetary systems, such as the Planning, Programming, Budgeting System being implemented in New York (State of New York Executive Department, 1968), will increasingly require establishment of institution-based research units to implement effectiveness studies.

Institutional administrators are finding that research not only adds to knowledge, but that it contributes significantly to care and treatment programs by helping to evaluate and refine techniques for training and treatment. Research programs also foster recruitment and retention of professional staff.

5. Institutions are increasingly affiliating with educational facilities, including universities, medical schools, colleges, community colleges, and others. Joint training programs—often including joint staff appointments—are becoming commonplace. Federal grant programs of all kinds, including the extensive programs for University Affiliated Centers (P.L. 90–170), are fostering expansion of such joint arrangements. States are liberalizing policies for paying their employees for educational leave, and affiliations with educational facilities are becoming an important aspect of the developing career ladders. Involvement of high school students with institutional retardates is being fostered through volunteer programs, as well as through a variety of federally funded employment programs (e.g., Student Work Experience and Training; Disadvantaged Youth).

These programs are proving valuable in upgrading the level of institutional staff and programming, in recruiting manpower for the field of mental retardation, and in educating the public regarding the mentally retarded.

6. Institutions are typically seeking avenues for reaching into communities and for serving community needs. Administrators are interested in articulating institutional programs with community services. A number of states have appointed superintendents of new institutions several years before completion of the facilities so that the emerging institution programs can contribute meaningfully to the total matrix of regional services (e.g., Georgia, Texas, New York). State long-range plans typically include residential facilities as an integral component of the developing comprehensive mental retardation regional services. In New York State, for example, a residential facility is planned as part of each of the proposed mental retardation centers serving a catchment area of 750,000 (New York State Planning Committee on Mental Disorders, 1965).

The traditional gap between institution and community is being bridged by three important developments:

Volunteers are being enlisted in ever-growing numbers to render direct services to the institution. They are increasingly being assimilated into treatment teams, where they function as extensions of the regular institution staff (Roos, 1964; Hinojosa, 1966, 1968).

Professional members of institutional staffs are offering consultation to agencies, private practitioners, and others in the communities. Frequently the institution has the highest concentration of professional talent within a considerable geographical area and serves as a manpower resource for surrounding communities.

Institutions are placing greater emphasis on involving parents in treatment planning. Parents are being invited to participate in training programs within the institution to equip them to handle their retarded children more effectively (Roos, 1965). Pre- and post-discharge parent counseling is becoming recognized as an essential facet of habilitation efforts.

Specific strategies for developing institutional community services differ widely among states and—to a lesser extent—among institutions within specific states. The following mechanisms seem to be gaining widest acceptance:

Some institutions are developing regularly budgeted community services. Because services to residents are usually not fully adequate, addition of community services typically requires additional funds if the institution's residents are not to be further deprived.

Several states are developing state-operated and funded regional centers, which assume a major role in supplying comprehensive services to the retarded in their regions (e.g., Connecticut). These centers do not necessarily negate the development of regional services by institutions or by local community agencies.

Support of community-operated mental retardation centers through state grants-in-aid is another common pattern (e.g., Texas, New York). Some states have not developed a grant-in-aid program but are able to purchase services from community centers (e.g., Kansas, Iowa). Some institutions have entered into cooperative arrangements with community centers and some have developed formal contractual arrangements for supplying the centers with specific services (e.g., Austin State School).

In some cases Federal funds have been used to establish institution-based regional services. Vocational Rehabilitation funds have frequently contributed to vocational workshops and to vocational counselor positions, and funds from the Children's Bureau have been used to establish diagnostic and evaluation clinics.

7. There is a growing emphasis on the development of specialized programs to meet the needs of individuals with special problems. Some institutions have established units for the blind retarded (e.g., Murdoch Center in North Carolina, Willowbrook State School in New York, Austin State School in Texas), the motor handicapped retarded (e.g., Gracewood State School in Georgia, West Seneca State School in New York), and the socially disruptive retarded (e.g., Rainier State School in Washington, Lynchburg Training School in Virginia, Austin State School).

A somewhat different approach to meeting the needs of special groups is the development of specialized institutions, as contrasted with the more common multi-purpose facility. Louisiana, for example, has established a facility for mildly retarded, school-aged children (Ruston State School) and

is planning a small facility to serve as a respite service to parents. Talla-
hassee and Orlando Sunland Centers, on the other hand, handle only profoundly retarded residents presenting serious nursing problems. Specialized
facilities may present serious problems in the larger states by removing retardates from geographical proximity to their families.

8. Because program implementation is often seriously limited by physical
facilities, emphasis is being placed on construction of new institutions. New
institutions are being developed to absorb growing waiting lists in some
states, whereas in others (e.g., New York) the primary emphasis is on reducing over-crowding in existing facilities. New construction to replace ill-
suited existing buildings has, in general, been more difficult to justify, in
spite of the President's Committee's findings in 1967 that three-quarters of
the institutionalized retarded live in buildings at least 50 years old (President's Committee on Mental Retardation, 1967). Development of new institutions is usually guided by the principles that institutions should be relatively small, usually a maximum of 500 residents, although some states—
such as New York and Texas—are planning new 1,000-bed facilities; institutions should be located as near as possible to the population served; and
the physical plant should incorporate maximum flexibility without compro-
mising suitability for program implementation. Architects are expressing
growing interest in the problems of institutional construction, and workshops and literature are beginning to appear (e.g., U.S. Department of
Health, Education, and Welfare, 1966; Bayes, K., 1967).

In view of what appears to be general agreement regarding desirable features of institutional facilities, it is surprising to note that new facilities vary
considerably from each other. Some new buildings differ but little in basic
concept from old facilities, consisting of large sleeping "dormitories" and
centralized large "day rooms." Other institutions, borrowing heavily from
the Danish programs, are being designed to house all residents, including
the profoundly retarded non-ambulant, in small home-like units of eight
beds each, arranged in two to four beds per room (e.g., New York).

The architecture of new institutions will have important staffing implications. In general, the smaller the living unit, the higher the staff-resident
ratio needed to supply basic supervision. Hence, institutions built on the
New York model of eight residents per unit will require large ward staffs
and, consequently, high per capita costs.

Emphasis on home-like, small living units is based on the philosophy that
such units facilitate return to the home as a result of generalization and increased resident-staff interaction. Perhaps less explicit reasons for design of
such units stem from the fact they are more pleasing to staff, parent, and
community representatives. There seems to be little doubt that the large
impersonal living units so common in older facilities contribute to de-hu-
manization and institutionalization.

Concern has occasionally been voiced that living conditions on some of the new "home-like" units may be unsuited to residents who will probably be discharged to lower socio-economic sub-cultures, in that they are considerably more desirable than the situation the dischargee is liable to find in the community, leading to disappointment, frustration, and possible return to the institution. Perhaps a more serious concern with this type of unit arises from its possible unsuitability for profoundly retarded or non-ambulatory residents. The necessary constant nursing care and careful supervision of the bed-fast resident may be impaired by small living units segmented into separate rooms. Ready accessibility to bathing, feeding, and crawling areas may be decreased, thereby impairing effective programming. Furthermore, privacy—which seems desirable for the less seriously retarded—may be less desirable for the profoundly retarded bed-fast person who may benefit from maximum stimulation (Doman, 1967). Approximating the home environment for the ambulant profoundly retarded individual may prove to be considerably less effective than engineering the environment to facilitate conditioning procedures, as has been suggested by behavior modifiers (e.g., Watson, 1967).

Administration and Management

Implementing changes within institutions is greatly dependent on the philosophies of top level administration. Historically, state institutions for the retarded have tended to operate under administrations whose strategies have fostered the *status quo*. In general, change has occurred slowly and painstakingly, particularly in long-established facilities. Klaber (1968) has presented data suggesting that the basic institutional "climate" tends to carry the imprint of philosophy and managerial style of its *first* administrator.

OBSTACLES TO IMPLEMENTING CHANGE

Long-established state residential institutions are typified by considerable inertia. A new administrator attempting to implement change in such a facility soon learns to anticipate—with a high degree of probability—that any suggestion for change will be met by the staff with lengthy explanations of reasons why the proposal will fail. Policies and procedures are often justified on the basis of tradition, past "successes" or mandates of long-departed former administrators. A case in point was reported by a new superintendent who, puzzled by the daily blowing of the institution siren at an odd hour, finally determined after much effort that the blowing of the siren had been timed to signal an obsolete change in shift.

Change increases vulnerability, and many members of institutional staffs —including top level managers—have learned to survive by minimizing this vulnerability. Clinging to past methods and procedures insures a certain basic degree of safety, inasmuch as these methods and procedures have demonstrated some survival value for those who compiled with them. Furthermore, current practices have the advantage over new practices in that they have more predictable results and, hence, offer less potential danger.

The importance to institutional staff of minimizing vulnerability becomes apparent when it is recognized that in most situations promotion has been a function of tenure (i.e., survival in the system) rather than a function of achievement; criticism has been a function of commission rather than of omission; and until recently, institutional staff—and particularly top administrators—had little job security. As recently as 1968, institution superintendents could be dismissed without definite "grounds" in a number of states (e.g., Texas), but dismissal is usually facilitated by some action on the administrator's part for which he can be criticized. The administrator who "doesn't make any waves" usually remains securely entrenched.

Most institutions can be viewed as in a state of tenuous internal equilibrium. The inter-relationship among staff and between staff and residents is extremely complex and usually involves constant power struggles and rivalries. Any change in the *status quo* threatens to change the balance among these forces, resulting in increasing internal tension within the system. Resistance to change may in part be a function, therefore, of the desire by administrators to minimize staff conflicts and to maintain a "smoothly functioning" institution. Members of the staff, who have managed to carve out a niche in the institution matrix, may feel threatened by any change that might disrupt the current homeostasis and, thereby, threaten their security.

Institutional change is further impeded by the fact that typically institutions contain a number of sub-cultures which function more or less autonomously. Communication among these sub-cultures is usually tenuous at best, and often changes initiated by one sub-culture are strongly resisted by another. To the residents at least the following three sub-cultures can usually be recognized in a typical state residential institution:

Top Level Administration, consisting of the superintendent and his key staff. This group has primary responsibility for operation of the facility, formulates broad policy, usually represents the institution to the community, and has formal authority over the rest of the staff. To the majority of employees, however, this group tends to be viewed as the "front office boys" who are relatively unaware of what really goes on in the institution because of their remoteness from the daily operation of the facility and because of their short tenure (the mean tenure of superintendents has been estimated at between two and four years). Hence, although the administration usually assumes that it "runs" the institution, in point of fact middle and lower management personnel probably have a much more direct influence on the details of operation. Administrative communications frequently do not reach the majority of the personnel or, if reaching them, are disregarded or misinterpreted.

Professional Staff, consisting of the professionals in the various disciplines represented in the institution and related assistants and students (e.g., psychology interns, social work students on field placement). This group is primarily responsible for performing specialized technical services, for serving as a source of expertise for the rest of the staff, and—to a greater or lesser degree—for assuming middle management functions. This group usually perceives itself as responsible for implementation of specialized programs serving the residents, including "treatment," "training," "education," "counseling." In most institutions, however, the actual contact between professional staff and residents is usually extremely limited, both in numbers of residents directly contacted and amount of time spent in direct contact. Professionals usually spend the majority of their time interacting among themselves, and translation of their efforts into direct services to residents is usually severely diluted by transmission through several levels of relatively untrained personnel. Because professional staff has usually operated from a discipline-oriented departmental structure, services have tended to be fragmented and often lacking in coordination.

"Sub-professional" Staff or "Workers," comprising the bulk of the institution personnel. This group includes both supportive staff such as laundry workers, maintenance staff, and food service workers, and resident care staff such as attendants and recreation aides. In spite of marked differences in function, these groups can usually be considered as members of the same sub-culture, in that they possess similar values and attitudes. Most programs for residents are implemented by this group, and in nearly all institutions the vast majority of contacts which residents have with staff members occur with members of this group.

Interactions among these three institutional sub-cultures are complex and typically characterized by misconceptions which impede effective communication. Although generalizations are hazardous, the following misconceptions have been observed in a number of institutions:

The administrators tend to perceive the professionals as impractical idealists whose aspirations are often "out of touch" with limitations imposed by fiscal, political, legal, and other realities. Often the professionals are also viewed as dissipating much of their energy in never-ending status and jurisdictional struggles which seriously interfere with delivery of services to the residents. The workers are viewed by the administrators as reactionary, traditional, and resistant to change. Not infrequently, administrators consider the workers as harboring a custodial orientation to resident care.

To the professionals, the administrators often appear reactionary, dog-matic, and paralyzed by red tape. Often the administrators seem to impede progress by clinging to the safe course of action and minimizing all possible sources of threat. The professionals tend to perceive the workers as ignorant, custodial, and in constant need of training and supervision.

Because, in general, the workers form a relatively stable and continuing sub-culture, they view the other groups as transients whose impact will be relatively short-lived. They consider both other groups as basically "out of touch" with what is really going on in institutions, and therefore as advocat-ing impractical and often potentially dangerous practices. The professionals, in particular, are viewed as harboring bizarre and unrealistic notions which, if implemented, would make operation of the institution impossible.

The difficulties introduced by such misconceptions are compounded by problems in communication. Each sub-culture has tended to develop its own rather unique terminology which is often meaningless to members of the other sub-cultures. Some of the professionals, in particular, have developed the fine art of couching ideas in terms meaningful only to members of a specific professional discipline. Differences in terminology often reflect basic differences in frames of reference and value systems. The administrators, for example, tend to evaluate things in terms of budgetary implications, effi-ciency, and public relations. The professionals tend to emphasize clinical and research implications, while the workers tend to emphasize the practical as-pects of day-to-day operations. Not infrequently, values and goals expounded by one group are in direct conflict with the values of another group. For instance, administrators often express the philosophy that the mildly retarded should not be institutionalized and that those already residing in institutions should be habilitated. Professionals tend to prefer working with the mildly retarded residents, however, and hence are often reluctant to lose their clientele. The workers often consider mildly retarded residents as necessary to the operation of the institution as "working" residents, and hence they are covertly opposed to programs aimed at habilitation.

The effect of sub-cultures often in conflict regarding basic issues of pro-gramming is particularly disturbing to those members of the staff whose identification with a particular sub-culture is unclear. Frequently building supervisors, who are charged with management of the ward personnel, are in constant conflict with regard to their identification. They are required to function as representatives of the administrators, implementing administra-tion programs and policies. Yet, they have usually been promoted from the ranks of the workers and continue to identify with this group. It is not un-usual, therefore, to find supervisors functioning in such a way as to remain in "the good graces" of the workers. Many are careful, for example, always to enter resident living units by the front entrance in a noisy manner, thereby effectively avoiding the possibility of confronting workers engaged in unsanctioned activities.

Implementing change may further be impeded by aspects of the formal "system" governing operation of state institutions. State bureaucracy frequently introduces a lengthy delay between formulation of a plan and its implementation. Program implementation often requires review and approval by state bureaus outside the agencies operating the mental retardation institutions, so that delays may be the product of inter-agency communication problems.[1] The following PERT network is illustrative of the time required for implementation of a new speech and language program in one of the larger states (T_E = estimated average time in weeks) (Figure 2–1).

The existence of merit or civil service systems in many states can be another obstacle to implementing change. Because such systems usually entail considerable rigidity regarding job descriptions and requirements, recruitment of hard-to-get professionals and establishment of new types of positions needed to develop novel programs are often lengthy and difficult processes. Merit systems have also tended to reward tenure rather than accomplishment, so that promotion into leadership positions has often resulted from longevity rather than demonstrated leadership capacity. As a result, some state systems encourage innovative and creative persons to leave in frustration while long-term, traditionally oriented employees have gradually emerged into supervisory and administrative positions. The establishment of so-called *career ladders* in many states (e.g., Illinois, New York) is a recent attempt to upgrade staff through continuing training and education rather than through tenure. The basic feature of these ladder programs is that they enable untrained employees to obtain additional training while working for the state, leading to promotions based on level of training completed. Frequently, the training sequence allows eventual completion of professional degrees.

Fiscal aspects of state systems also may prove to be impediments to program innovation. In some states the financial structure is based on a rigid line item budget which prevents any significant modification in use of funds during the budget period. In many states the executive budget office exercises considerable control over expenditures, so that any departure from the budget requires detailed justification. These restrictions are particularly crippling in those states which operate on a biennial budget, because they often practically delay changes for as long as three years. The budgeting process itself has tended to delay change by requiring vast amounts of professional time, which might otherwise be devoted to program development and implementation.

---

1. Program Evaluation and Review Technique.

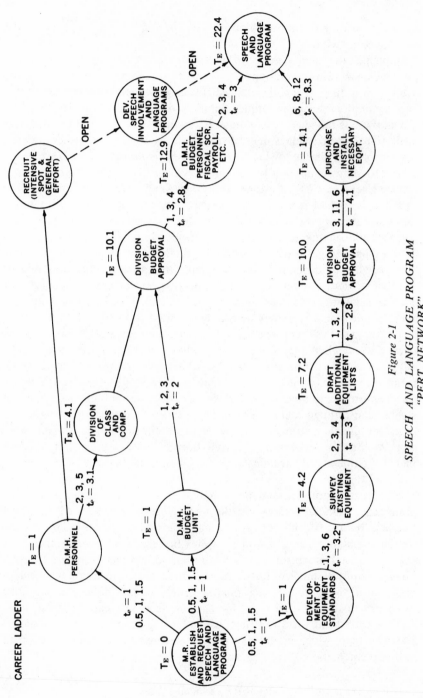

Figure 2-1

SPEECH AND LANGUAGE PROGRAM
"PERT NETWORK"

Styles of Administration

Administration strategies vary considerably among the states. In general, the superintendent of each state institution is responsible to a centralized office under the direction of one top-level administrator. Usually, the mental retardation programs are included with other programs, such as mental health, welfare, or social services, under a department where the administrator is directly responsible to the governor or a central board. South Carolina, however, in 1967 established a separate department of mental retardation, and some other states have been considering a similar arrangement. A recent survey (National Association of State Mental Health Program Directors, 1968) reveals wide differences in salaries of state top-level administrators of mental retardation programs, as well as considerable variation in their professional disciplines. Again, the degree of control exerted by the state-level administrator over the institution superintendents varies considerably. In some states, institution superintendents operate almost autonomously, whereas in others they do little more than implement central office policy. In some states, superintendents have their own governing or advisory boards. Although tenure of superintendents is usually short, some states include them in the civil service system (e.g., New York) and, hence, rather effectively protect them from discharge by state-level administration.

Probably the universal institutional administrative pattern in the United States is that of a single superintendent in charge of the total institution. The pattern of multiple administrators, prevalent in Denmark for example, has not been used in this country. Although there is considerable variability among institutions, the general table of organization included the following features: Overall administration by a superintendent and one or more assistants, a "clinical" or "medical" director responsible for all or part of the clinical programs, and a business administrator responsible for fiscal and supportive services. Professional disciplines usually are organized into departments, responsible either to the clinical director or to an assistant superintendent. Ward staff are often dichotomized into a nursing service for the most seriously impaired residents and a cottage life or student life service for the least seriously impaired residents. The former service tends toward a heavy medical emphasis, whereas the latter has an educational and training focus. In some states (e.g., New York), all ward staff are under nursing direction.

The relationship between ward staff and professional staff is often unclear. Frequently, although the professional departments are formally assigned a staff relationship to ward staff, they function as if in a line relationship. Consequently, ward staff tend to be exposed to conflicting directives, resulting in confusion. Institution administrators often have been frustrated by the difficulty of bringing professional resources to bear effectively on resident programming. Coordination of the various department-based disciplines is usually difficult, and probably in most institutions programming for the individual resident is basically the function of the ward attendant. Professional departments tend to develop specialized programs (e.g., special education classes, group therapy, parent counseling, speech therapy) for selected residents, and not infrequently they compete for the most "desirable" residents. As a result, the most impaired residents are often seriously neglected, while a handful of mildly retarded residents are overwhelmed with professional attention. Development of comprehensive programming for institutional residents has been further complicated by the tendency of departments to compete for status, prestige, and power.

A number of institutions have recently abandoned the traditional departmental structure for a "unitized" organization. Essentially, the approach consists of sub-dividing the resident population into several groups, each of which is assigned to a multi-disciplinary team. These teams become the basic programming unit of the institution, and they have full responsibility for all residents assigned to them. Under this arrangement, departments are de-centralized and department heads usually serve in a staff capacity to the teams and to the administration. Although details of operation differ, the unit approach seems effective in minimizing many of the problems associated with the departmental organization. Professionals work directly with ward staff and residents on a daily basis, and their affiliation is with the team rather than with the professional department.

Unitization of institutions reflects a general shift in managerial style in many facilities. Traditionally, institutions have operated as monolithic, autocratic management systems, stressing vertical rather than horizontal organization. In terms of Blake & Mouton's "Managerial Grid" model (Blake & Mouton, 1964), the prevailing managerial style has been of the 9–1 or "task management" variety, reflecting primary concern with production and de-emphasis on the human relations aspects of management. Often, superintendents have adopted the "paternalistic" pattern described by Blake & Mouton, whereby they have attempted to offset the autocratic climate they have created by attempting to develop a benevolent style of personal interaction with their employees. Decision-making has typically been autocratic and unilateral, with formal power vested in the superintendent and sparingly delegated to a few key administrators.

Communication within institutions has been characterized by heavy reliance on written memoranda and unilateral information flow. Directives have been handed down the administrative chain, and reports have travelled back up the chain. Typically, exposure (i.e., information presented by supervisors to subordinates) has overshadowed feedback (i.e., information presented by subordinates to supervisors), resulting in what has been described as a sizable "managerial blindspot" (Hall and O'Leary, 1966); that is, management remains unaware of considerable information possessed by subordinates.

The managerial style, use of power, and handling of communication just described are not well suited to current concepts of unitization and multi-disciplinary teams. Until the basic management matrix of an institution is changed, the success of the multi-disciplinary teams and of attempts at administrative decentralization will probably not succeed. Many institutions are, in fact, modifying significantly their management style in the direction of Blake & Mouton's 9–9 managerial style (i.e., simultaneous concern for production and for human relations), shared or democratic use of power, and greater sharing of information (i.e., increased exposure and feedback). These institutions have usually instituted formal management training programs for their managers, including use of "sensitivity training" and other forms of laboratory workshops (Schein and Bennis, 1965; Robins and Burns, 1968).

A potent factor in delaying the modification of institutional management climates has been the wide-spread operation of institutions as technocracies. Administrative power has been distributed on the basis of specific professional affiliation rather than by administrative skill. Usually medicine—and often a specific medical specialty—has been the basis for this position. The typical rationale involved consists of defining mental retardation restrictively in terms of the profession's own area of expertise (e.g., "mental retardation is an educational problem," "mental retardation is a medical problem"); claiming that, therefore, only members of the profession can—or should— manage professional services to the retarded (e.g., "only educators can fully understand the retarded and train them"); and concluding that because of their unique professional expertise, only members of the profession are able to—or should—administer programs for the retarded.

This type of strategy to maintain professional control of institutional administration is illustrated by the following quotes taken from a recent position paper prepared by the New York State Mental Hygiene Physicians (1968) as a formal stance regarding the New York State Department of Mental Hygiene's proposal to establish "Non-Medical Chiefs of Service" on selected services in some of its newer facilities:

"... The Association takes the basic position that mental retardation is a psychiatric problem. The general treatment program for mental retardation should, therefore, be under the supervision of a psychiatrist ... Whatever the cause, experience in dealing with even the mildest levels of retardation has shown that all retardates suffer from emotional problems ... Each retardate must be evaluated individually, taking into consideration all the relevant neurological, social, cultural, familial, and psychological factors. The breadth of this analysis requires the experience and training of a psychiatrist . . . A physician or psychiatrist can understand and appreciate the non-medical aspects of it (mental retardation), but the trained educator or social worker would be hard pressed to deal with the medical problems involved . . . The individual placed in the position of Chief of Service will, by the very nature of that position, be forced to make medical diagnosis; therefore, this person should be a psychiatrist."

This type of argument can, of course, be used by any of the disciplines relevant to mental retardation by adopting a suitable definition of mental retardation. From the standpoint of administration theory, this position confuses line authority with functional authority (Bailey, 1966). Expertise in a profession is valid grounds for functional authority, and decentralized multi-disciplinary approaches recognize this concept, in that members of each profession remain functionally responsible to their department head with regard to all matters pertaining to the technical aspects of professional practice.

The trend during recent years has been away from restricting administrative positions to members of specific professions. Legislative statutes limiting institution superintendents to members of the medical profession have recently been eliminated in a number of states (e.g., Kansas, New York). A recent national survey revealed that of 49 states responding, 29 employed non-medical institution superintendents (National Association of State Mental Health Program Directors, 1968).

Extra-Institutional Problems

Institutions can best be understood within the total context in which they operate. Pressures originating from outside the institution may strongly influence the quality and rate of institutional change. Hence, the institution's geographic location, its relative proximity to centers of professional resources, its availability to its catchment area, accessibility of manpower, and numerous other variables play a potent role in shaping its programs.

The geographic isolation of older facilities tended to foster relative separation from the communities served by the institution. Such institutions often have had difficulty in recruitment and retention of specialized professional staff, while having ready access to a more or less captive pool of unskilled or semi-skilled personnel. The current tendency to locate institutions in population centers near professional resources, while facilitating professional recruitment and retention, often leads to serious shortages in available unskilled and semi-skilled staff. (For example, Willowbrook State School, located on Staten Island, reported 286 attendant vacancies in October 1968.)

One of the major justifications for locating mental retardation institutions in population centers is the assumption that proximity to the families being served will increase the amount of parent contact and involvement with their institutionalized children. Although the desirability of this goal is generally shared by current experts, the validity of the premise is questioned by Klaber's Connecticut study (Klaber, 1968) which revealed no significant relationship between families' distance from institutions and frequency of visits. Because the study was limited to families living within a 50-mile radius of each facility, the results may not be applicable to larger catchment areas.

The National Association for Retarded Children, a parents' organization established in 1950, and its state and local units, has had a major impact on revolutionizing institutional programs. Parent groups have influenced institutional programs principally by stimulating legislative changes, supporting progressive institution programs, publicly criticizing shortcomings, educating the public, and contributing directly to institutions financially and through volunteer services. Parent associations (ARC's) have not only acted as catalysts for program development, but they have often developed their own programs, including sheltered workshops, day care centers, diagnostic and evaluation centers, special classes, and even "comprehensive centers." The National Association for Retarded Children has held the policy that operation of direct services by local Associations should be limited to demonstration programs aimed at stimulating development of similar programs by local and state public agencies. In some cases, however, the programs and facilities developed by local ARC's rival or even surpass state operations.

Professionals have gradually begun to recognize parents as potential allies rather than as obstacles in the habilitation process. Parent counseling has become the focus of professional attention, and there has been increasing recognition that parents need realistic information and help in practical aspects of child training rather than "treatment for psychopathology" (e.g., Roos, 1965; Casse, 1968).

Innovative volunteer programs have demonstrated that volunteers—including parents—can function effectively as extensions of the professional staff, implementing specialized educational, training, and treatment programs (Roos, 1964; Hinojosa, 1966, 1968).

The institution's relationship to the central state agency can also exert a significant influence on its development. In the past, institutions have often operated relatively autonomously, at times without a central office. Recent years have witnessed a trend toward increasing central office influence over institutions. Central office staffs have increased in size and have assumed more responsibility for development and implementation of institution programs. The New York State Department of Mental Hygiene has recently established central office Program Analysis teams, for example, charged with the development, implementation, and evaluation of institution programs. The types of demands from central offices on institutions tend to include demands for information, such as activity reports, budget preparations, and population movement data; demands for new programs or program changes, such as establishment of physiotherapy, family care, or screening procedures; demands for procedural or organizational changes, such as unitization or restricting admissions to severely and profoundly retarded; and demands for "political favors," such as admission of specific applicants or hiring of specific employees. The types of demands made obviously can have strong impact on the institution.

The relationship between central office and institution is at times clouded by the tendency of central office staff directors to operate as if they had line authority over the institutions. For example, disciplinary consultants may issue administrative directives to institutional members of their own discipline, or central office specialists in support services (e.g., business, fiscal affairs, engineering, food service) may issue direct orders to their institutional counterparts. The result of such confusion of line and staff functions is that line administrators (such as the superintendent or clinical director) may not be involved in critical decision-making. A further complication arises when institution personnel receive conflicting directives from central office staff consultants and from their institution line supervisors. To minimize such difficulties, superintendents frequently insist that all administrative line transactions between the institution and the central office be channeled through their office.

Mechanisms of fiscal control may have serious implications regarding the amount of flexibility afforded institution administrators. In some states the state budget agency (and often other agencies) must approve almost any proposed modification in deployment of resources. Because almost all decision-making in such systems becomes virtually the prerogative of the budget agency, the institution and central office administrators essentially operate in a consultant, or staff, capacity to the budget agency. In other states, however, lump sum budgets allow institutions considerable flexibility in use of resources, and hence program changes are greatly facilitated.

Other agencies serving the retarded or shaping the institution's future are also important. Considerable long-range institutional planning is predicted on the development of other community programs. New York, for example, is projecting that 10,000 retardates will be housed in community-operated hostels by 1989, and a gradual reduction in need for institutional beds is, therefore, anticipated. The degree to which alternatives to institutionalization are developed will be reflected by institutional changes.

Conclusions

With the increasing emphasis on long-range planning and planning-programming-budgeting-systems, institutions are being forced to formulate program goals. The lack of empirical data to substantiate widely accepted positions emphasizes the urgent need for research aimed at validating our current assumptions. There seems to be general agreement, for example, that institutions should be relatively small (although there is disagreement as to the specific size), that institutions should be located in or near population centers, that community programs will have a major impact on the composition and size of institutional populations, and that special disability groups should be housed in special units or facilities. There is little or no research evidence bearing directly on these crucial issues; however, long-range planning and commitment of substantial funding are proceeding as if these assumptions had been fully validated.

There are even more basic questions, however, which are seldom asked and which are not amenable to research. Answers to these questions are basically dependent on ethical values. For example, is the basic goal to increase the retarded person's happiness or to decrease the economic burden imposed on society or to minimize the differences between his behavior and society's? These goals may be mutually incompatible, and each would very likely lead to markedly different programs.

References

American Association on Mental Deficiency. Standards for state residential institutions for the mentally retarded. *American Journal of Mental Deficiency, Monograph Supplement*, 68, 1964.

Association of New York State Mental Hygiene Physicians. Position paper presented to the New York State Department of Mental Hygiene, New York, 1968.

Bailey, J. K. The organizing function: An overview. Unpublished manuscript, University of Hawaii, 1966.

Bayes, K. *The therapeutic effect of environment on emotionally disturbed and mentally subnormal children*. London: Unwin Brothers Ltd., 1967.

Bensberg, G. J., C. D. Barnett, and W. P. Hurder. Training of attendant personnel in residential facilities for the mentally retarded. *Mental Retardation*, 1964, 2, 144–151.

Blake, R. R. and J. S. Mouton. *The managerial grid*. Houston: Gulf Publishing Co., 1964.

Butterfield, E. C. and E. Zigler. The effects of differing institutional climates on the effectiveness of social reinforcement in the mentally retarded. *American Journal of Mental Deficiency*, 1966, 70, 48–56.

Casse, R. M. Jr. The professional's responsibility in aiding parental adjustment. *Mental Retardation*, 1968, 6, 49–51.

Cleland, C. C., W. F. Patton, and W. L. Dickerson. Sustained versus interrupted institutionalization: II. *American Journal of Mental Deficiency*, 1968, 72, 815–827.

Davies, S. P. *The mentally retarded in society*. New York: Columbia University Press, 1959.

Dayan, M. Toilet training retarded children in a state residential institution. *American Journal of Mental Deficiency*, 1964, 2, 116–117.

Doll, E. A. The essentials of an inclusive concept of mental deficiency. *American Journal of Mental Deficiency*, 1941, 46, 214–219.

Doman, G. *A summary of concepts, procedures and organizations*. Philadelphia: Institutes for the achievement of human potential, 1967.

Ellis, N. R. Toilet training the severely defective patient: An S-R reinforcement analysis. *American Journal of Mental Deficiency*, 1963, 68, 98–103.

Gardner, W. I. and H. W. Nisonger. A manual on program development in mental retardation. *American Journal of Mental Deficiency*, Monograph Supplement 66, 1962.

Goddard, H. H. *Feeblemindedness: Its Causes and Consequences*. New York: Macmillan, 1914.

Goldfarb, W. The effects of early institutional care on adolescent personality. *Journal of Experimental Education*, 1943, 12, 107–129.

————. Psychological privation in infancy and subsequent adjustment. *American Journal of Orthopsychiatry*, 1945, 15, 247–255.

Hall, J. and V. O'Leary. The manager as an agent of change. In *Executive development program for managers in the Department of Mental Health and Mental Retardation*. Austin: The University of Texas, 1966.

Harlow, H. F., G. L. Rowland, and B. Gary. The effect of total social deprivation on the development of monkey behavior. *Recent research on schizophrenia*, 1964, Rep. No. 19, 116–135.

Harlow, H. F. Total isolation: Effects on macaque monkey behavior. *Science*, 1965, 148, 666.

Hinojosa, V. Volunteer research and training project. Unpublished manuscript, Austin: Austin State School, 1966.

————. Programmed learning and volunteers. *Programs Report*. Austin: Behavioral Development Center, Austin State School, 1968, I, 10–14.

Institutes for the Achievement of Human Potential. *Treatment procedures utilizing principles of Neurological organization*. Philadelphia: Institutes for the Achievement of Human Potential, 1963.

Klaber, M. M. Paper presented to National Association of State Mental Retardation Program Coordinators. Hartford, 1968.

Klaber, M. M. and E. C. Butterfield. Stereotyped rocking—a measure of institution and ward effectiveness. *American Journal of Mental Deficiency*, 1968, 73, 13–20.

McCandless, B. R. Environment and intellectual functioning. In R. Heber & H. Stevens (Eds.), *Mental retardation*. Chicago: University of Chicago Press, 1964.

Montessori, M. *Montessori method.* Trans. A. F. George. New York: F. A. Stokes, 1912.

Moore, O. K. Autotelic responsive environments and exceptional children. Hamden, Conn.: Responsive Environments Foundation, Inc., 1963.

National Association of State Mental Health Program Directors. Non-medical administrators of public institutions for the mentally handicapped. *Studies,* 1968, 93.

————. Salaries: State MH-MR programs. *Studies,* 1968, 120.

New York State Planning Committee on Mental Disorders. *A plan for a comprehensive mental health and mental retardation program for New York State.* Vol. V. Albany, New York, 1965.

President's Committee on Mental Retardation. *MR 67: A first report to the president on the nation's progress and remaining great needs in the campaign to combat mental retardation.* Washington, D.C.: Superintendent of Documents, U.S. Government Printing Office, 1967.

————. *MR 68: The edge of change.* Washington, D.C.: Superintendent of Documents, U.S. Government, U.S. Government Printing Office, 1968.

President's Panel on Mental Retardation. *A proposed program for national action to combat mental retardation.* Washington, D.C.: Superintendent of Documents, U.S. Government Printing Office, 1962.

Provence, S. and R. C. Lipton. *Infants in institutions.* New York: International University Press, 1962.

Robins, S. and W. Burns. A staff development laboratory in a state hospital. Unpublished manuscript, New York: Pilgrim State Hospital, 1968.

Roos, P. Mental retardation—a challenge to volunteers. Paper presented at the annual meeting of the Mental Hospital Institute of the American Psychiatric Association. Dallas, Texas, 1964.

————. Development of an intensive habit-training unit at Austin State School. *Mental Retardation,* 1965, 3, 12–15.

————. Initiating socialization programs for socially inept adolescents. *Mental Retardation,* 1968, 6, 13–17.

Rosenzweig, M. R., D. Krech, and E. L. Bennett. A search for relations between brain chemistry and behavior. *Psychological Bulletin,* 1960, 57, 476–492.

Scheerenberger, R. C. A current census of state institutions for the mentally retarded. *Mental Retardation,* 1965, 3, 4–6.

Schein, E. H. and W. G. Bennis. *Personal and organizational change through group methods.* New York: John Wiley and Sons, 1965.

Seguïn, E. *Idiocy and its treatment by the physiological method.* Albany: Columbia University, Brandow Printing Co., 1907.

Shotwell, A. M. and D. Shipe. Effect of out-of-home care on the intellectual and social development of mongoloid children. *American Journal of Mental Deficiency,* 1964, 68, 693–699.

Skodak, M. and H. M. Skeels. A final follow-up study of one hundred adopted children. *Journal of Genetic Psychology,* 1949, 75, 85–125.

Spitz, R. A. Hospitalism: An inquiry into the genesis of psychiatric conditions in early childhood. In Freud, A., *et al.* (Eds.), *The psychoanalytic study of the child.* Vol. I. New York: International Universities Press, 1945, 53–74.

————. The role of ecological factors in emotional development in infancy. *Child Development,* 1949, 20, 145–156.

State of New York Executive Department. *Guidelines for planning programming budgeting.* Albany, New York, 1968.

Stedman, D. J. and D. H. Eichorn. A comparison of the growth and development of institutionalized and home reared mongoloids during infancy and early childhood. *American Journal of Mental Deficiency,* 1964, 69, 391–401.

Thorne, G. *Modifying attendant behavior.* Paper presented to National Association of State Mental Retardation Program Coordinators. Hartford, 1968.

United States Department of Health, Education, and Welfare. *Design of facilities for the mentally retarded.* Washington, D.C.: Public Health Service Publication No. 1181-C-1, 1966.

Watson, L. S. Application of operant conditioning techniques to institutionalized severely and profoundly retarded children. *Mental Retardation Abstracts,* 1967, 4, 1–18.

Zigler, E. and J. Williams. Institutionalization and the effectiveness of social reinforcement: A three-year follow-up. *Journal of Abnormal and Social Psychology,* 1963, 66, 197–205.

Planning a Residential Facility
for the Mentally Retarded

The mentally retarded person whether he is an infant, a child, an adolescent or an adult, is first a human being and only secondarily retarded. Though he may require specialized services, his basic needs are similar to those of other people in our society (Tarjan, 1966).

A commitment and an appreciation of the fact that the retarded person is indeed, first a human being should be the underlying and overriding consideration in all aspects of planning facilities for the mentally retarded. It should be the one thread which ties together all the planning efforts, the design of the facility and the services programmed for that facility.

Changing Concepts in Residential Care

Certain historical developments and current trends in residential care for the mentally retarded should be considered at the onset of planning. For many years, the residential facility has been the principal source of services for mentally retarded individuals (Task force . . ., 1964). The new concept, which is becoming increasingly popular with professional and laymen alike, is that the residential facility is but one of a number of resources in the management of mental retardation and that it best meets the needs of only a small percentage of the mentally retarded (Task force . . ., 1962). This concept has not yet been realized in the United States. While many states are moving more actively into the establishment of community services, currently these services probably fall below those being offered by residential facilities. Eventually these community services will serve the needs of most of the mentally retarded in each state; but these services are not generally available at present. This does not mean, however, that those community services which are currently available and those projected in the State Comprehensive Mental Retardation Plans should not be taken into account in planning a new residential facility. To be truly comprehensive, residential and community services must complement each other and the role of each must be carefully delineated so that one does not duplicate, complicate, nor handicap the other.

Residential facilities have been the most visible service provided for the mentally retarded. They represent the greatest investment in planning, manpower, buildings, and dollars of any provisions made for the mentally retarded. It is mandatory that new facilities be planned which complete knowledge of the strengths and weaknesses of existing facilities and in the light of current trends and future needs. The questions of size, location, whether to be multi-purpose or, whether to develop further institutional facilities at all will confront the planning team. Some of these issues may be of vital importance. Others may not represent the real problem in planning services but will screen and submerge the critical issues. None of these questions has been satisfactorily resolved (Task force . . ., 1962).

Historically, residential institutions have been supported by governments. Legislators have a tendency to favor appropriations for buildings rather than for programs or personnel, one-time expenditures rather than recurrent expenses. As an example, when federal funds became available for the construction of Community Mental Health Centers and Community Mental Retardation Facilities, no provisions were made for staffing. Yet the program is the primary goal. Personnel, as well as buildings, must be considered early in the planning efforts (Proceedings of institute. . . ., 1967).

Current Trends in Residential Care

As recommended by the President's Plan on Mental Retardation (1962), traditional institutions will probably house fewer residents in the future. Overcrowding may disappear. Space standards will be raised. New organizational patterns will evolve, creating smaller more home-like units within the large institution. But the real challenge will be to improve personnel (MR Workshop, 1965).

There will probably be a greater diversity of institutional programs. Greater emphasis should be placed on extramural activities, on part-time and short-stay residential care. Research and professional training are becoming essential components of residential programs. Realistic and meaningful affiliations with community resources, with medical schools and universities will become the accepted rather than the exception (MR workshop, 1965).

The entire system of institutional care in this country is now in transition (Tarjan, 1966). The full-time residential facility is increasingly used for the severely retarded and those with concomitant physical and mental handicaps. New concepts emphasize greater flexibility and increased utilization and include residential care only on weekdays, placement in small cottage-type units, combined work-institutional programs, and short-term placement with readmission to society as a goal (Covert, 1965; Task force . . ., 1964; Rogers, 1962).

The "Why" of Planning

The need for increased services and facilities in the face of the many pressing problems calls for planning. Planning is a dynamic and continuous process for translating available resources into effective patterns of action. The process consists of a series of activities for developing, releasing, and guiding cooperative effort (Areawide planning . . ., 1963). The local situation as it now exists in each state must be taken into careful consideration by those individuals planning residential facilities for the mentally retarded. It is utterly absurd to make far-ranging and lofty plans in a state whose pocketbook will not even afford the simplest facility. It is absurd to build a large and potentially sophisticated physical plant if funds are not available for staffing it for its best utilization.

Planning is important because many of the services now being provided for the mentally retarded are comparatively new, especially those at the community level. Although public interest in the mentally retarded in this country dates back more than 150 years, interest in this problem during the past decade exceeds that of any similar period in history. During this period many new services have been established (Planning of facilities . . ., 1964). Most of these services have been established independently with little consideration given to the important task of fitting them into a statewide plan for meeting the total needs of the mentally retarded.

A great number of agencies, public and private, at both state and local levels, administer services for the mentally retarded. There has been comparatively little meaningful and realistic joint planning and coordination among the agencies in the development of services for the mentally retarded (Manual on program development . . ., 1962).

Cross-agency Planning

Complexities in planning residential facilities arise because of the involvement of many agencies, private, volunteer, and government, with responsibilities for many of the program components both in and out of the facility. For instance, many of the residents, both the educable and the trainable, require special education classes at the elementary and secondary level. How are these services to be provided? Vocational rehabilitation programs (evaluation, pre-vocational training, training stations, and rehabilitation residences) must be planned and responsibility for their administration must be determined. Vocational rehabilitation departments sometimes will construct needed facilities on the grounds of residential facilities to provide professional training for their own staffs as well as to provide services in the community, to other residential facilities, or to specialized diagnostic clinics, such as might be established in the state's medical schools (Proposed program . . ., 1962). Other community programs such as day care, recreation, and religious programs should also be involved in a well-rounded residential program and must be given consideration in total planning.

It is evident that the agencies responsible for providing these programs in the residential facility must also be involved in planning for them (Planning of facilities . . ., 1964). Joint planning by agencies—state, local, private, and volunteer—which have or will have administrative responsibilities for providing these services is the best single assurance that the needed network of services will be truly effective as it is developed and expanded. The planning process serves the valuable purposes of simultaneously laying the foundation for program development and of communication among those who will later be the administrators of the services.

Whenever related services are administered by several different agencies a coordinated approach to planning is essential. Cross-agency planners should consider programs at all levels—federal, state, and local. They must be aware of which federal programs will support construction and staffing. Local or county governments may also be involved, particularly if they are to provide special education programs for residents of the facility. Effective coordination among administrative agencies or their subdivisions is often difficult to achieve; but coordination is necessary to guarantee that the mentally retarded receive adequate services of all needed types (Planning of facilities . . ., 1964).

Through the years recommendations have been made by a variety of groups and organizations about how to achieve a coordinated approach to planning services for the mentally retarded. In 1968 a National Conference on Mental Retardation was called by the Council of State Governments.

This conference recommended "that each state establish an interdepartmental agency, such as an interdepartmental committee, council or board for joint planning and coordination of state services for the mentally retarded."

In 1960 the sixth White House Conference on Children and Youth recommended that "each state establish a permanent structure to coordinate all public and private services for the mentally handicapped, to review legislation, and to carry out overall long-range planning in relation to other services."

Again in 1962 the President's Panel on Mental Retardation, having studied the complex problem of multi-agency responsibility in services for the mentally retarded, recommended . . . "each state should make arrangements through such means as an interdepartmental committee, council, or board for the joint planning and coordination of state services for the mentally retarded."

Further support for such interagency planning can be found in the recommendations of the Comprehensive Mental Retardation Plans developed by all states under the mental retardation planning grants provided through Public Law 88–156. The Mental Retardation Planning and Implementation Projects established under these grants in every state developed a long-range blueprint for services for the mentally retarded. Every state recognized the need for some type of interagency coordinating body and made recommendations for its establishment.

When plans are being made for programs and services in a residential facility, the interagency coordinating committee should be utilized to its fullest extent. A plan can be evolved in which all parts are based on the same goals and assumptions for the future; events can be planned in their proper sequence; and those planning will not only have complete information about their own areas of concern, but will be aware of the overall goals, policies, and plans of other agencies.

The interagency coordinating committee will usually be comprised of the top personnel in the agencies concerned with programs for the mentally retarded. It serves as an executive-level policy-making body. To assist this group, there should also be established a representative advisory committee comprised of both official and voluntary agency personnel who have direct responsibility for the implementation of programs and policies. These are the "firing line" people in the concerned agencies. Studies and reports from this group will aid the interagency coordinating committee in making long-range plans and decisions. Both groups need to be actively involved in the planning process to insure that decisions for programs can be implemented.

All these details must be carefully thought out, agreements made, funds and personnel committed before designing a facility.

Preliminary Steps in Planning

The first steps in the procedure of planning for a residential facility are: to determine what services are to be provided, for whom, in what quantity, and of what quality; to project the cost of both construction and operation; to project the manpower needed for staffing; to coordinate with other services in the community or service area; to select site location, restrictions, and accessibility (Proceedings of institute . . ., 1968).

THE COLLECTION OF DATA

Both public and private agencies engaged in the planning of services and facilities for the retarded face many situations which can impede their success and effectiveness. Lack of precise data is probably the first obstacle encountered; others include a lack of realistic standards for programming and the unavailability of certain services for particular levels and age groupings of the retarded (Planning of facilities . . ., 1964). Standards recommended by the American Association on Mental Deficiency are, at best, preliminary and tentative and need further refinement and updating (a Manual on program development . . ., 1962; Standards for state residential institutes . . ., 1964).

Adequate data should be developed to provide a base for projecting the extent, character, and location of services and facilities which are needed to provide a comprehensive program. The data that should be collected are:

> Size of the population group for which services are to be planned (Tizard, 1964)
> Levels of retardation and age groups to be served
> Extent of community support
> Socioeconomic and cultural characteristics of the service area
> Availability of community health, education, and welfare services for the retarded
> Relative need for specialized services
> Contribution by other groups to the comprehensiveness of programming within the area
> Extent of cooperation of services with other mental retardation facilities for programs
> Extent to which funds (or facilities) will permit the mentally retarded to live in own home, in own community, or outside the community (Planning of facilities . . ., 1964).

RELATION TO OTHER STATE PLANS

In the early planning stages it is important to develop a thorough knowledge of the State's Comprehensive Mental Retardation Plan and the State's Plan for the Construction of Community Mental Health Centers and Facilities for the Mentally Retarded. The planning of services and facilities for the mentally retarded should be consistent with the basic principles in the State's Comprehensive Mental Retardation Plan and correlated with the State Construction Plan (Planning of facilities . . ., 1964).

The State's Comprehensive Mental Retardation Plan in most cases has outlined the need for additional facilities and the State's Construction Plan has frequently determined the placement of the facility and the geographic area to be served.

Basic Considerations in Planning

The ultimate test of all planning for services and facilities for the retarded is the effectiveness of the action taken on the recommendations of the planning team. The recommendations must be understood by the key leaders of the planning area and be capable of implementation with the current and future resources of the area. It is at this point that the differentiation between short-range programming and long-range goals comes clearly into focus. The recommendations of the planning group involving short-range programming must be amenable to immediate action. Those involving long-range objectives should be based on the anticipated successful resolution of problems requiring first attention.

Effective action on the recommendations of a planning group regarding the needs for construction of facilities for the retarded involves, among many things, the following:

Establishment of a realistic program to carry out recommendations. The program should be well conceived, practical, and its goals and objectives accepted by the community and planning authority.

Gaining and maintaining full support of community and professional leaders. Full support is essential and must be sustained over a long period of time to accomplish the results anticipated in the recommendations.

Securing and maintaining adequate and sound financial support. Continuing financial support for both capital outlays and operating funds must be secured.

Developing professional staff necessary to provide quality services. Qualified and experienced professional personnel should be available in sufficient numbers to meet current and potential staffing requirements of existing and programmed services and facilities (Planning of facilities . . ., 1964).

TIME FOR PLANNING

It has been repeatedly emphasized by planning groups that they never have enough time nor enough information to plan thoroughly (Proceedings of institute . . ., 1967). Not only should enough time be allowed to study the situation, but all available information should be accumulated and thoroughly digested before planning efforts begin. If a marked departure from the usual type of facility is anticipated, surveys of existing practices should ordinarily be followed by experiment on new concepts before radical changes in policy are introduced on a wide scale (Tizard, 1967).

ESTABLISHING THE PLANNING TEAM

Composition of the planning team will be dependent upon local situations as related to the agencies responsible for planning and constructing the facility and operating the programs within the facility. Continuity of planning must be assured. It usually takes four to eight years from the time the need for a new institutional facility is officially recognized until the institution is ready for occupancy (a Manual on program development . . ., 1962).

The basic planning team might be comprised of: a program coordinator, a director of the responsible agency or his representative, a representative for fiscal affairs, a representative from the building authority, representatives from the architectural firm, and consultants knowledgeable in a variety of fields related to programs and services.

The program coordinator should represent the agency responsible for planning and operating the facility. He has responsibility for the coordination of efforts including projection of the proposed programs (Proceedings of an institute . . ., 1967), writing the program plan, relating facility design to proposed programming of services, maintaining contact with appropriate agencies involved in the planning, and proper utilization of the consultants.

The director of the responsible agency should be initially and continuously involved on the planning team as an interpreter of policy, procedures, administrative directives, and, in general, be the final authority for approval of decisions related to the planning process. He will determine what amounts of authority to delegate to the program coordinator and the architect.

The person representing fiscal affairs must be constantly aware of decisions being made in order to coordinate plans for construction and operation with the state's financial capabilities. He must know how much money is needed, when it is needed, how much is going to be available and when it will become available. This individual should also advise and monitor contracts, agreements, purchases, and so forth.

If construction is done through a building authority separate and distinct from the planning and operating agency, this authority should be represented on the planning team. If the planning agency is responsible for supervising and financing construction, its fiscal affairs agent should appropriately fill this spot on the planning team.

In mental retardation, more than most other fields, the architect needs to share in developing the program. Through the experience of developing programs, he learns some of the characteristics of those for whom he is planning. While everyone knows from experience generally what goes on in a theater, school, or airport terminal, there are relatively few who can testify about building for the mentally retarded. Time spent with the planning team will be invaluable to the architect when he begins his preliminary designs for the facility. He will probably want to visit other facilities for the retarded and consult with professionals in the field. He should read "Design of Facilities for the Mentally Retarded," "Planning for Facilities for the Mentally Retarded," and other such publications; they are "musts" for the architect.

Harold Horowitz, a member of the American Institute of Architects and head of the Architectural Services Staff of the National Science Foundation, lists eleven basic points which the architect should use as a guideline in his design for facilities:

1. Objectives of the Master Plan
2. Special restrictions and limitations on design
3. Characteristics of the site
4. Site development requirements
5. Functional requirements for the facility
6. Characteristics of the occupants
7. Specific facility requirements
8. Relative location and interrelationship of spaces
9. Budget
10. Flexibility for future growth and changes in function
11. Priority of need among the various requirements (Proceedings of institute . . ., 1967)

By being a part of the planning team, the architect can achieve a complete understanding of these points and utilize them in the design of the facility.

In addition to regular members of the planning team, experienced consultants should also be utilized. Qualified consultants may be found among professional personnel of established facilities and in organizations and agencies involved in the planning of medical, education, vocational, and related health and welfare services for the retarded. These consultants should be skilled in the various techniques of planning services and facilities to meet area-wide needs, have an understanding of the problems faced by the mentally retarded, and have the ability to translate this knowledge into a program of action (Planning of facilities . . ., 1964).

Ideally the program coordinator, the consultants and the architect work closely together. When they do, communications open up, ideas develop, problems are stated and questioned from different points of view. The program planner expresses his hopes and concerns. The consultants share their experience and judgments. The architect translates these into designs which are more likely to meet the needs of the mentally retarded.

Additional Steps in Planning

Once the planning team has been assembled and the duties and responsibilities of each member carefully defined, a guide to both program development and architectural design can be developed. This plan should be an effort of the whole planning team. The program coordinator, however, will have the responsibility for putting together the many ideas evolved and actually writing the program plan.

What will be the optimal size of the facility? This question usually has already been answered either in the state comprehensive mental retardation plan or the state construction plan. Reference to these two documents should help to settle the matter. The current favorite is one which has 500 beds, perhaps because most institutions are larger than that today.

Other special concerns of the group should be discussed, elaborated, and decisions made concerning the role of this institution in a total care program. For example, residential care has been a significant element in the overall program for the retarded. Major changes in the management of mental retardation can now be expected. If the emphasis is to be on community care, will the roles of the residential institution shift (Tarjan, 1966)? Should a residential facility have the purpose of providing for the retarded individual only those services which cannot be obtained in the community, such as supervision, protection, and intensive, diagnostic, evaluation treatment and training activities which require specialized manpower, equipment, and facilities? Should it be the goal of the institution to admit only those in need of such special services and to return them to the community as soon as the individual is no longer in need of these (Task force . . ., 1962)? Or will certain individuals be admitted for lifetime care? Will this facility be multipurpose or special purpose? Will training of professional personnel be a major program of the facility? Will research be one of its primary goals? Will diagnostic and evaluation services be provided for prospective residents as well as for the community in general? How will the facility relate to existing community programs?

Lip service is usually paid to the idea of relying on "outside" agencies and community resources for certain services, but the complexity of the organization required to board, lodge, bring up, educate, care for, and occupy a large number of handicapped people can easily seduce planners into broadening the scope of the activities to be provided by the facility itself. Should the institution have its own theater, its own fire brigade, its own EEG and

X-ray laboratories, its own surgery, its own mortuary? Should there be one or two full-time chaplains, four or only two psychologists? Does a 500 bed institution require, as the AAMD Project on Technical Planning in Mental Retardation (1964) recommends, "consultant in pediatrics, psychiatry (including child psychiatry), electroencephalography, neurology, neurosurgery, orthopedic surgery, physical medicine and rehabilitation, internal medicine, general surgery, anesthesiology, opthamology, otorhinolarnygology, radiology, and pathology?" Is it necessary for all these specialists to make regular visits to the institution and to conduct clinics and ward rounds? Or could the neurology surgeon and the anesthetist perhaps be eliminated from the list? These will be the kinds of knotty problems to be considered (Tizard, 1968).

FINANCING

It would be a novel experience if every idea suggested and every program component desirable could be incorporated into the final program plan for the facility. Financial limitations, however, might seriously curtail inclusion of many elements. The plans and design of a residential facility usually hinge on the predetermined funds available for construction of such a facility (PCMR Message, April 1968). While this method has been used many, many times, it is undesirable. It cannot be overemphasized that a number of steps should be taken before the cost of construction is set. Facilities of this type do basically two things: They house retarded persons for whom programs must be developed and operated, and they house some employees who care for and provide programs of treatment for the retarded. A tentative estimate of the construction cost should be given only after one knows how many are to be housed, the number of employees necessary for the operation, the scope of the programs, the square footage required, the furnishings and equipment necessary, and estimated construction costs in the area for the next five years.

The method of finance varies greatly from one state to another. In certain states, construction is financed out of a budget appropriated by the state legislature. In other states, residental facilities for the retarded are financed by a building authority on bond issue and are leased to the operating agency for a period of years until the money for which the bonds were issued is repaid. In both cases, planning of the facility requires determination of individuals to be housed, programs to be run, and employees necessary to run these programs before any attempt can be made to estimate this cost. A figure should not be quoted nor estimated until this information is compiled. Only then can a tentative cost estimate be made. It is vitally important that the funding agency be assured of the availability of sufficient funds before contract documents are begun.

Preliminary Statement of Philosophy and Goals

The above are all important considerations and must be dealt with before the program plan can be developed. Once these issues are resolved, a statement of the philosophies and goals projected should be drafted for official approval before further planning proceeds (Task force . . ., 1965). Such a statement might say:

1. This facility should be concerned primarily with:
    (a) Residential care, diagnosis and therapy (A proposed program . . ., 1962; Mercer, 1968; Tizard, 1964).
    (b) Rehabilitation—both inpatient and outpatient for individuals and families (Tarjan, 1966).
    (c) Training of professional and subprofessional workers in the field of mental retardation. Close coordination with educational institutions should be initiated in the planning stage (PCMR Message, May 1968).
    (d) Research—basic research, applied research, perhaps an institute for the study of human behavior.
    (e) Coordination of a total state program for the mentally retarded—perhaps a referral center for smaller community clinics and other agencies might be developed.
    (f) Providing diagnostic, evaluation, rehabilitation, and counseling services for the community at large.
    (g) Training and rehabilitation of the minimally retarded and those individuals with I.Q.'s of 70 to 85—as they tend to become the school drop-outs, youthful offenders of the law, and welfare dependents.
2. This facility should provide:
    (a) Social and moral training (Rogers, 1962).
    (b) Pre-vocational and vocational training.
    (c) Counseling and guidance services for residents, families, and community agencies.
    (d) Genetic study and counseling.
    (e) Placement and after-care services—continuity of management of problem until adequate solution.
    (f) Programs administered for the needs of individuals, i.e., tailored programs.
    (g) A day care center for service and training purposes (Dybwad, 1968).
3. Consideration should be given to developing:
    (a) A physical plant based on requirements of residents and personnel.

(b) Homelike environment blending into surrounding community. Wards and ward-like situations are to be avoided. Emphasis should be placed on respect for privacy, development of individuals, and independent living. Facilities must have realism of community living (Tizard, 1966; King et al., 1968; Dittman, 1962; Tarjan, 1966).

(c) Outdoor spaces that serve as extensions of living areas. They should be attractive. The beauty of the surroundings should encourage visits, pride, and community participation (Roselle, 1954).

(d) Buildings that fit appropriately into landscape and blend with buildings of surrounding community. Construction should convey warmth, dignity, stability, and an atmosphere of professional competence.

(e) Contractual maintenance services—water, sewerage, laundry, food, steam.

(f) Landscaping, curbings, gutters, and roads that are appropriate for use by the physically handicapped.

(g) A master plan should be developed at the onset, regardless of whether the entire plan should proceed at once or in stages.

(h) A site as near as possible to a university campus—with easy access to public utility and bus lines for transportation of both residents and employees.

(i) Outstanding classroom and audiovisual areas for resident, student and professional classroom teaching.

(j) A scale model of plant to help avoid planning errors.

(k) A plan to select personnel to administer therapy, teach, and conduct research.

(l) Appointments during planning stages of a director, personnel officer, budget officer, administrator, maintenance engineer, clinical director, director of cottage life, and appropriate program directors. Within the early construction phases the director of in-service training, director of volunteer workers, and public relations officer should be recruited. Other resident-care personnel should be "on the job" at least six months before admission of residents.

(m) An evaluation and rehabilitation center as the first service. All potential admissions should be screened and pre-admission programming done through this center before admission. Educators, physicians, psychologists and social workers should be available at this time.

(n) Following activation of the evaluation and rehabilitation center the hospital and medical services should begin operation,

followed quickly by operation of services for the non-ambulatory.

(o) School, recreation, and pre-vocational training programs
should begin operation at the time of admission of the first
ambulatory patient. The possibility of residents attending
public schools should be investigated.

(p) All plans and programs should be carefully and repeatedly
reviewed as to compliance with both county, state and federal plans, regulations and philosophy.

Outline of the Program Plan

The statement of the philosophy and goals for the facility sets the tenor
and directions for the remainder of the planning. The statement should be
approved by the entire planning team and then delivered for review to the
officials who make the final program and budget decisions. Once approved,
the actual development of the program plan will begin. An outline of the
program plan might include the following:

I. Name of Sponsor of the Proposed Project
    A. Number, selection, and tenure of the governing board
    B. Officers of the board and committees appointed
    C. Community interests represented on the board
    D. Relationship of sponsor to state government
II. Need for the Proposed Facility
    A. Types of mentally retarded individuals to be served
    B. Adequacy of existing state facilities
        1. Age and type of construction
        2. Number and types of beds (Private, semi-private, wards)
        3. Site, area, and location
        4. Licensure report on existing facilities
    C. Other facilities for the mentally retarded
    D. Adequacy and availability of personnel
    E. Description of service area
        1. Counties and population of area to be served
        2. Geographic distribution of patients to be served
        3. New industries, population trends, and character of the
           area
    F. Relationship of proposed facility to the existing and pro-
       posed state programs on mental retardation
    G. Need for improved and expanded services
        1. Unmet needs for wider variety of services

       2. Extent of community demand for improved services
       3. Existing services nearby
III. A Description of the Proposed Program of Service
    A. A statement of standards and philosophy
    B. Goals and programs of the modern institution
    C. Projected population of the facility
    D. Physical facilities as related to proposed programs
IV. Staffing of the Proposed Facility
 V. Description of Construction Project
VI. Description of Site
VII. Demonstration of Specialized Services
VIII. Clinical Training of Personnel
    A. General operation of proposed training program
    B. Specific training programs
       1. Medicine
       2. Dentistry
       3. Nursing
       4. Speech and Hearing
       5. Psychology.
       6. Social Work
       7. Special Education
       8. Sociology
       9. Child Development
     10. Physical Therapy
     11. Occupational Therapy
     12. Recreation of Handicapped
     13. Guidance and Counseling
     14. Religious Therapy
     15. Vocational Rehabilitation
     16. Hospital Administration
IX. Research

Writing the Program Plan

Once the outline of the program plan has been approved, each area must then be elaborated and carefully described in terms that are understood by both the planning team (including the architect) and the responsible official agency.

Some of the information necessary for the development of the program plan, particularly statistical data, will already be available from various official agencies. Additional help can be gained from the state's comprehensive mental retardation plan and the state's construction plan. It is the responsibility of the program coordinator to assemble this information and utilize it as he writes the program plan. In completing the information he will, of course, be assisted by other members of the planning team, the architect, and various consultants.

The program plan should follow the outline previously approved. The following will be the kinds of information to be included under each heading (Where appropriate, examples utilizing the information from "A Program Plan for the Georgia Retardation Center," [1965] has been given for illustration.):

Name of Sponsor of the Proposed Project

Detailed information should be given about the agency which has requested that the facility be built, about the agency responsible for the construction of the facility, any lease agreements between agencies, title to the property on which the facility is being built, bonds issued for the construction, how the bonds are to be retired, rental agreements, and any other information to clearly define areas of responsibility for construction and occupancy. Administrative channels of ownership and responsibilities must be clearly defined at the onset.

Need for the Proposed Facility

The following information justifies a proposed facility and it needs to be as clear and complete as possible.

Types of Individual to be Served. Carefully describe the types of individuals to be served as well as those who will not be served, with appropriate reasons for each. Include admission policies; the extent of diagnostic and evaluation services to be offered; circumstances for temporary admissions; day-care, night hospital care, and after-care services to be provided.

Adequacy of Existing State Facilities. Complete information should be given about existing residential services in the state, the extent of overcrowding, the waiting list for admissions, and the projected numbers of retarded to need services. The role of the proposed residential facility in meeting the current and projected needs for services should be clearly stated.

Other Facilities for the Mentally Retarded. Since the trend in this country is toward expanded community programs, an inventory of existing community services, both day-care and private residential programs, should be outlined. Location of these facilities and the numbers being served will be essential. These can usually be found in the state's construction plan or the state's comprehensive mental retardation plan.

Adequacy and Availability of Personnel. Some indication of the adequacy and availability of personnel to staff the facility should be explained. If adequate staff is not immediately available, from what sources will they be drawn? How will the facility help to train personnel? What can the facility do to help utilize the available personnel to its maximum and to train sub-professionals to help relieve the inevitable shortage?

Description of the Service Area. The description of the service area will take into account the geographical area of the state to be served by the proposed facility, the present and projected population of the area, and characteristics of the area which may influence population trends, industrial growth, and similar indications that will affect the facility and its services.

Relationship of Proposed Facility to Existing and Proposed State Programs. The relationship of the proposed facility to the existing and proposed state program on mental retardation takes into account the differences and the similarities of this facility to those which exist and are proposed. All of the proposed programs including residential care, man-power training and development, research, and public education should be compared and evaluated. This will show how the new facility can complement existing and proposed programs and how it can fit into the state program of comprehensive care for the mentally retarded.

Need for Improved and Expanded Services. The need for improved and expanded services for the mentally retarded cannot be viewed in proper prospective if the provision of residential care is the only consideration. Residential care and the need for expansion of these facilities are a part of a program and are not to be viewed as a total program or service.

It would be helpful to relate how the proposed facility can help to implement some of the recommendations outlined by the President's Panel on Mental Retardation. The publication, "A Proposed Program for National Action to Combat Mental Retardation," lists the following needs for improvement and expansion of services for the mentally retarded:

1. Research in the causes of mental retardation and in methods of care, rehabilitation, and learning.
2. Preventive health measures:
   (a) Maternal and infant care
   (b) Protection against known hazards of pregnancy
   (c) Extended diagnostic and screening services
3. Strengthened educational programs generally and extended and enriched programs of special education.
4. More comprehensive and improved clinical and social services.
5. Improved methods and facilities for care, with emphasis on the home and the wide range of local community facilities.
6. A new legal as well as social concept of the retarded including protection of their civil rights; life guardianship provisions when needed; and enlightened attitude on the part of the law and the

courts; and clarification of the theory of responsibility in criminal acts.

7. Helping overcome the serious problems of manpower as they affect the field of science and every type of service through extended programs of recruiting with fellowships, and increased opportunities for graduate students, and those preparing for the professions to observe and learn at firsthand about the phenomenon of retardation —emphasis is placed on the need for more volunteers in health, recreation, and welfare activities, and for a domestic peace corps to stimulate volunteer service.

8. Programs of education and information to increase public awareness of the problem of mental retardation.

Beyond the strong emphasis on research and prevention, the Panel recommends:

(a) That programs for the retarded, including modern day care, recreational, residential services, and ample educational and vocational opportunities be *comprehensive*.

(b) That they operate in or close to the communities where the retarded live—that is, they be *community centered*.

(c) That services be organized to provide a central or fixed point for the guidance, assistance, and protection of retarded persons if and when needed, and to assure a sufficient array or continuum of services to meet different types of need (Tizard, 1968).

(d) That private as well as municipal, state and federal agencies continue to provide and increase services for this worthy purpose. While the Federal Government can assist, the principal responsibility for financing and improving services for the mentally retarded must continue to be borne by states and local communities.

The planned facility may meet only a part of the total need; but it should help guide, initiate and implement a total program for the retarded.

A Description of the Proposed Program of Service

This description should begin with a statement of the standards and philosophy of the proposed institution. The planning group should develop a positive statement of the role of the residential facility, making sure that the various components proposed are compatible with the state's total program of comprehensive care for the mentally retarded. Some of the points covered earlier will help to amplify the statement about what this residential facility should be. However, there are other positive features of residential facilities as well as some problems which can interfere in the achievement of objectives, and they should be realistically considered at this point.

Residential facilities include services for the severely retarded and totally dependent, for those who cannot be maintained in the home or community because of emotional or behavior problems, and for members of communities unable to support financially the services required, or for those persons whose placement in generic services or facilities such as foster homes is impractical or inadequate (Planning facilities . . ., 1964). Every institution for the mentally retarded should be therapeutic. It should actually foster the development of the mentally retarded to their maximum capacity and thus bring them as close as possible to the main stream of independence and "normalcy" and provide some accommodation or adjustment in society for those disabilities which cannot be overcome.

The challenge of the modern institution for the retarded is how to replace the old concept of custodial care with modern programs of therapy, education, training, rehabilitation, and research (a Manual on program development . . ., 1962). Institutions have over extended their programs so that personal attention has been lost in mass impersonal services. Traditional institutional living prepares one for institutional living rather than preparing one to return to the community. More able patients have sometimes been exploited at the expense of their rehabilitation. Much of the direct service is provided by untrained attendants while the professionally trained personnel are engaged in administrative tasks. Citizens are genuinely interested in the welfare of the handicapped, but institutions have long been thought of as places of misery, tragic happenings, and unattractive settings. They should be so inviting, interesting, and progressive that citizens will think of them as places they like to know, to understand, and promote their goals and functions, and desire to help. Moreover, the creation of both attractive and functionally efficient plants is fundamental for operation of a progressive program. Beauty and efficiency influence the behavior and accomplishments of everyone.

Children have the right to demand of those who control their early years the opportunity for a maximum development of all innate abilities. They have the right to live in homes and communities which approach as nearly as possible the desirable standards of normal homes and communities (Humphrey, 1968).

Diagnosis and evaluation should take place before admission and a definite program for the retarded person developed and made available at the time of admission (Task force . . ., 1962). The institution should extend its services beyond its traditional boundaries and reach out to assist the retarded person and family before admission. There should be a flexible admission and release policy (Gove). No child or adult should remain in the institution longer than necessary. The institution is responsible for the care of persons returned to the community until proper assistance is assured by community agencies.

Community education is a part of an institutional program. Programs utilizing volunteer services are necessary. Staff development programs are mandatory. Cooperative programs with colleges and universities for training in many disciplines should receive high priority. Institutions for the retarded, community agencies, and educational institutions must develop coordinated planning and demonstrations of new methods of therapy, teaching, research, and vocational rehabilitation (Areawide planning . . ., 1963).

Goals and Programs of the Modern Institution

Once the statement of the standards and philosophy is developed, the next logical step is to define specifically what the proposed institution will do toward reaching the goals and programs of the modern residential institution. These include its role in care, treatment, training, manpower development, research, and public education.

CARE

A clearly outlined, clearly understood, administratively enforced, and financially practical program with demonstrable results is fundamental to success in dealing with the complex, often life-time symptom of mental retardation. The symptom of mental retardation is frequently complexly and irrevocably associated or fused with physical and personality disability.

The emphasis in care should be on *health,* not on disease. The emphasis should be on individual care, not on assembly line regimentation. Only when results are unmistakenly demonstrated will facilities for the retarded be accorded the same respect and public support as general hospitals and schools. Only when health, not disease, is emphasized will financial support and public acceptance be a fact. Programs, personnel, and physical facilities for the mentally retarded have been and still are financially poor, half-heartedly supported, and dimly understood by the public *because the programs have demonstrated inadequate results.*

The mentally retarded have the same needs as other growing and developing individuals; for appropriate stimulation—biological, emotional, social, and intellectual—but, in addition, they need special services appropriate to their particular disability and stage of development.

TREATMENT

Treatment includes the prevention of potential disabilities as well as the amelioration, cure, and rehabilitation of physical, mental, educational, social, and personality disorders. It includes the total ranges of diagnostic and therapeutic services necessary for the promotion of health. It should be viewed in relationship to the total individual, not as an isolated part. The social health should be at least as important as physical health. The goal of treatment should be an improvement of function and not a focus on dysfunction. If an individual has a handicap that cannot be ameliorated, the emphasis must be on helping him function in spite of this handicap. His assets, not his liabilities, should gain attention.

TRAINING

The amount, degree, and range of training should be limited only by the potentials of the population involved. Each individual should be viewed as having potential for growth and development. Each individual should be involved in a training program tailored to his own needs. It is important to view the individual not only in light of his currently recognized potential, but also in light of the lack of scientific knowledge on the part of those working with him. This potential, therefore, should not be viewed as static or having fixed limits. For those who will not be able to return independently to the community, training should be directed toward self-help skills, recreation, socialization, use of leisure time and, in some instances, profitable skills. For those who will return to the community, training should be directed toward acceptable socialization, skills in communication, and occupational skills.

MANPOWER DEVELOPMENT

The institution represents a broad spectrum of areas of specialization and services, and has, as a result a rich potential for training. Although training of individuals for work within mental retardation programs is primary, participation in other state and community programs is acceptable, justifiable, and should not be discouraged. Orientation, seminars, and specialized short-term courses should be a part of the manpower development program. Continuing in-service education is a vital part of the program. Career development should be emphasized. A close relationship with educational institutions is mandatory for success of this program (Dybwad, 1968).

Volunteers of all ages should be challenged. Retired persons should be recruited to place their rich experience and special talents at the service of the mentally retarded.

With additional training and experience, certain minimally retarded individuals can help care for the more severely retarded on the community level.

Training of parents and other community leaders in the care, understanding, and rehabilitation of the mentally retarded should be a vital and continuing program of the institution.

RESEARCH

Research must be incorporated into institutions for the mentally retarded if the ageold gap between knowledge and its application is to be narrowed.

Research may take several forms in an institution for the mentally retarded: Research dependent upon the study of the mentally retarded individual; research upon problems of immediate concern toward improved operation of a facility; basic or pure research, both diagnostic and therapeutic.

The goals of the institution as they apply to research should be to provide
for the administration of an organized program of research and seek funds
for this purpose; to encourage and support institutional personnel with
demonstrated research interests and ideas to carry on research by making
the necessary resources (time and money) available to them; to cooperate
with universities, departments of rehabilitation, and other research agencies
in making materials and facilities available; to stimulate research efforts
which will contribute, not only to the improvement of diagnosis, treatment,
training, and care facilities within the institution, but to new knowledge
about mental retardation.

As a matter of policy, no research should be done that might endanger or
cause undue discomfort to the resident. All applications for research must
be reviewed and acted upon by the proper authority.

PUBLIC EDUCATION

Public support, and more basically, public acceptance, understanding, and
empathy for those individuals with the symptom of mental retardation will
come only through public education and knowledge. From the earliest stages
of planning through its entire operation, communications with individuals
and groups should be established, fostered, and continued (Planning for
mental health services . . ., 1963).

Every good channel of communication should be established to improve
understanding. The involvement of the institution with other social institutions involving all aspects of community life will help to promote understanding and to enlist the support of lay and professional persons in the
institution's mission. The institution should take the initiative in establishing
an exchange of information, manpower, facilities, leadership, and services
with the larger community.

Projected Population of the Facility

To project personnel requirements, develop an organizational structure, and
design the physical plant, the population to be served—residents, day care
students, and personnel—must be determined. While employing criteria of
age, I.Q., and ambulation is at best superficial, it is a beginning in the concept of providing programs for people. Much statistical data is available and
must be utilized as it applies to the facility under consideration.

In dealing with people, statistics should be used with care. A group of
people might be compared with a collection of marbles of all sizes, composi-

tions, and colors of the rainbow. If one attempts to "average" their color by mounting them on a circular disk and rotating it rapidly, the color visualized is dirty gray. But there isn't a dirty gray marble in the lot. People are as distinctive as marbles, and when one attempts to average them, the result is dirty gray people. Averaging when applied to people in this careless way can be vicious and deceptive. Each person is a unique specimen (Williams, 1967).

Projecting a population by ability and age groupings for design concept purposes does not preclude the "mixing" of ages, sexes, and ability levels into "family type" units once the program is in operation.

However, some statistical breakdown is necessary, and the breakdown should include a basic statement about the characteristics of the groups described. The following from "A Program Plan for the Georgia Retardation Center" is illustrative of the type of information to be developed:

AMBULATORY

I.Q. 0–35. PROFOUNDLY AND SEVERELY RETARDED
Long-term residential care requiring complete and constant care. Emphasis on simple self-help skill, more acceptable behavior, socialization, and recreation. There should be constant and continuous introduction of new experiences and stimuli.

AGES	NUMBER OF RESIDENTS
0–10 years	60
11–15 years	110
15–40 years	130
40+ years	20

I.Q. 35–50. MODERATELY RETARDED
Potential for return to the community on limited and supervised basis. Emphasis on socialization, self-help, and simple vocational skills, recreation and very simple classroom situations.

AGES	NUMBER OF RESIDENTS
6–10 years	20
11–15 years	40
15–20 years	160

I.Q. 50–70. MILDLY RETARDED WITHOUT REFERRAL FOR PARTICULAR ANTI-SOCIAL BEHAVIOR Good rehabilitation potential. Emphasis on normal living, modified academic education, vocational skills, and socialization techniques. Repeated exposure to community will be needed. Responsibilities of independence must be imparted.

AGES	NUMBER OF RESIDENTS
6–10 years	20
11–15 years	40
15–20 years	40
20–40 years	20

I.Q. 50–90. MILDLY RETARDED OR WITH BEHAVIOR DISORDERS
Usually institutionalized because of overt anti-social behavior. Probably will
need additional special education and vocational training. Excellent candidates
for vocational rehabilitation. Of special interest will be guidance in acceptable
social behavior. Psychiatric help will be needed with many. Proper use of
leisure time will be stressed. Responsibilities of independence must be imparted.

AGES	NUMBER OF RESIDENTS
14–20+ years	40

I.Q. 40–70. MODERATELY-MILDLY RETARDED These individuals are
primarily here for "geriatric" or nursing home care. Can be taught self-help
skills as well as techniques for care of less able residents. Leisure time activities will be important. Physical rehabilitation will be a necessary program
component.

AGES	NUMBER OF RESIDENTS
20+ years	80

NON-AMBULATORY

*I.Q. 0–35. PROFOUNDLY AND SEVERELY MENTALLY AND PHYSI-
CALLY HANDICAPPED* Demands primarily nursing care. Some self-help
skills and recreation, physical therapy. Emphasis on communications.

AGES	NUMBER OF RESIDENTS
0–6 years	30
6–10 years	40
11–20 years	70
20+ years	40

I.Q. 35–50. MODERATELY RETARDED. Nursing care with emphasis
on as much self-help as residents' potential permits. Active recreation and
leisure programs. Constant exposure to new situations and stimuli. Occupational and physical therapy.

AGES	NUMBER OF RESIDENTS
10–40 years	20

*I.Q. 50–70. MINIMALLY RETARDED BUT SEVERELY PHYSICALLY
HANDICAPPED* Nursing care plus academic education, strong programs
of self-help, socialization, communications, recreation. Occupational and
physical therapy.

AGES	NUMBER OF RESIDENTS
10–40 years	20

TEMPORARY ADMISSIONS

The person admitted temporarily is to be admitted by referral from other
state or community sponsored programs for a specific and special purpose

that this facility can best meet. At the end of a previously determined time, these individuals will return to the referring agency. In no instance should this service be used as a route for permanent admission.

DAY OR NIGHT HOSPITAL CARE

Day or night hospital care refers to individuals who reside in the surrounding community and come to the institution for training during the day while living at home, or individuals living within the institution at night who go into the surrounding community during the day for work or training. This is mainly a demonstration for technique development and manpower development.

FOSTER HOME SUPERVISION

Certain individuals who are being sent back to the community will need continued supervision for a period of time in foster home or boarding house environment. The institution should continue some degree of supervision until discharge from the program. Foster home placement directly from the community should not be a function of the institution, but of the community or other state programs.

OUT-PATIENT EVALUATION

Each resident, before admission and on referral from another agency, should be completely evaluated and a program designed for his individual needs. Certain diagnostic referrals may be accepted from the community if community facilities are not available, even though the individual is not a candidate for admission. In general, the bulk of evaluations will be pre-admission evaluations. For easy reference the above information is summarized in Table 3–1.

Physical Facilities as Related to Proposed Programs

The facet of planning that requires the most time to develop deals with the physical facilities and their relationship to the proposed program goals. Those involved in writing a program plan for a proposed facility might profitably refer to documents such as "A Program Plan for the Georgia Retardation Center" for guidance and to help avoid omission of specific details which may easily be eliminated without some sort of check list to follow. In general, distinct program areas must be devised and constructed to accommodate the "average" individual in each group, with enough flexibility to serve exceptional needs, abilities, disabilities, ages, and personality assets or liabilities (Planning the patient care unit . . ., 1962; Tizard, 1964). For example, a six-year-old hemiplegic child of I.Q. 50 with a convulsive

Table 3–1. *Summary of Projected Georgia Retardation*
Center Population

Ambulatory			
I.Q. 0–35			
Age	0–10	years	60
	11–15	years	110
	15–40	years	130
	40 +	years	20
I.Q. 35–50			
Age	6–10	years	20
	11–15	years	40
	15–40	years	160
I.Q. 50–90			
Age	6–10	years	20
	11–15	years	40
	15–20	years	40
	20–40	years	20
I.Q. 50–70 (Primarily Social Problems)			
Age	14–20 +	years	40
I.Q. 40–70 (Physically Infirm)			
Age	20 +	years	80
Non-Ambulatory			
I.Q. 0–35			
Age	0– 6	years	30
	6–10	years	40
	11–20	years	70
	20 +	years	40
I.Q. 35–50	(all ages)		20
I.Q. 50–70	(all ages)		20

disorder has certain similar program needs as a six-year-old child, I.Q. 50, without added disabilities. Yet, there are specific, different, and special program needs for the physically disabled child with a convulsive disorder.

In addition to living areas, consideration must also be given to planning for administrative offices, records library, laboratories, pharmacy, X-ray rooms, infirmary, adjunctive therapies (physical therapy, music therapy, dentistry, psychology, occupational therapy, religion, physical medicine, speech and hearing, social work), research facilities, food service, laundry, housekeeping, maintenance, and all of the supportive services necessary to operate the facility. Consideration should be given in each area to expansion and growth in order that the space will remain adequate as service demands increase.

To illustrate the kinds of minimum preliminary detail that must go into this part of the program plan, the following are examples of two areas described in "A Program Plan for the Georgia Retardation Center."

Example I. (Housing)

Cottage for Profoundly and Severely Retarded Ambulatory Individuals

There will be 320 people of this category divided approximately equally between the sexes (refer to section on projected population for program needs and age variations). A maximum of four (4) units should comprise a building but the units within the building should remain autonomous as family groupings except for certain common utilities, administrative space, and bulk storage. This group of buildings should be located near the hospital, infirmary, administration building and readily accessible to outdoor play areas.

Units should contain:

1. Entrance hall.
2. Coat and boot storage in hall closet.
3. A family training room (off entrance hall with bath and closet facilities for overnight visits by parents) and extended stay of family for training purposes. This space may also be used for "temporary" admissions.
4. Dining room to accommodate 10–25 people, both residents and personnel.
5. Housekeeping storage.
6. Soiled linen room with double soak tub located convenient to laundry pick-up area.
7. Clean linen storage near bath and bedrooms.
8. Trunk, suitcase, and seasonal storage area.
9. Indoors activity room adjacent to outdoor enclosed play yard. A shower, sink, and water closet should be provided in this area.
10. Sleeping quarters. The two-bed rooms should contain a minimum of 80 square feet per person and the single-bed rooms 100 square feet per person.
11. There should be a locked closet for each in each room. Closets should contain space for hanging clothes, drawers for personal linens, shoerack, and open shelving for toys and other personal belongings.
12. One bath per cottage unit. Each bath to contain tubs, (no showers over tub), shower stalls separated by partial partition, water closets with ceramic barrier between water closets. All tubs and showers must have remote thermostatic controls. Each bath should have

appropriate floor drains to prevent flooding. Provisions for the individual's privacy should be included.

13. Restricted area outdoor recreation space for minimum of 10 persons.
14. Closed circuit television reception for instructional purposes and to receive commercial programs located in indoor activities room.
15. Houseparents apartment. Should include an entrance hall with coat closet, combination living room-dinette-kitchenette, bedroom for two beds, bath, two closets. Should have access to residents' sleeping areas as well as outside entrance.
16. Each building with minimum of two offices for administrative personnel. Include sink and medicine storage and preparation.
17. Each building to contain office and work space appropriate for number of university trainees scheduled for building.

Example II.

Facilities for Biological Research

  (1) Animal housing
  (2) Unusual and varying rates of air conditioning, ventilation, and humidity
  (3) Special furniture and equipment
  (4) Fume hoods
  (5) Cabinet work
  (6) Compact storage
  (7) Flexible space
  (8) Multiple flexible services—water, waste, gas, vacuum, electricity
  (9) Heavy equipment
(10) Future additions
(11) Access to clinical areas
(12) Auxiliary exit in fire hazard areas
(13) Emergency showers
(14) Emergency and fire fighting equipment
(15) Elevators if necessary
(16) No recirculation of air
(17) Tremendous storage areas
(18) Shielding for radioactive areas
(19) Some degree of separation between water used in laboratory and domestic water
(20) Consider problem of dumping corrosive waste into domestic sewer line. Check codes.
(21) Central source distilled water
(22) Consider problem of loss of conditioned air through hoods and exhaust
(23) Large volume air must be brought in without causing draft
(24) Allow for future increase of power; need fairly accurate voltage regulation

(25) Alcoves for vending equipment
(26) Offices
(27) Small reception
(28) Conference areas
(29) Classrooms or classroom-auditorium
(30) Supply and equipment entrance-exit
(31) Microscopy
(32) Constant temperature rooms
(33) Constant humidity room(s)
(34) Chromotography
(35) Glass washing
(36) Storage
       Equipment
       Glassware
       Supplies
       Files
       Chemicals
       Animal Food
(37) Computer room (space for)
(38) Water distillation
(39) Balance room
(40) Protective devices
       Fire
       Gas (fuel)
       Vacuum
       Compressed gas
       Electricity
       Steam
       Liquids (various)
       Gases (various)
(41) Waste disposal systems
(42) Animal quarters
(43) Refrigeration
(44) Communications
(45) Library
(46) Janitorial services
(47) Rest rooms, toilets, lockers, etc.
(48) Spectrophotometry
(49) Photography

Staffing of the Proposed Facility

The determining factors in the development of the personnel pattern for a facility are the objectives of the facility as expressed through administrative philosophy (Task force . . ., 1962; Tizard, 1968). Regardless of existing philosophies outside the organization or the definition of personnel administration, the objectives, organization, and function of the personnel within the facility must stem from and support its objectives and goals. If this is not the case, conflicts will develop over interpretation of administrative philosophy and the institution will be impeded in attaining its objectives.

Clearly, then, in planning for a new facility, care must be taken not only to develop well defined statements of organizational goals and objectives but also a clear and comprehensive administrative philosophy (King et al., 1967; Hallenbeck et al., 1967; Pearson, 1965; Tarjan, 1966).

The major functional areas of the facility as determined from the objectives must be defined and delineated.

An initial staffing pattern can be projected and an organizational chart developed taking into account the physical aspects of the facility, and following staffing ratios such as those suggested by the American Association on Mental Deficiency and the advice of various professionals in their area of specialty.

There must be an actual listing of employees by number and category necessary for operation of the facility. This will determine office space and work areas required for the performance of the employees' duties. Table 3–2 shows an example from "A Program Plan for the Georgia Retardation Center" listing several specific professional programs.

Table 3–2 helps the planner to think realistically in terms of the individual space needs of the staff and can be utilized by the architect in designing adequate facilities to house both programs and staff.

Description of the Construction Project

It is necessary to specify the estimated costs for the land, construction, equipping, and furnishing the proposed facility. If the project is being constructed in phases, the planner must give the cost figures for each phase of construction and specify whether there will be one or more contract documents developed for the construction.

A schedule for completion of the project as a part of the contract document is a good idea. No two would ever be alike, but the following from "A Program Plan for the Georgia Retardation Center" provides a guideline:

Schedule for Completion: In order to facilitate staffing and occupancy of the Georgia Retardation Center, the contractor shall so schedule the work that the owner may accept beneficial occupancy of various elements of the project in accordance with the following schedule:

    (1) Site work – all grading, walks, and parking areas in the vicinity of the accepted units, and all roads throughout the project;

    (2) Central power plant and power house and involved distribution;

    (3) Administration building;

Table 3–2

Speech and Hearing	
*2–245	Speech Pathologist and Training Coordinator
2–247	Instructors (University Faculty)
2–263	Intermediate Stenographer (Secretary and Receptionist)
2–241	Interns (2)
2–248	Interns (2)
2–268 and 270	Interns (4)
2–278	Sr. Speech Therapist
2–279	Speech Therapist
Physical Therapy	
1–15	Physical Medicine Specialist
1–13	Intermediate Stenographer (Secretary and Receptionist)
1–17	Physical Therapist Intern (2)
1–18	Physical Medicine Intern (2)
1–20	Sr. Physical Therapist
1–21	Physical Therapist
1–38 and 39	Orthotics Technician
1–30	Instructors (University Faculty)
Occupational Therapy	
1–69	Occupational Therapy Director and Training Coordinator
1–68	Intermediate Stenographer
1–71	Instructors (University Faculty)
1–72 and 73	Occupational Therapy Interns (4)
1–74	Sr. Occupational Therapist and Occupational Therapist
Music Therapy	
1–107	Music Therapy Director and Training Coordinator
1–108	Intermediate Stenographer
1–109	Instructors (University Faculty)
1–112	Sr. Music Therapist
1–113 and 114	Interns
1–115	Music Therapist

*Indicates floor of building and room number where staff will work.

This will enable the initial basic program staff to begin implementing operation of the facility.

Description of the Site

A description of the site where the facility is to be constructed might include all or part of the following details:

(1) Specific location such as city, county, parish, and street address

(2) Size of the tract in acres and whether or not it is wooded, hilly, has creeks or streams, etc.

(3) Availability of utilities such as water, gas, sewage

(4) Buffer zone between property and existing residential area, business, industry, etc.

(5) Land characteristics such as kind of soil, sub-surface rock, amount of usable land for construction, and sub-surface water

(6) Zoning of property if zoning ordinances are in effect

(7) Location of nearby airports (private or commercial), highways, expressways, railroads, etc.

Specialized Services

In certain cases specialized services such as a University-Affiliated Training Program fall within the overall program and activities of a facility for the mentally retarded. If so, a basic description of the administrative mechanism for the operation of such a program should be included in the program plan.

Future progress in the prevention of mental retardation and in the care and treatment of the mentally retarded depend upon an adequate number of professionals trained in the broad area of mental retardation (Areawide planning . . ., 1963). Service facilities cannot proceed alone; institutions of higher learning must also be closely involved in this endeavor. In fact, the role of the service agency in the educational process is primarily that of providing the treatment setting and population for use in educational programs more appropriately the prerogative of public and private colleges and universities. However, although they may have the same objectives there are obstacles to effective cooperation and collaboration between academic and service institutions.

There exists a difference in organization, outlook, and perspective of the two institutions. The college or university is sharply compartmentalized into disciplines, with each discipline primarily defined for the transmission of its specific knowledge and with the development of new knowledge regarding itself. People in a particular discipline are not necessarily concerned with the application of such knowledge to concrete situations or conditions nor with developments in other areas. In a sense, then, the professional discipline is provincial in nature and concerned with its own aggrandizement. The service agency has as its primary mission the application of available knowledge to specific human situations and conditions to eliminate or ameliorate the condition. While the service agency should be concerned with the continuing development of all disciplines which apply to the mentally retarded, its first interest must be the retarded individual and the judicious use of all knowledge and expertise which will benefit this person. This difference in orientation poses a continuing threat to the smooth functioning of a joint undertaking between the two facilities, and those responsible for planning of such an enterprise must be constantly aware of it.

Because of the differences in objectives the academic community and the service agency have not found much common ground for partnership in the past. This lack of tradition and experience in collaboration is another barrier to overcome. Effective cooperation comes from practice and collaboration between such disparate organizations and requires a whole-hearted effort by all parties involved.

Before there can be meaningful participation in a joint enterprise, channels for communication must be established, and the needs and desires of each party must be fully explored. Lack of experience in joint enterprises and lack of serious communication are deterrents which hamper judgment in determining the scope of the program to be undertaken and the requirements to be imposed on each party. Consequently, the obligations assumed may be too ambitious and beyond the needs and resources of either party. They may also lead to a failure to recognize the true needs of each party and the resources which each can contribute. A miscalculation of this nature may thwart the entire program.

From the beginning those responsible for planning the training and research program must work to overcome these obstacles or to circumvent them.

In a new service facility the planning for a training and research program should be done as a part of the planning for the physical facilities. This is necessary so the service institution can plan to accommodate the training program and for the academic institutions to be assured of the adequacy of training facilities and clinical material.

The detailed planning for a clinical training program must include the following:

A candid assessment by the top-level administrators of the attitude of the facility and the larger organization of which it may be a part. In addition, these officials should have a clear understanding of the resources in terms of space, personnel, and financial support which such a program entails, and of the fact that it is a long-term continuing obligation. Unless the training program is firmly supported in concept and needs by management it will tend to be mediocre even if it survives, but probably it will die a natural death.

The determination of the academic institution or institutions to be approached for such an enterprise. To receive the greatest contributions to and returns from the training program there must be an assessment of what an academic institution is best prepared to do, and the approach must follow that purpose. This determination involves a candid evaluation of the academic program. The college or university must have a sincere interest in and need for participating in such an endeavor on a continuing basis, and the commitment to it should come from the top administrative office of the institution.

Planning for the training program of the facility should be a joint enterprise. Each party contemplating collaboration should spell out very clearly their interests, needs, and resources. For the university this entails the disciplines to be involved, the number and types of students for which clinical experience is needed, and the types and levels of clinical experience desired. The service institution must make clear the facilities and population available for the program.

Such a joint undertaking requires a clear understanding of the responsibilities which each party has assumed. The areas of responsibility include planning, the preparation of teaching material, the guidance of students, schedule requirements, and the conduct of the training program.

The participants should agree on the procedure to be followed in implementing the training program. This includes the procedure to be followed in establishing or revising training programs in the facility, the standards which such programs must meet, the administration of programs when established, and the defraying of costs connected with the program. These factors should be clearly enunciated, for neither party should promise more than it can deliver.

Administrative machinery must be provided for the implementation of the program. Clear channels for communication and feedback between the service institution and the academic community must be available. Responsibility for the overall training program must be clearly delegated both to the service agency and to the affiliating educational institutions, and such assignment should be made to a person high in the administrative hierarchy of both organizations.

SPECIAL EDUCATION TRAINING PROGRAM

In Special Education, graduate students will be prepared for career work with the retarded. Teachers will be trained for work in public schools, private schools, and institutions for educable children at both elementary and secondary levels.

The facility will be used for observation by both graduate and undergraduate students for identification of clinical types, variations in learning, problems in the evaluation and testing of the mentally retarded. Students will be required to spend time in observation (See Table 3–3). Supervised practice teaching at the facility will be available for special education baccalaureate candidates. A full-year internship following course work will be available at the facility for those in graduate programs.

Although most educable retarded children at the facility will be in public school programs in the community, special areas should be designed to provide the full range of training desired by the affiliating colleges and universities. Practice teaching classrooms with observation areas and a specially designated unit for the severely handicapped educable retarded should be available. The physically handicapped are often not accepted in public school programs. New approaches should be tested to develop ways for these residents to be accepted into the school system.

The Special Education program will work closely with the Vocational Rehabilitation Services in order that students can understand the joint responsibilities in curriculum planning and counseling that occur at the secondary school level.

The teacher will have the opportunity to work in a setting which demonstrates the full range of professional resources that can be available in the diagnostic, treatment, and rehabilitation process, and he will learn the role he plays as a member of this team (Program plan . . ., 1965).

In-Service Training of Personnel

A .detailed outline of training for all new personnel to be employed is a necessary part of planning for construction and operation of the facility. As Tizard and others have pointed out, attitudes and techniques of personnel in their relationship to the retarded individual probably have a more profound affect on the retarded than size of facility, size of unit, staff ratios, or other considerations.

Before the first service employees are recruited, detailed outlines of the in-service training procedure must be formulated. Elements suggested for inclusion are:

    a. Training
    b. General orientation
    c. Training objective
    d. Personnel policies
    e. Attitudes toward the mentally retarded
    f. Attitudes toward job and associates
    g. Specific work oriented training
    h. Continuing education

Each of these units must, of course, be expanded—listing, for example, specific course materials, time involved, faculty, and location. Certain care information should be supplied to each employee, and each employee must be given specific information as it directly relates to his job performance.

Table 3–3. Specific Training Program—Special Education (Educable Retarded)

Type of Training	Affiliating Institution and Department	Length of Time per Contact per Student	Frequency of Contact per Student	Number of Students per year	Number of Instructors per year
	Georgia State College Department of Education				
1. Observation (undergraduate student) (graduate-masters)		2 years at junior and senior levels; one year	intermittant; intermittant	20–25; 15–20	¼; ¼
2. Short-term Experience (student teaching baccalaureate)		one quarter	daily	30–40	1
3. Long-term Experience (internship-masters level)		three quarters	daily	10–15	1
	Atlanta University				
1. Observation (masters) regular program summer program		one week; one week	once a year; once a year	15; 75– 8	1 full-time for all level of training
2. Short-term Experience (5th year level) regular program summer program		one quarter; 3–6 weeks	daily; daily	15; 12	

Research Programs

Certain types of research may be done by the staff of the facility, but most research might be carried out more properly through affiliations with research oriented facilities such as nearby colleges and universities. The institution for the mentally retarded would supply the subjects of study and allocate appropriate space for the conduct of research, while the colleges and universities would supply research personnel, equipment, supplies, and so on. Careful contractural agreements should be enunicated to satisfy and protect both parties before such a project is initiated.

Presentation of Program Plan

The writing of the program plan includes information, ideas, and suggestions from many sources and individuals. It must be submitted to the entire planning team for review and approval. There may be extensive revisions; so rough draft copies would probably be best at this stage. Later, after consensus by the entire planning team, finished copies should be prepared for submission to appropriate officials, boards, and authorities for final approval.

Design

It is only when the program plan has been developed to this extent and approved that initial design of the facility can realistically begin. One proven method by which this process may be accomplished is the establishment of a "marriage" between the client and architect (Planning of facilities . . ., 1964). The principal components in this partnership are the program coordinator representing the owner or sponsoring agency and the project director representing the architectural firm. The program plan governs the actions of this partnership as it is their guide in directing the project to a successful conclusion by definite stages.

During the development of the schematic drawings the program coordinator might well move his working quarters into the architect's office. To achieve a successful design, the coordinator must get to know the people with whom he will be working, who later will be his partners in pursuing the course of construction and working with changes necessary as construction progresses. He must be able to communicate successfully with all individuals involved in design, whether it is the architectural draftsman or the chief mechanical engineer. He must know when and how to utilize professional consultants and translate their recommendations into design. He must be able to relate to and evaluate the professional judgements of the architectural firm and work with technical consultants utilized by them. He must interpret program needs and translate the recommendations of consultants into language meaningful to the designers. This cannot be done successfully without frequent contact. Once basic concepts are worked out, design proceeds with frightening speed, and decisions must be made in the proper sequence at the appropriate time.

After completion of schematic drawings, the program coordinator and the architectural firm must present design and projected cost of construction for approval of the planning committee and the sponor of the project. If approved, contract documents can proceed. Any changes have to be incorporated before final design (contract documents) can begin.

By this time basic floor plans of buildings and design of outdoor spaces and structures are essentially fixed. A careful and close check of these documents against the requirements of standards and licensure, population, personnel, and programs is necessary.

Selection of Equipment and Furnishings

Ideally, selection of the equipment and furnishings is a joint endeavor between the program coordinator and the interior designer. Architectural spaces are designed for use by the retardates and by the personnel who will conduct the projected programs. The interior designer who chooses the equipment and furnishings should be a part of the architectural firm. He too must be familiar with the philosophy, goals, and projected programs, and be knowledgeable of the occupants of the particular spaces under consideration. It is important that the interior designer become thoroughly familiar with the interior finishes of each of the buildings.

The planning and preparation of an equipment list is a full-time job requiring the undivided time and attention of one individual. It is an arduous painstaking task. In addition to the actual listing of equipment, sufficient time is needed to:

1. Acquire a comprehensive knowledge of the architect's blueprints and specifications;
2. Hold conferences with the director or chief of each of the professional areas and with the administrative officer of each of the service areas, or if not known at the time, with the counterpart of each in established facilities;
3. See as many salesmen and visit as many showrooms as time will permit. (New products are coming on the market almost daily and much can be learned from a good salesman.) (Planning a patient care unit . . ., 1962);
4. Visit as many facilities caring for the retarded as can be arranged;

5. Evaluate all equipment considered;
6. Determine whether a given area can accommodate all the equipment desired;
7. Contact the appropriate agency if the facility is being constructed in whole or in part with grant funds because it may have specific procedures for the development of the equipment listing;
8. Contact the state agency administering the Hill-Burton Construction Program because in all probability it has material for distribution including guide material and check lists which are very helpful.[1]
9. Start a catalog library and establish files according to professional and service areas for the accumulation of notations and memoranda to be used for reference when the actual equipment listing begins.

It is almost essential that a comprehensive knowledge of the blueprints and specifications be acquired before any other steps are taken. One way to start is to list each room in numerical order and by the title appearing on the architect's "Finish Schedule," and then by checking each room listed against the floor plans. One should not assume that they are always in agreement. Next, the architect's specifications should be reviewed and notations made of the items included, or not included, in the general construction contract which will affect the equipment listing. For example:

1. Provisions for residents' clothing;
2. Venetian blinds or other window treatment;
3. Cubicle rods and curtains;
4. Lockers for employee locker rooms;
5. Shelving for storage areas not designated for transfer carts;
6. Refrigerators—ice makers—food carts;
7. Piped-in oxygen and numerous other items.

From this point on, the steps previously listed will fall into place as circumstances dictate. During this process ideas will become crystalized, and in all probability agreements will be reached on the general type, style, and make of most of the major items of equipment.

Before any purchases are made, however, an itemized budgetary equipment listing should be prepared to avoid duplications and numerous omissions and to assure equitable distribution of the funds allocated for equipment. This listing should be prepared in a systematic manner, so that each item listed can readily be traced through all the channels it will have to pass

1. One can order a copy of "Public Health Service Publication No. 930-D-4" from the Superintendent of Documents, Government Printing Office, Washington, D.C., 20402. The price is 50 cents. Although prepared for general hospitals, much of it is applicable to a facility for the retarded also.

from the time it is originally entered to the time it is received, placed, paid for and its location, specifications, and other data entered on the inventory control.

It is best to select all the major items of equipment first and list on a room-by-room basis. The items such as small office accessories, linens, small instruments, china, and the like should be left until last and listed in categorical order. Supply items usually requisitioned on a regular basis from the central supply storeroom are *not* considered part of the equipment listing.

No matter who prepares the equipment listing, some things are going to be overlooked. Therefore, it is best to delay the purchase of some of the items which are desirable but not necessarily essential until the facility has been in operation long enough for it to be known that all the essential items of equipment have been provided.

Before purchase of furnishings and equipment, but after the final listing is finished, certain considerations will have to be given to style of furnishings, special fabrics, finishes, and so on that will be commensurate to the needs and limitations for which the particular items are specified.

Once a realistic date of completion for construction is established by the contractor and a date of occupancy of the facility determined equipment and furnishings can be placed on order. In general, orders should be placed with vendors six months before predetermined need. Usually a 30-day delivery notice is requested. Requests earlier than six months before expected delivery are unrealistic because of price changes and assembly requirements of the furnishings.

The Contract Documents

The development of the final blueprints of design or the contract documents are primarily the responsibility of the architect. During this stage of design the project coordinator acts essentially as a consultant to the architectural firm.

Certain specific areas will affect design at this stage and careful consideration must be given to the development of procedures and operational details that affect final drawings.

FINISH SURFACES

Finish surface dictates the internal atmosphere and greatly affects the cost of maintenance of these structures. The designation of the materials for use on floors, walls, and ceilings cannot be left entirely to the architect. The program coordinator, knowing the levels, abilities, handicaps, etc. of men-

Table 3–4

Code 20.2 Item #	Quan.	Item Reception Area 2–260		Unit	Total
20–1	1 ea.	Sofa—3 seater			415.00
20–3	2 ea.	Tables, End		90.00	180.00
20–4	2 ea.	Chairs—Lounge, open arms		115.00	230.00
20–25	1 ea.	Table, Window 42 x 18 x 23	Bernard/ Simmonds 1011		106.00
20–12	2 ea.	Chairs, Side		45.00	90.00
		#2–260 Sub Total			(1,021.00)
		Waiting Area 2–267			
20–1	1 ea.	Sofa, 3 seat			415.00
20–3	2 ea.	Tables, end		90.00	180.00
20–26	1 ea.	Tables, end 18 x 27 x 22	Directional WL127	85.00	85.00
20–4	4 ea.	Chair, Open Arm Lounge		115.00	460.00
20–14	1 ea.	Chest, 4 Dr.			87.00
20–15	2 ea.	Chair—Side		39.00	78.00
		#2–267 Sub Total			(1,305.00)
		Reception 2–263			
20–27	2 ea.	Sofa, 2 seat 55 x 30 x 30½	Directional WL–422	318.00	636.00
20–3	2 ea.	Tables, end		90.00	180.00
20–4	3 ea.	Chairs—Open arm Lounge		115.00	345.00
20–28	1 ea.	Desk 42 x 21 x 30	Statton 1807		79.00
20–12	1 ea.	Chair—side			45.00
20–7	1 ea.	Table 45" D.			137.00
20–6	4 ea.	Chairs, arm		148.00	592.00
		#2–263 Sub Total			(2,014.00)
		Code 20.2 Total 3 Units			4,340.00

Code 20.2

tally retarded people must assist the architect in these details. The architect must advise the program coordinator on quality and durability of materials, general use of materials, building codes, and so on.

Each room of the facility requires individual and detailed consideration. As these materials are being selected the interior designer must list patterns, color, etc. of the materials to be used. An example of this type of listing is in Table 3–5 taken from the contract documents of the Georgia Retardation Center.

Table 3–5

Section Three Continued 2nd. Flr.

No.	Stain	Color	No.	Name	Material	Type	Pattern	Color
	Doors			**Room**		**Floor**		
E217A	Walnut		2–236	Janitor	C.H.			
—	"		2–237	Waiting Rm.	Carpet	1	Zenith	1019
F218	"		2–238	Toilet (Womens)	Carpet	1*	"	1075
F220	"		2–239	Storage	Carpet	1	"	1019
F217A	"		2–240	Observation	Carpet	3	"	3A
D205	"		2–241	Therapy	Carpet	3	"	3A
—			2–241A	Storage	Carpet	3	"	3A
—			2–242	Record	Carpet	1	"	1019
D204B	"		2–243	Toilet (Womens)	Carpet	1*	"	1075
D204C	"		2–243A	Toilet (Mens)	Carpet	1*	"	1075
D204A	"		2–244	Storage	Carpet	1	"	1019
D200	"		2–245	Speech Path.	Carpet	3	"	3B
D204	"		2–246	Lounge	Carpet	1	"	1019
D202	"		2–247	Instructor	Carpet	1	"	1019
—			2–247A	Storage	Carpet	1	"	1019
D206	"		2–248	Therapy	Carpet	3	"	3A
—			2–248A	Storage	Carpet	3	"	3A
—			2–249	Mechanical Rm.	C.H.			
F219A	"		2–250	Testing	Carpet	3	"	3A
F219	"		2–251	Testing	Carpet	3	"	3A
—			2–119A	Storage	Carpet	3	"	3D
C201D	"		2–252	Mechanical Equip.	C.H.			
C201B	"		2–253	Records	Carpet	3	"	3B
F221	"		2–254	Toilet (Mens)	Carpet	1*	"	1075
C201A	"		2–255	Clerical Pool	Carpet	3	"	3A

Base	Ht.	Material	Type	Pattern	Color	Material	Type	Pattern	Color
			Wainscot				**North Wall**		
A					2208	P P	2208		
A					2259				
E	4'–0"	C.T.	1702	Dove	White	V W C	2	44.387	Design
A					2278	P P	2278		
A					2280	P P	2280		
A					White	V W C	1	52.575	White
A					"	P P	White		
A					2019	P P	2019		
E	4'–0"	C.T.	1702	Dove	White	V W C	2	44.363	Design
E	4'–0"	C.T.	6455	Fawn	"	V W C	2	66.200	Design
A-J					2278	P P	2278		
A-J					2709	V W C	1	52.557	White
A					2019	V W C	1	52.574	Gold Ess.

Table 3–5 (*continued*)

Base	Ht.	Material	Type	Pattern	Color	Material	Type	Pattern	Color
					Wainscot			North Wall	
A					"	W P	Walnut		
A					"	P P	2277		
A					White	V W C	1	52.575	White
A					"	P P	White		
A					2208	P P	2208		
A					2280	P P	2280		
A					"	P C A			
A					2278	P P	2278		
A					2208	P P	2200		
A					2019	P P	2019		
E	4'–0"	C.T.	6455	Fawn	White	V W C	2	39.790	Design
A	3'–0"	W.B.			Walnut	V W C	1	52.569	Prov. Gold

Material	Type	Pattern	Color	Material	Type	Pattern	Color
	East Wall				South Wall		
P P	S. A. N.			P P	S. A. N.		
V W C	3	madagaska	Natural				
V W C	2	44.387	Design	V W C	2	44.387	Design
P P	S. A. N.			P P	S. A. N.		
P P	"			P P	"		
V W C	1	52.575	White	V W C	1	52.568	Mellon
P P	S. A. N.			P P	S. A. N.		
P P	"			P P	S. A. N.		
V W C	2	44.363	Design	V W C	2	44.363	Design
V W C	2	66.200	Design	V W C	2	66.200	Design
P P	S. A. N.			P P	S. A. N.		
E B				V W C	1	52.557	White
W P	Walnut						
CWS & VWC	1	52.574	Gold Essence	V W C	1	52.574	Gold Ess.
P P				P P			
V W C	1	52.575	White	V W C	1	52.568	Mellon
P P	S. A. N.			P P	S. A. N.		
P P	"			P P	"		
P C A				P C A			
P C A				P P	2280		
P P	S. A. N.			P P	S. A. N.		
P P	"			P P	"		
P P	"			P P	"		
V W C	2	39.790	Design	V W C	2	39.790	Design
P P	2280	Paint		V W C	1	52.569	Prov. Gold

Table 3–5 (continued)

Material	Type	West Wall Pattern	Color	Ceiling Ht.	Type	Shelving
P P	S. A. N.			9'–0"	P P	
W P	Walnut			8'–0"	A-2	
V W C	2	44.387	Design	7'–6"	P P	
P P	S. A. N.			8'–0"	A-5	As Det.
P P	"			9'–0"	A-2	
V W C	1	52.575	White	9'–0"	A-1	
P P	S. A. N.			9'–0"	P P	E
P P	"			7'–0"	P P	
V W C	2	44.363	Design	9'–0"	P P	
V W C	2	66.200	Design	9'–0"	P P	
P P	S. A. N.			9'–0"	A-5	As Det.
V W C	1	52.557	White	9'–0"	A-1	
V W C	1	52.574	Gold Essence	9'–0"	A-1	
W P	Walnut			9'–0"	A-1	
P P				9'–0"	P P	H & E
V W C	1	52.575	White	9'–0"	A-1	
P P	S. A. N.			9'–0"	P P	
P P	"			9'–0"	A-5	
P P	"			9'–0"	A-2	
P P	2280			9'–0"	A-2	
P P	S. A. N.			8'–0"	P P	D
P P	"			9'–0"	A-5	
P P	"			9'–0"	A-1	
V W C	2	39.790	Design	7'–6"	P P	
P P				9'–0"	A-1	

Special Lighting	Trim	Remarks
	2208	C.T. Wainscot 4'–0" @ Wash Area
	2259	
	White Tile & Fixtures	Grab Bar 550
	2278	
	2280	
	White	
	"	
	2019	Furred Clg. as Shown
	White Tile & Fixtures	White Tile & Fixtures
	2278	
	2709	
	2019	
	"	
	"	
	White	
	"	

Table 3–5 (continued)

Special Lighting	Trim	Remarks
	2208	
	2280	
	"	
	2278	
	2208	
	2019	
	White Tile & Fixtures	
	2280	N & S Wall Wainscot with Chair

BASIC SUPPORTIVE SYSTEMS

Laundry

To determine the equipment, spatial, and staffing requirements for the laundry it is first essential to determine the quantity of linens, wearing apparel, and other items that must be processed in each time period in which the laundry is to operate.

The quantity to be processed for the patient population is estimated from knowledge of the population and the program plan. Many variables are involved such as the types of patient clothing to be laundered, the frequency with which bed linens are to be changed, and the use of linens in outpatient services, physical therapy, recreation, and other programs. Drawing on the collective experiences of the planners and verifying their determinations wherever possible against published standards and the experiences of similar facilities, the laundry requirements for each category of individuals is projected, extended, and the totals for all categories are summed.

To the quantity of laundry to be processed for residents should be added all other laundry that is to be processed for operating units or employees. The total laundry requirements for the facility must then be analyzed according to the volumes and types of operations to be performed—amounts hand ironed, machine ironed, drip dry, etc. This analysis will provide a basis for determining the method to be used and for selecting appropriate laundry equipment and determining spatial needs.

Staffing may be developed from the preceding analyses and should represent supervisory personnel, equipment operators, and persons to perform operations such as sorting, marking, checking, sewing, and linen handling.

Grounds Care

Planning for grounds care will include consideration of the extent of the landscaping, the use made of the grounds, and the geographical location of the facility. The great variety of conditions that may be encountered do not, however, preclude the use of logical methods of analysis. The maintenance activities should be analyzed according to the types and quantities of operations to be performed. Equipment of various manufacturers is then evaluated to determine its suitability in performing required tasks. From these analyses, equipment can be selected and staffing requirements determined.

Food Service

Careful planning of the food service is important because of the effect it will have on the morale and well being of the residents of the facility. Some pertinent factors influencing the planning process are the resident population, the place food service is to fill in the programming of the facility, the food choices available to the resident, where he is to eat his food, the serving of nourishments, and the food services for employees.

Once these factors are known they can be translated into operations to be performed in the food service program and the approximate volume to be processed in each operation. Then the appropriate equipment can be selected. Its arrangement should be planned to permit the most efficient operation possible. Spatial and staff requirements may be determined directly from these analyses.

Procurement of Basic Support Services

Certain areas of operation of a residential facility can become so time consuming that they divert the administration's attention away from the primary goals of therapy for the residents of the facility. The goal is to provide a system of delivery of food, rather than operation of a kitchen; provision of clean laundry wherever it is needed, rather than the mechanics of running a laundry; and having attractive and useful outdoor spaces, rather than driving a grass mowing machine.

Traditionally the above services have been provided by employees of the facility, and if this is the plan, employees, equipment storage space, and supplies will have to be provided to get the job done. Today, however there are numerous private business firms which are prepared to furnish various basic support services under contract. Food and housekeeping services and grounds care are quite commonly provided by highly specialized contractors. The contractor may provide services for a fixed fee, or services may be provided under a cost plus contract. The contractor performing under the cost plus contract usually employs the staff and purchases supplies or other items that are utilized in providing the service. The contractor is reimbursed for his expenditures plus a management fee from which he takes his profit.

If one is planning to contract for these services this must be known during the planning stages because less space and equipment will be necessary if the contract method is to be utilized. While no mental retardation facility has yet fully exploited this system, many facilities are finding that services procured in this manner are less expensive and help to free managerial time for greater concentration on the individual retardate's needs. Whether to provide services with its own staff or to contract for services is a matter that must be decided under the circumstances existing in each facility.

Implementation of the Program Plan

Once the contract documents have been completed and a contract is negotiated with a contractor for construction of the facility, the role of the program coordinator radically changes. He then concerns himself as a professional program advisor to the construction project and later, hopefully, as director of the facility. Many questions will arise during the construction that will require decisions that could affect operations of the programs within the facility. The questions are basically concerned with change orders, errors, and omissions of details in the contract documents.

HANDLING CHANGE ORDERS

Many contracts are bid on the basis of alternates to the base contract, either additive or deductive. For example, if the base bid is higher than the funds currently available for construction, a decision will have to be made on what part of the construction to delete to keep the contract within the available funds. In general, it is preferable in this circumstance to delete buildings or sections of buildings rather than to strip essential elements of a building and forever handicap program development scheduled for that particular area.

ERRORS AND OMISSIONS IN CONTRACTS

No matter how carefully planned and drawn, no set of contract documents will be without error. There is no way to predict where errors might occur or how they might ultimately affect programming. The height of grab bars, the location of sinks, and the positioning of windows, for example, while seemingly rather minor details can profoundly affect operations at a later date. Many of these details are inadvertently omitted on the contract documents, and decisions must be made about them during construction. Additionally, some details are best held for decision until the construction is underway. Someone, preferably the project coordinator working with the architect, should make these decisions at the appropriate times.

Scheduling for People and Programs

Much more difficult than planning and financing the facility and supervising the construction is the recruitment of employees for the facility's programs. Low in supply, high in demand—employees at every level are difficult to obtain. Depending on the location of the facility—state, urban or rural—certain employees are more difficult to obtain than others. Long before the facility is scheduled for occupancy, a study of the availability of projected employees must be made and certain key staff employed. A schedule of employment of personnel must be tied in with actual need—planning, out-patient evaluation, receiving of equipment and supplies, and admission of residents. Then budgetary support for their employment must be obtained. An example of this type of planning and detail is shown in Table 3–5 and Exhibit 3–1.

Table 3–6. Georgia Retardation Center Budget Projection and Schedule for Personnel Recruitment

Current Program Level (FY 1969)		*Agency Funds*	*State Funds*	*Total*
Personal Services			659,714	659,714
Operating Expense		29,394	211,036	240,430
Total		29,394	870,750	900,144
Proposed Increases in Priority Order:				
1. *Fixed Increases*	*Cost*			
a. Current Salaries		1,671	539,247	540,918
(1) Regular within-grade increases and related costs	23,001			
(2) Annualization of part-year salaries and related costs	515,991			
Positions in FY 1969 budget were included for an average period of 6.81 months.				
(3) Increases in consultant's fees	1,926			
b. Operating Expense			138,411	138,411
Justification: Increase in operating expenses for new facility being placed in operation:				
(1) Power, water and natural gas	99,986			
(2) Service contracts for elevators and other new equipment	11,805			
(3) Operation of telephone switchboards for full year	16,620			
(4) Travel funds	10,000			
2. Adjustments to Merit System Classification Plan		3,830	495,015	498,845
To provide for adjustments in the pay plan to upgrade certain classes such as Nursing, Engineering, Medical and to eliminate overlaps and inequities in other classes.				

Table 3–6 (*continued*)

Current Program Level (FY 1969)	Agency Funds	State Funds	Total

Program Expansion or Other Increases

3. Chamblee, Georgia: New positions in the medical, para-medical, adjunctive therapies, and support services to open the Center to receive patients on 10/1/69.

a. 78 new positions, including within-grade increases and net of lapse factor	—	412,435	412,435
b. Fringe benefits	—	55,679	55,679
c. Supplies	—	107,087	107,087
		575,201	575,201

4. Athens, Georgia: New positions to receive forty (40) patients into the residential facilities of the Training Branch on 9/1/69, and operating funds to provide adequate care.*

a. 32 new positions, including within-grade increases and net of lapse factor	—	94,015	94,015
b. Fringe benefits	—	12,692	12,692
c. Supplies	—	6,500	6,500
d. Travel	—	1,200	1,200
e. Repairs	—	4,700	4,700
f. Transactions with University of Georgia	—	120,430	120,430
g. Hospitalization of patients	—	1,800	1,800
h. Garbage disposal	—	720	720
i. Communications	—	3,990	3,990
j. Power, water and natural gas	—	18,750	18,750
	—	264,797	264,797

5. Chamblee, Georgia: New positions in professional and support services to receive twenty (20) severely retarded non-ambulatory patients on 10/1/69. The 1st and 2nd wards of the General Infirmary will receive ten (10) patients each.

a. 145 new positions, including within-grade increases and net of lapse factor	—	456,134	456,134
b. Fringe benefits	—	61,578	61,578
c. Supplies	—	113,206	113,206
d. Motor vehicle expense	—	1,000	1,000
e. Hospitalization of patients	—	10,000	10,000
	—	641,918	641,918

6. Chamblee, Georgia: New positions to receive twenty (20) severely retarded non-ambulatory patients on 11/1/69. The 3rd and 4th wards of the General Infirmary will receive ten (10) patients each.

a. 39 new positions, including within-grade increases and net of lapse factor	—	126,652	126,652
b. Fringe benefits	—	17,098	17,098
c. Supplies	—	31,434	31,434
	—	175,184	175,184

Table 3–6 *(continued)*

Current Program Level (FY 1969)	Agency Funds	State Funds	Total

7. Chamblee, Georgia: New positions to receive twenty (20) severely retarded non-ambulatory patients on 12/1/69. The 5th and 6th wards of the General Infirmary will receive ten (10) patients each.

a. 39 new positions, including within-grade increases and net of lapse factor	—	113,064	113,064
b. Fringe benefits	—	15,264	15,264
c. Supplies	—	28,061	28,061
	—	156,389	156,398

8. Chamblee, Georgia: New positions to receive twenty (20) severely retarded non-ambulatory patients on 1/1/70. The 7th and 1st wards of the General Infirmary will receive ten (10) patients each.

a. 30 new positions, including within-grade increases and net of lapse factor	—	73,942	73,942
b. Fringe benefits	—	9,982	9,982
c. Supplies	—	18,352	18,352
	—	102,276	102,276

9. Chamblee, Georgia: New positions in professional and support services to provide management in the Community Living Program to place the Community Center in operation, and to open Cottage No. 6 to receive sixty (60) severely retarded patients, as follows:

2–1–70	20 patients
6–1–70	20 patients
10–1–70	20 patients

a. 121 new positions, including within-grade increases and net of lapse factor	—	278,706	278,706
b. Fringe benefits	—	37,625	37,625
c. Supplies	—	64,442	64,442
	—	380,773	380,773

10. Chamblee, Georgia: New positions to receive twenty (20) severely retarded non-ambulatory patients on 3/1/70. The 2nd and 3rd wards of the General Infirmary will receive ten (10) patients each.

a. 27 new positions, including within-grade increases and net of lapse factor	—	43,647	43,647
b. Fringe benefits	—	5,892	5,892
c. Supplies	—	10,833	10,833
	—	60,372	60,372

11. Chamblee, Georgia: New positions in professional and support services to open Cottage No. 7 to receive sixty (60) severely retarded patients, as follows:

4–1–70	20 patients
8–1–70	20 patients
12–1–70	20 patients

Table 3–6 (continued)

Current Program Level (FY 1969)	Agency Funds	State Funds	Total
a. 71 new positions, including within-grade increases and net of lapse factor	—	94,895	94,895
b. Fringe benefits	—	12,811	12,811
c. Supplies	—	23,552	23,552
	—	131,258	131,258

12. Chamblee, Georgia: New positions to receive twenty (20) severely retarded non-ambulatory patients on 5/1/70. The 4th and 5th wards of the General Infirmary will receive ten (10) patients each.

a. 20 new positions, including within-grade increases and net of lapse factor	—	21,961	21,961
b. Fringe benefits	—	2,965	2,965
c. Supplies	—	5,451	5,451
	—	30,377	30,377

13. Chamblee, Georgia: New positions to receive twenty (20) severely retarded non-ambulatory patients on 7/1/70. The 6th and 7th wards of the General Infirmary will receive ten (10) patients each.

a. 21 new positions, including within-grade increases and net of lapse factor	—	12,436	12,436
b. Fringe benefits	—	1,680	1,680
c. Supplies	—	3,086	3,086
	—	17,202	17,202

14. Increase in stipends to assist prospective employees in obtaining training in disciplines required in operation of the facility. — 33,480 33,480

15. Increase in labor cost—temporary labor to be utilized in equipping the new facilities. — 2,000 2,000

TOTAL PROPOSED INCREASES	5,501	3,743,900	3,749,401

TOTAL PROPOSED BUDGET—1970

Personal Services	—	3,696,110	3,696,110
Operating Expense	34,895	918,540	953,435
Total	34,895	4,614,650	4,649,545

PROGRAM STATISTICS	1969 Level	Proposed 1970 Level
No. of Positions in Budget	128	751
No. of Employee Man Years (FTE)	78	525
No. of Inpatients Staffed for in Budget		
Chamblee	—	260
Athens	—	40

Table 3–6 (continued)

PROGRAM STATISTICS	1969 Level	Proposed 1970 Level
No. of Outpatients		
Chamblee	—	—
Athens (Day Care Patients)	40	40
Employee Inpatient Ratio	—	2.5:1
No. of Inpatient Days	–0–	39,000
No. of Day Care Patient Days		
Chamblee	—	—
Athens	1,200	14,600
Average Inpatient Per Diem Cost	—	51
Average Day Care Patient Per Diem Cost	—	25

SCHEDULE FOR BEGINNING PATIENT SERVICES

Training Branch, Athens, Georgia

The Training Branch has a capacity of forty (40) day care patients and forty (40) inpatients. The day care patients will be admitted in June, 1969, and the inpatients will be admitted in September, 1969.

Georgia Retardation Center, Chamblee, Georgia

At the completion of the 1st phase of construction the facility at Chamblee, Georgia, will have 480 beds available for the admission of patients. Beginning in October, 1969, patients will be admitted at the rate of twenty (20) per month until all beds are filled in September, 1971.

BASIC SERVICES

The primary facility at Chamblee, Georgia, will house 1,000 patients upon completion of the second phase of construction and basic services are sized for this patient load. This necessitates proportionately more personnel to operate these service units initially, but economies of scale may be expected to materialize as the size of the operation increases.

NEGOTIATING CONTRACTS WITH OTHER AGENCIES

Contracts with other agencies such as vocational rehabilitation and education must be carefully worked out in advance of occupancy so that these agencies have adequate time to recruit and train employees and to schedule their anticipated work loads.

PRE-ADMISSION EVALUATIONS

Many individuals admitted to a facility for the mentally retarded are subjected to a programming delay following admission. This is especially true of the larger facilities. Each prospective patient should be thoroughly evalu-

Exhibit 3–1

Athens, Georgia: New positions to receive forty (40) patients into the residential facilities of the Training Branch on 9–1–69, and operating funds to provide adequate care.

1	Social Worker II	17–4	10,380	
4	Stenographer I	8–1	14,880	
1	Cottage Life Supervisor	14–1	5,580	
10	Cottage Mother	12–1	45,900	
3	Houseparent II	9–1	10,260	
3	Staff Nurse II	13–1	15,180	
10	Student Employee	4–5	5,100	
32	Subtotal—Regular Salaries		107,280	
	Merit Increments		5,364	
	Subtotal		112,644	
	Lapse Factor		−18,629	
	Adjusted Salaries		94,015	
	Fringe Benefits		12,692	
	Supplies		6,500	
	Travel		1,200	
	Repairs		4,700	
	Transactions with Univ. of Georgia		120,430	
	Hospitalization of Patients		1,800	
	Garbage Disposal		720	
	Communications		3,990	
	Power, Water and Natural Gas		18,750	264,797

ated before admission, an individual program plan written for his treatment, and a determination made regarding the adequacy of the facility and its programs for the individual before he is admitted.

DEVELOPMENT OF A SCHEDULE FOR ADMISSIONS

The new facility and its staff are untried. A certain time period is needed to get the problems of the physical plant corrected and to give the staff a "shake down cruise" before large numbers of retarded individuals are admitted. Therefore, admissions should begin on a limited basis. No more than 10 to 20 individuals should be admitted per month in the beginning. It is preferable not to admit all of these to one unit but to several units so as not to overload inexperienced and unsure staff. See Table 3–7 for an example of a schedule of projected staff needs in relation to admissions.

Conclusion

Planning is only a beginning step toward a predetermined goal. Therefore, each problem under consideration must be planned. While experiences of

*Table 3–7. Schedule of Projected Staff Needs
in Relation to Admissions*

Staff for a 60-bed Cottage for Severely Retarded—4 Units

A. Professional and Technical Staff

Stationed at Cottage	Shift I	Shift II	Shift III
Clinical Psychologist II	1		
Social Worker III	1		
Recreation Therapist	1		
Speech Therapist	1		
Psychological Technician	1	1	
Recreation Leader II	4	4	
Physical Therapy Technician	2	2	
Speech and Hearing Technician	1	1	
Music Therapy Technician	1		
Occupational Therapy Technician	1		
Stenographer II	2		

Frequent Visit

Physical Therapist	1	(will be utilized during different shifts)
Occupational Therapist II	1	(will be utilized during different shifts)
Sociology Consultant	1	(will be utilized during different shifts)
Music Therapist II	1	(will be utilized during different shifts)

Visiting or Periodic Schedule

Clinical Chaplain	1	(will be utilized during different shifts)
Nutritionist	1	(will be utilized during different shifts)
Dentist	1	(will be utilized during different shifts)
Dental Hygienist	1	(will be utilized during different shifts)
Dental Aide	2	(will be utilized during different shifts)
Dental Assistant	1	(will be utilized during different shifts)
Staff Physician I	1	(will be utilized during different shifts)

Table 3–7—(Continued)

B. Sub-Professional Staff

Unit I	Unit II	Unit III	Unit IV
12–1–69	12–16–69	1–1–70	1–16–70
	Houseparent		Houseparent
Shift I	*Shift I*	*Shift I*	*Shift I*
1 Child Development Technician	1 Child Development Technician	1 Child Development Technician	1 Child Development Technician
2 Cottage Aides	2 Cottage Aides	2 Cottage Aides	2 Cottage Aides
Shift II	*Shift II*	*Shift II*	*Shift II*
1 Child Development Technician	1 Child Development Technician	1 Child Development Technician	1 Child Development Technician
1 Cottage Aide	1 Cottage Aide	1 Cottage Aide	1 Cottage Aide

Table 3–7 (continued)

Shift III	Shift III	Shift III	Shift III
1 Child Development Technician 1 Cottage Aide	1 Cottage Aide	1 Cottage Aide	1 Cottage Aide
Shift IV	Shift IV	Shift IV	Shift IV
2 Child Development Technicians 2 Cottage Aides	1 Child Development Technician 2 Cottage Aides	1 Child Development Technician 2 Cottage Aides	1 Child Development Technician 2 Cottage Aides
2–1–70	2–1–70	2–1–70	2–1–70
Shift I	Shift I	Shift I	Shift I
1 Cottage Aide	1 Cottage Aide	1 Cottage Aide	1 Cottage Aide
Shift II	Shift II	Shift II	Shift II
1 Cottage Aide	1 Cottage Aide	1 Cottage Aide	1 Cottage Aide
Sub-totals			
5 Child Development Technicians 8 Cottage Aides	3 Child Development Technicians 8 Cottage Aides 1 Houseparent	3 Child Development Technicians 8 Cottage Aides	3 Child Development Technicians 8 Cottage Aides 1 Houseparent

Totals

14 Child Development Technicians
32 Cottage Aides
 2 Houseparents

other groups with similar goals and aspirations may prove to be invaluable aids, each planning body must be highly individualistic and must solve their problem with the solution best meeting their own needs. This chapter merely outlines a procedure.

References

Areawide planning of facilities for rehabilitation services. Report of the Joint Committee of the Public Health Service and the Vocational Rehabilitation Administration, 1963.

Covert, C. Mental Retardation—a handbook for the primary physician. *Journal of the American Medical Association,* 1965, 191, 3, 82.

Dittman, L. L. The family of the child in an institution. *American Journal of Mental Deficiency,* 1962, 66, 5, 759–765.

Dybwad, G. The mentally handicapped child under five. Oxford and District Society for the Mentally Handicapped, 1968.

Ecob, K. G. The retarded child in the community. The New York State Society for Mental Health, 1955, 8.

Facilities for training to meet the needs of the mentally retarded. U.S. Department of Health, Education and Welfare, 1967, 5.

Factors to be considered in setting up a new state institution for mentally retarded children. Cost estimates for state institutions in North Carolina and Tennessee. An unpublished paper.

Gove, R. M. Large residential institutions versus smaller regional facilities. A paper, publication date unknown.

Hallenbeck, P. N. and D. A. Behrens. Clothing problems of the retarded.

Humphrey, Mrs. H. H. Better institutional planning. *Newsletter of the President's Committee on Mental Retardation,* March, 1968.

Jackson, J. Toward the comparative study of mental hospitals: characteristics of the treatment environment. A research report supported by NIMH, produced by the Comparative Studies of Mental Health Organization, The University of Kansas, August, 1962.

Jacobs, W. New hope for the retarded child. Public Affairs Committee Inc. 1964, 14.

Kimbrell, D. L., F. Kidwell, and G. Hallum. Institutional environment developed for training severely and profoundly retarded. *Mental Retardation,* 1967, 5, 1, 34–37.

King, R. D. and N. V. Raynes. Patterns of institutional care for the severely subnormal. *American Journal of Mental Deficiency,* 1968, 72, 5, 700–709.

————. An operational measure of inmate management in residential institutions. Social Science and Medicine, 1968, 2, 41–53.

————. The determinants of patterns of residential care. Paper presented at the First Congress of the International Association for the Scientific Study of Mental Deficiency, September, 1967.

A manual on program development in mental retardation. Monograph Supplement to *American Journal of Mental Deficiency,* 1962, 66, 4.

Mental retardation—improving resident care for the retarded. Proceedings of an American Association on Mental Deficiency workshop, December, 1965.

Mental Retardation 67: A first report to the president on the nation's progress and remaining great needs in the campaign to combat mental retardation. The President's Committee on Mental Retardation, 1967.

Mercer, M. Why mentally retarded persons come to a mental hospital. *Mental Retardation,* 1968, 6, 3, 3–7.

O'Connor, G. and R. M. Hunter. Regional data collection as an aid to institutional administration and program planning. *Mental Retardation.* 1967, 5, 4, 3–6.

Pearson, Paul H. The forgotten patient: medical management of the multiple handicapped retarded. *Public Health Reports,* 1965, 80, 10, 915–918.

Planning of facilities for the mentally retarded. Report of a U. S. Public Health Service Committee on Planning Facilities for the Mentally Retarded, 1964.

Planning the patient care unit in the general hospital. U. S. Department of Health, Education, and Welfare, 1962.

Planning for statewide mental health services. Georgia Department of Public Health, June, 1963.

President's Committee on Mental Retardation Message, *Newsletter of the President's Committee on Mental Retardation,* April, 1968.

————. May, 1968.

A proposed program for national action to combat mental retardation. The President's Panel on Mental Retardation, 1962.

Proceedings of an institute, Architectural Contributions to Effective Program Achievement in Mental Retardation, sponsored by American Association on Mental Deficiency, et al, Denver, Colorado, May, 1967.

A program plan for the Georgia Retardation Center. Georgia Department of Public Health, 1965.

Raynes, N. V. and R. D. King. The measurement of child management in residential institutions for the retarded. Paper presented at the First Congress of the International Association for the Scientific Study of Mental Deficiency, September, 1967.

Rogers, D. P. Development of a state-wide program for the vocational rehabilitation of the mentally retarded. Report of an Office of Vocational Rehabilitation demonstration grant, West Virginia Division of Vocational Rehabilitation, February, 1962.

Roselle, E. N. Some principles and philosophy in the planning and development of institutional plants with particular reference to institutions for the mentally retarded. *American Journal of Mental Deficiency,* 1954, 58, 4, 595–624.

Seminar for medical personnel in residential settings. Gracewood State School and Hospital, Gracewood, Georgia, February, 1968.

Standards for state residential institutions for the mentally retarded. Monograph supplement to American Journal of Mental Deficiency, 1964, 68, 4.

Tarjan, G. The role of residential care—past, present and future. *Mental Retardation,* 1966, 5, 6, 4–8.

Tarjan, G. S., W. Wright, H. F. Dingman, and R. F. Eyman. Natural history of mental deficiency in a state hospital. *American Journal of Diseases of Children,* 1961, 101, 195–205.

Task force on behavioral and social research. The President's Panel on Mental Retardation, 1964.

Task force on clinical services. Mental Retardation Planning Project, Georgia Department of Public Health, 1965.

Task force on prevention, clinical services and residential care. The President's Panel on Mental Retardation, 1962.

The problem of mental retardation. U. S. Department of Health, Education and Welfare, 1966, 8.

Time Magazine, Building for the year 2000, August 2, 1968.

Tizard, J. The experimental approach to the treatment and upbringing of handicapped children. *Developmental Medicine and Child Neurology,* 1966, 8, 3, 310–321.

————. The care and treatment of subnormal children in residential institutions. Reprinted from the proceedings of the First International Conference for Special Education, July 25–28, 1966.

————. *Community services for the mentally handicapped.* London: Oxford University Press, 1964.

————. The role of social institutions in the causation, prevention and alleviation of mental retardation. Paper prepared for Peabody-NIMH Conference on Socio-Cultural Aspects of Mental Retardation, June, 1968.

Tizard, J. and B. Litt. Residential care for the mentally retarded. Paper presented at the First Congress of the International Association for the Scientific Study of Mental Deficiency, September, 1967.

Williams, R. J. *You are extraordinary*. New York: Random House, 1967.

Wishik, S. M. *Georgia study of handicapped children*. Georgia Department of Public Health, 1964, 104–105.

CHAPTER FOUR

HARVEY F. DINGMAN,
AND RICHARD K. EYMAN

Statistics in Institutions for the Mentally Retarded

Introduction: Records in Institutions

"Mental Hospitals, like other organizations for work, are established to fill a set of recognized social needs. That is to say, the justification for their existence lies in their serving a variety of instrumental functions for patients and for society at large. To implement these goals each hospital develops certain structures and modes of operation that comprise its maintenance organizations" (Smith and Levinson, 1957). Because most institutions have the multiple goals of patient care, staff training, and research, relevant statistics based on hospital records comprise an integral resource for establishing and evaluating these goals.

Tarjan (1966) has described other reasons these statistics are needed. "Historically, residential institutions have been supported by governments. Legislators have a tendency to favor appropriations for buildings rather than for programs or personnel. Today we are preoccupied with the bigness of institutions. It is expected that, as recommended by the President's Panel on Mental Retardation (1962), the traditional institutions will be reduced in their populations. During the next decade much time will be spent on

NOTE: This investigation was supported by Public Health Service Research Grant No. MH–08667 from the National Institute of Mental Health, Department of Health, Education and Welfare, and Public Health Service General Research Support Grant No. 1–S01–FR–05632–02, from the Department of Health, Education and Welfare.

Computing assistance was obtained from the Health Sciences Computing Facility, UCLA, sponsored by NIH Grant FR–3.

117

debating which type of institution is the 'ideal' one. Many decisions will be made. Most will probably reflect emotionality or armchair thinking rather than scientific considerations. There are very few data available to pass judgment on the comparative efficiency of small or large, generic or specialized facilities. It is rather easy to say that institutions are not needed; if this assumption was correct, residential services would be sought with decreasing frequency and the waiting lists would disappear. One should ask, therefore, of those who advocate the closing of institutions that they first create the community resources which might make institutions unnecessary, then prove that, in fact, institutions are no longer needed."

Intelligent answers to many of the problems about the optimum treatment of the mentally retarded must be based on data. Institutional statistics should be a part of that data.

Similar to the data that is gathered routinely in any public institution, the adequacy, sufficiency and accuracy of data gathered in hospitals for the mentally retarded have been challenged repeatedly (Zubin and Jervis, 1967). Time and again critics have suggested that data from institution records are unsatisfactory for treatment, training, or research; that such data are incomplete, or, assuming that the data are accurate and complete for that institution, that they do not give a clear picture of the significance of mental retardation in the total community. Considering such complaints, it is surprising to find that much research has been based on institutional records and statistics (Windle, 1962).

Historical Records

There seem at least three reasons why research based on hospital records continues to be utilized by many scientists and administrators.

The data is on hand and has been available in hospital records for many years. It is not unusual to find patient records encompassing half a century or more of institutional residence. A scientist or administrator who is interested in biometric studies of the mentally retarded would be somewhat less than remotely opportunistic if he did not take advantage of existing hospital records. After all, little other data are open to this kind of investigation. Despite their lack of quality the obvious difficulties of analyzing this type of data, many scientists continue to use them simply because they are available and suitable for longitudinal studies of the institution in a society (Tarjan *et al.*, 1958).

The data in hospital records are derived from a well-defined retardate population for which the problem of settling on one or another arbitrary definition of who is retarded can be avoided. Obviously, mentally retarded hospitalized patients offer a convenient study group by virtue of their institutionalization. The investigator does not have to face all the controversy in this area (Stevens and Heber, 1960; Windle, 1962; Brison, 1967; But- terfield, 1967; Baumeister, 1967). As Butterfield (1967) and Baumeister (1967) have pointed out, institutionalized retardates also have more serious adjustment problems and have been studied to a much greater extent than non-institutionalized retardates.

A third reason for basing investigations on records of mental institutions is that some of them are of necessity quite accurate because they are related in some way to the economics of the institution. If an individual is admitted to an institution and placed on its rolls, that agency assumes the responsi- bility for him, and his presence is recorded because of the requirement of a reimbursement file. Other types of basic records, such as medication, are systematically recorded because they too support the financial reports which involve reimbursement to the institution. Records on death in the institu- tion are also likely to be accurate.

This is not to conclude that the financial necessities of life automatically create good and usable records; as a matter of fact, they can be quite in- adequate. However, institutional personnel who collect numbers and report summary statistics to the proper authorities (i.e., the Hospital Business Administrator or Accounting Officer) probably produce important and re- liable data. Thus, records generated by the accounting office are frequently found to be excellent sources of data for statistical studies of institutions.

The appropriate study of mental retardation in an institution must start with some consideration of the institutional record-keeping system and the way in which these records are stored, updated, and utilized. The most use- ful way to summarize voluminous institutional records is to construct a model institutional process. This model cannot be developed directly from empirical data, but will ultimately depend on such data for its validation.

Release-return Models

In a series of studies, Tarjan *et al.* (1958, 1959a, 1960, 1961) investi- gated the natural history of mental deficiency at Pacific State Hospital (a California hospital for the mentally retarded). These studies focused on patient characteristics related to admission and subsequent probabilities of release, retention, or death. These studies employed a net change model developed by Kramer (1957) to estimate the probability of specified out- comes at fixed intervals after admission to the institution. An admission cohort of patients was collected and followed to their first significant release (e.g., home leave, foster care, death). Subsequent returns to, release from, the hospital, time on release, and so on were not considered. Cumulative probability curves, for release or death only, of specified groups of retardates were provided, Kramer (1957) has stated that although this model oversimplifies the phenomena under study, nevertheless, it points up problems that need attention and can predict trends in the composition of the institutional population.

An alternative method for description of specified release, discharge, or death has the advantage over the Kramer net change model that time on release and subsequent returns to the hospital are taken into account. A release-return index is used to summarize release incidents and their duration for predefined periods of time (e.g., six months, one year). The index (I_{rr}) is the average number of releases per individual studied $(\bar{R}_n)$, multiplied by the average duration of the release $(\bar{R}_d)$ expressed in units of so many fractions of the time period used.

The index takes into account the size of population available for leave, the time at risk, the frequency and duration of releases. It represents the number of days the average patient spent on leave during some specified time period. Thus, the index is a probability measure and, when multiplied by the size of the total population, it provides an estimate of future releases and their duration. Consider the following example: 100 patients less than 12 years old with I.Q.'s below 30 are followed for six months after their admission. A patient who lives through this half-year period is given one unit; if a patient survives in the hospital three months during the six-month period, he is given a score of ½ unit. Individuals may be dropped from the sample for a number of reasons (e.g., death, transfer, discharge), and no longer be available to participate in a release-return program. Thus, the index will also depend upon the probability of the patient remaining on the hospital books (P_{hb}) as well as upon the average number and duration of releases. Table 4–1 provides an outline for the calculation of the release-return index.

The example given in Table 4–1 was based on an assumption of no deaths, discharges, and so on. Depending on the purpose of the study, these experiences may be analyzed separately or they may be included in the release-return index. For example, the investigator may wish to interpret discharge as a successful release and include it in the computation of the index. Hence, a patient discharged could be considered as released for the entire study period.

The majority of follow-up studies are for a period of three or four years (Windle, 1962). In the example presented a separate index could be calculated for each one half-year period, following the admission of the patient. In this instance, the index could be graphed over one half-year periods up to the total follow-up period. The major advantage of this approach is the efficiency of reducing data without losing much of the information contained therein.

Table 1. Definition and Computation of the Release-Return Index (I_{rr})

Definitions:

$I_{rr} = P_{hb} \times \bar{R}_n \times \bar{R}_d$ where

$$P_{hb} = \frac{\text{Person Years}}{\text{Sample Size x Study Period}} = \begin{array}{l}\text{proportion of time during which}\\\text{cohort members are eligible for release.}\end{array}$$

where;

Person Years = | Sample Size x Study Period | — | Death time + discharge time, etc. |
= correction of cohort size by deducting time lost due to death or direct discharge; these patients cannot re-enter the cohort.

Illustrative
Data:

A

Admission Cohort	0	1	2	3	4	Total
		Number of releases for specified ½ year period				
100	80	10	5	3	2	100

B

Admission Cohort	1	2	3	4	5	6	Total Releases
	Months* out on release for specified ½ year period						
100	10	10	10	3	3	1	37

C Deaths, discharges, transfers for 6 month follow-up period of 100 admissions = 0

*In the interest of brevity months were substituted for 183 entries representing days in the 6-month period.

Computations:

$$P_{hb} = \frac{[100 \text{ persons x } 183 \text{ days}] - [0 \text{ death, discharge, etc., time}]}{100 \text{ persons x } 183 \text{ days}}$$

= 1 wherever there are no deaths, transfers, etc.
(See row C)

$$\bar{R}_n = \frac{1 \times 10 + 2 \times 5 + 3 \times 3 + 4 \times 2}{100} = \begin{array}{l}.37 \text{ releases per patient}\\ \text{per ½ year period}\end{array}$$

(See row A)

$$\bar{R}_d = \frac{1 \times 10 + 2 \times 10 + 3 \times 10 + 4 \times 3 + 5 \times 3 + 6 \times 1}{37}$$

(See row B)

= 2.513 months per release for 6-month study period

= 75.39 days per release for 6-month study period

$I_{rr} = 1 \times .37 \times 75.39 = 27.8943$ days out on release per patient for ½ year study period

Muench (1959) has stated, "In the application of mathematics to science our chief aim is the creation of a mathematical model or picture which will contain the essential relations under study." In discussing catalytic models in biometrics, Muench develops some interesting parallels with the chemists' picture of catalysis in which the catalyst has become a force of infection, measurable in terms of the fraction of all individuals it strikes each year and which it attacks if it finds them susceptible.

Stimulated by Muench (1959), we visualized an institution for the mentally retarded as an electro-chemical process. The institution is surrounded by a semi-permeable membrane, and mentally retarded individuals flow into the institution, are kept there for a specified period of time, and then released into the surrounding area. If those persons who are being admitted to the institution possess different electric charges or ions (e.g., some individuals have a greater charge than others), a differential rate of admission of individuals to the institution would result. Similarly, if the flow from the institution depends on the dissipation of the electrical charges of ions before the individual's return across the semi-permeable membrane, one, then, could study a differential return rate in terms of the characteristics that seem to be related to a differential admission rate (Tarjan *et al.,* 1959b).

Individuals who are admitted to institutions for the mentally retarded have intelligence quotients that fall two or three standard deviations below average. The lower his I.Q., the earlier the individual is likely to be placed in an institution (Tarjan *et al.,* 1966), provided his age is not a condition of admission and his family can communicate successfully with hospital staff (Sabagh *et al.,* 1966; Eyman *et al.,* 1966). In many parts of the United States a minimum age, ranging anywhere from two or three weeks to ten or twelve years, is a prerequisite for admission to public institutions. Nevertheless, it is probably generally true that the more severely retarded are placed in institutions earlier (Tarjan *et al.,* 1966).

Individuals whose I.Q.'s are higher tend to be released before those whose I.Q.'s are lower. Thus we can visualize, via our model (Dingman *et al.,* 1964b), a severely retarded individual as having a high ionic charge, so that he is passed across the semi-permeable membrane earliest and stays in the institution the longest because it is difficult, if not impossible, to dissipate the high ionic charge which propelled him into the institution in the first place. The individual who has a very small ionic charge (a mildly retarded person) can be found to more easily cross the semi-permeable membrane back to the community. He stays in the institution for a very short period and soon returns to the community. Having little charge to begin with, it did not take long to dissipate this charge.

Other variables show similar relationships. While it is difficult to study degree of handicap from physical traits, individuals with physical handicaps come to the institution somewhat sooner than those with no physical problems (Tarjan *et al.,* 1960; Sabagh *et al.,* 1966). Other evidence suggests that retardates can be placed out of the institution as soon as they acquire physical skills such as walking, toileting, and speaking.

To estimate future bed utilization, the ionic model has been built into a computer program (Dingman *et al.,* 1964b; Dingman *et al.,* 1965; Tarjan *et al.,* 1966). The computer logic states that the hospital, which is surrounded by a semi-permeable membrane, is a closed system and is composed of different types of patients. These types may be defined in any way convenient to the investigation. Patients may come into this closed system from the *waiting list,* which can be any size (versus the hospital, which is assumed to be at capacity); or patients may be released outright from the hospital, die, or go on *aftercare* status. The aftercare pool may also be of any size, and patients may return to the hospital.

Using this rationale, the major factor affecting hospital composition is hospital policy concerning who will be admitted. Certain types of patients may be given preference over others. The hospital might prefer a certain diagnostic category: severe retardation, those who have waited a long time for admission, or it may admit on a first-come, first-served basis. Furthermore, the waiting-list itself has "discharge" and death losses because patients are removed from the list for reasons beyond hospital control.

The program takes the following aspects into consideration: The number of each type patient in the hospital and on the waiting list; the number of individuals added to the waiting list each month; death and discharge rates for the waiting list and hospital patient types; function values (polynomial) for placement on aftercare programs; and weights to apply to each patient type on the waiting list. The program uses a polynomial function for aftercare programs because of placement rate increases over time as more aftercare settings become available. Suitable values for the function may be used to cancel this part of the computer logic. The weights for the waiting list override the first-come, first-served rule, which applies if no weights are used. The program assumes that the composition of *new* additions to the waiting list remains the same over time.

By changing the values of the various aspects of the program, for example, death rate, it can be used to simulate a hospital for the mentally retarded with specific characteristics and specific admission policies. Thus, the program can be used to determine the effect of various admission and release policies and to provide a basis for administrative decisions.

Many complex factors affect movement in and out of institutions for the retarded. Studies indicate that the more intelligent as well as the more mature retarded are more skillful (Windle, 1962; Lohmann *et al.,* 1967; Tarjan *et al.,* 1966). Therefore, flow rates across the semi-permeable membrane will not vary linearly with length of institutional residence, because placement rate is a function of the various capacities and incapacities of the population being studied. Some strange factors affect movement across this boundary. Shafter and Coe (1956) reported that the replacement of large farm homes with smaller cottage-type dwellings is one of the major factors in reducing placement opportunities of retardates in the rural areas of one farming state. When an old large family-type farm house is replaced by a smaller house that is constructed for only the immediate family of the farmer, there is no space to house a retardate eligible for leave from an institution. Similarly, it has been found that the placement rate from an institution varies inversely with the square of the distance from the institution (Zipf, 1949). One could draw a circle around an institution and by determining its catchment area, predict roughly its placement rate. All of these important factors should be taken into account in some model, even though there are a variety of methods to study each of these kinds of variables in isolation.

Model Appropriate for Institutional Programs

The model of the semi-permeable membrane separating the community from the institution can also be used to study processes within the institution. Certainly any program of activities in the institution depends, to a large extent, on the selection of individuals who will participate in the program and the effect of their participation in the hope of their eventual release. The patients who participate in a program in an institution do not necessarily go directly to the community. A great many of them graduate to some other program in the institution. Thus, it is possible to characterize movement in and out of institution programs in the same way in which movement in and out of the model institution can be characterized.

Most institutions operate highly visible school programs. Not every patient in each institution can or should participate in the institution's formal school. Children do move into the school group, however, either through aging and/or acquisition of skills. Movement out of the school group may occur for a wide variety of reasons. Frequently, a retardate leaves school because he is older and progressing more slowly than his school mates. Patients are also expelled from school for misbehaving. Although school teachers in institutions for the mentally retarded are frequently unwilling to maintain objective records of individual progress, they are, nevertheless, sensitive to the failures of the program and make strong efforts to retain those in the school who benefit from the program.

One of the most apparent deficiencies of institutions for the retarded is that they do not evaluate themselves objectively. A similar deficiency of classes for the retarded in the community was accurately described by Kirk (1964) and Stevens and Heber (1964): "It is the reviewer's opinion that research in this area was initiated without adequate preparation in terms of structure, theory, adequate hypothesis or adequate instruments."

Bereiter (1963) and Lord (1963), among others, emphasize the methodological difficulties of evaluating programs or beneficial change in subjects over time. Bereiter commented, "Although it is commonplace for research to be stymied by some difficulty in experimental methodology, there are really not many instances in the behavioral sciences going unresearched because of deficiencies in statistical methodology. Questions dealing with psychological change may well constitute the most important exceptions. It is in relation to such questions that the writer has even heard colleagues admit to having abandoned major research objectives solely because the statistical problems seemed to be insurmountable."

Eyman *et al.* (1967) demonstrate how a simplified version of time dependent Markov Chains can be used to study change and to evaluate a school program. Residents admitted to Pacific State Hospital between 1958 and 1962 were followed for a four-year period. Two groups were selected for study. The first group was comprised of those patients selected to be in school within three months after admission; the second group included those patients not selected to be in school. The two groups were then matched on age, I.Q. toilet training, and other variables known to be important in selection for the school program. For both school and non-school samples, the status of each patient was checked each year after admission according to the scheme described in Table 4–2.

Figure 4–1 shows the possible results of these yearly checks. By three months after admission, a patient is either in the school group or non-school group, and each year after admission he can be in status E_1, E_2, or E_3 (see Table 4–2). Designating patient "transitions" in this manner, it is possible to construct a "transition frequency matrix" which is essentially a cross tab-

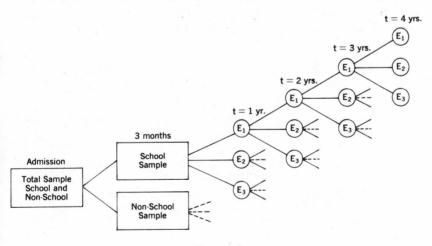

Figure 4-1

*Table 4–2. A Set of Mutually Exclusive and Exhaustive States
Used for Evaluating the School Program*

For School Sample

   E_3 Most preferable outcome
        Released on Indefinite Leave to Home, Foster Care, Work Placement, or
        Discharged

   E_2 Satisfactory outcome
        In Hospital; still in Day School, or no longer in Day School, but in In-
        dustrial or Therapy Night School

   E_1 Unsatisfactory outcome
        In Hospital; dropped from school because of lack of progress or behavior
        problems and neither in Industrial Therapy nor in Night School

For Non-School Sample

   E_3 Most preferable outcome
        Released on Indefinite Leave to Home, Foster Care, Work Placement, or
        Discharged

   E_2 Satisfactory outcome
        In Hospital; enrolled in Industrial Therapy

   E_1 Unsatisfactory outcome
        In Hospital; not participating in Industrial Therapy

ulation of patients in terms of their status at one time against their status a
year earlier.

In Table 4–3, column designations refer to the patient's status one year
later than row designations. Diagonal numbers (N_{11}, N_{22}, N_{33}) represent
patients who did not experience change in status from one year to the next
year. The upper right entries (to right of diagonal) characterize an improving trend in status, and the lower left entries (left of diagonal) depict a

*Table 4–3. Transition Frequency Matrix for Change
in Status from One Year after Admission to
Two Years after Admission*

		$E_1(t)$	$E_2(t)$	$E_3(t)$
	Years (1, 2) t = time of determination of status, i.e., two years after admission.			
t–1 = yr.	$E_1(t$–1)	N_{11}	N_{12}	N_{13}
after	$E_2(t$–1)	N_{21}	N_{22}	N_{23}
admission	$E_3(t$–1)	N_{31}	N_{32}	N_{33}

retrogressing trend. From the data in such a transition frequency matrix, a Markov transition probability matrix may be derived. (See Table 4–4)

The model equation for the Markov chain takes the form of

Eq 1: $P\ [\text{an individual in } E_i\ (t-1) \rightarrow E_j(t)] = P_{ij}(t-1, t)$

$$ij = 1, 2, 3$$
$$t = 1, 2, 3, 4$$

and reads, "the probability of transition from E_i to E_j, given that the individual is in E_i at time $t-1$," is $P_{ij}\ (t-1, t)$; or, equivalently, the transition probability matrix is given in Table 4–4.

Table 4–4. Probability Matrix for Change in Status from One Year after Admission to Two Years after Admission

	$E_1\ (t)$	$E_2\ (t)$	$E_3\ (t)$
$E_1\ (t-1)$	P_{11}	P_{12}	P_{13}
$E_2\ (t-1)$	P_{21}	P_{22}	P_{23}
$E_3\ (t-1)$	P_{31}	P_{32}	P_{33}

The sum of probabilities in each row equal to one

$$\sum_{J=1}^{3} P_{ij} = 1$$

and the estimated probabilities computed by

Eq 2: $P_{ij}(t-1, t) = \dfrac{N_{ij}(t-1, t)}{N_i(t-1, t)}.$

N_{ij} is the number of patients in cell$_{ij}$; N_i is the row total.

Each P_{ij}, with the probability of being in a given state at a given time, is calculated as a proportion of the row total and gives an estimate of a conditional probability. It is conditional to the extent that an outcome at time t depends only on what happened at t–1. It is based on the assumption that the outcome of the third year depends on the outcome of the second year, but not on that of the first year.

Two types of hypotheses can be tested with this kind of study. First, it can be hypothesized that the conditional probability of release is different for two groups of residents, in this case the school and non-school groups. Hence, one is interested in assessing whether the two sets of transition matrices could have come from a common universe. If the null hypothesis in this situation is confirmed and the transition probability matrices for the school group are similar to the probability matrices for the non-school group, it is best to combine both groups and reestimate the conditional probabilities based on the total sample using Equation 3.

$$\text{Eq 3:} \qquad P_{ij}(t) = \frac{N_{ij}^{(1)}(t) \& N_{ij}^{(2)}(t)}{N_{i.}^{(1)}(t{-}1) \& N_{i.}^{(2)}(t{-}1)}$$

This is particularly suggested when the cell frequencies in the subgroups are small so that the use of these probabilities, based on the common universe, will provide the best estimates for prediction within the institution studied. If the transitions of the two groups prove to be different, the best estimates of probabilities would be calculated separately for each group using Equation 2.

The second hypothesis is concerned with the effect of schooling, or non-schooling experience over time. To test this hypothesis it is necessary to determine whether there is an appreciable change in transition rates over the study period. The null hypothesis states that no time trend exists so that the conditional probabilities over the follow-up period are essentially the same; i.e., any transition probability at any time point equals the transition probabilities for that same call (P_{ij}) at other points in time.

The statistical test for this hypothesis assesses the probability that the transition matrices at each point in time could have come by random selection from a common universe of all time points. The probabilities in this common universe are estimated by

$$\text{Eq 4:} \qquad P_{ij} = \frac{\sum_{t=1}^{3} N_{ij}(t)}{\sum_{t=1}^{3} N_{i}\cdot(t{-}1)}$$

and are the best predictors of transition probabilities if the null hypothesis is supported. If the null hypothesis is rejected, the probabilities are again estimated from Equation 2, for each separate time period. Where a time trend is evident, this approach also enables the identification of the time point at which maximum improvement occurs in the group under study. It is that time point which coincides with the maximal rate of transition.

The log likelihood ratio test (Kullback *et al.,* 1962) is an appropriate test to examine both hypotheses. In the study by Eyman *et al.* (1967), it was demonstrated that a version of the Markov Chain provides a sensitive and fair test under circumstances where a more common-sense approach would not take into account the fact that at the end of the first year most school patients were in school whereas most non-school patients were neither in school nor Industrial Therapy.

While it is important to study the flow into a particular program and the flow out of the program as a characterization of the success of the program, the fact that institutions often have many inter-related programs makes it difficult to interpret the examination of any one of them. Fortunately, most institutional programs are heirarchical in that they serve residents of different intellectual levels. By ordering programs according to the type of resident they serve, it is theoretically possible to set up a Markov Chain to investigate their success by studying the extent to which patients move from program to program. Such a model can be generalized from the preceding discussion of the Markov Chain in connection with institutional school programs. An alternative approach is presented by Tarjan *et al.* (1967) for the evaluation of hospital programs based on differentiation between participants and non-participants in each program. Regardless of the specific method employed, total evaluation of the programs of an institution is much more promising than attempts to restrict evaluation to individual programs for a selected number of patients.

The prevalence of institutional programs depends largely upon funds which have been given to the institution for that purpose, as well as the interest and motivation of the professional staff. Typically, funds are provided on a short-term basis. After a program has been initiated, it is assumed that the program will be self-maintaining; however, this outcome is generally not true. In actuality new programs are developed which usually absorb patients from the old programs.

If the program has been successful within the institutional framework, the individual who developed and operated the program is recognized as an outstanding employee and may be promoted to a position where he no longer has direct control of his program or any other program. Employees who are less motivated or less capable may then be asked to institute replacement programs. It is at this point that problems occur and programs falter. Thus, there exists the interesting paradox that the success of the initial program with respect to some of the criteria discussed, often leads to its eventual termination. An evaluation of the total institution would be necessary for any administrator to be able to examine realistically the reasons and details for the success of programs. While the records of 20 or 30 patients in a program may be lost, a formal evaluation of a complex of programs for an institution of two to four thousand individuals is not likely to be lost. And as long as an evaluation is placed on the interrelationships in the flow between programs, hospital staff have some chance of seeing a total assessment of programs that can insure success for the total rehabilitation effort in a single facility.

The Multivariate Approach

More recent efforts to deal with patient movement between programs within or outside the hospital have emphasized the complexity of such efforts (Tarjan *et al.,* 1967; Eyman, 1967) and the need to include a large number of patient-related variables for adequate study of such phenomena. Any effort to include more than two or three variables will require a multivariate approach, based on techniques for handling 12 to 50 variables in a specified analysis.

The combination of variables for further analyses immediately poses new problems. This procedure is based on the presumption that the study population is sufficiently large to accommodate nesting tabulations without seriously jeopardizing the reliability of the results. Because any attempt to nest more than three or four variables generally produces too few cases in too many categories, more sophisticated multivariate techniques become necessary. Multiple regression analyses, discriminant analyses, factor analyses, principal component analyses, Guttman scale analyses, pattern analyses and latent class analyses are among those used extensively for this purpose.

A detailed discussion of each of these techniques is not possible here. It is sufficient to say that multiple regression, principal component and discriminant analyses have been very useful in isolating subsets of three or four variables which relate to a specific aspect of prognosis i.e., release, and which can be nested and used to further specify subgroups of patients with a particular prognosis.

In a study by O'Connor and Hunter (1967) factor analyses and latent class analyses were used to identify subgroups of patients on a larger set of variables, irrespective of prognosis. The prognosis of retardates, with a given profile of factor scores or assigned to a specified latent class, could then be determined.

The latent class model has provided the most promising results concerning the prediction of mortality and morbidity (Miller *et al.,* 1962; Kim, 1968) among institutionalized retardates. This model has two advantages. Latent class analysis (Lazersfeld, 1950) assumes the statistical independence of variables within each latent class. When this premise is met, variable interactions within each class can be ignored and pattern differences (if one wishes to interpret them) are more meaningful. Interpretation can proceed on both a microscopic pattern level or macroscopic class level with equal ease. Secondly, the most commonly used latent class model was developed for dichotomized variables and is particularly suited to the inclusion of qualitative information such as sex, diagnosis, and so on, and the crude category scales currently in use for rating the retardates' abilities and background characteristics.

Latent class analysis is most helpful when the subgroups that are identified statistically correspond to subgroups formed from other data. For example, Dingman (1959) validated statistically the notion that there are two major types of mentally retarded, a notion that has been held for many years by workers in the field. The advantage of such validation goes beyond simple confirmation. Utilizing probability techniques, it is possible to objectively and routinely assign patients their most likely classification.

The utility of such statistically derived typologies for administrative and medical purposes can be illustrated by two examples. Sabagh *et al.* (1959) computed mortality rates using age, sex, race, and other variables and clearly demonstrated that there are distinct differences in such rates, depending on the characteristics of the patients. Because of the limited number of deaths, however, it was possible to compute mortality rates for only a few cross-classifications, and the effects of interaction among the variables were difficult to assess. Accordingly, Miller *et al.* (1962) utilized the latent class model to classify patients into two groups. One of these groups contained almost all of the patients who would be likely to die within the first year after admission; membership in this group was predictive of a greater chance of death. Predictions of those newly admitted patients who were most in danger of dying were then sent to the hospital staff for a seven-month period. Four patients who were admitted during this period died—all from the high-risk group. Because it was expected that 13 patients would die, the experiment could be considered a success. The medical staff had been alerted to the patients who might die and were able to take preventive action. In fact, certain staff members verbally reported that they regarded the prediction of mortality a challenge to their medical skills. The physicians felt that the study was at least a partial success because it had alerted them to the patients who required special attention and enabled them to provide such attention. The overall well being of the patients had been improved. This hypothesis received further unfortunate support by the fact that after the predictions were no longer made, the mortality rates returned to their former levels.

A second example of a typology with utility is provided by the work of Dingman *et al.* (1946b). The transmission enteric diseases is known to be oral-fecal in nature. It should have been possible to identify those patients who were likely to contract diseases such as shigellosis and amebiasis by statistically combining information about their degree of toilet training, whether they are fed by others, are ambulatory and use their arms and hands, their age and diagnosis. Dingman *et al.* dichotomized these variables to maximally predict contraction of shigellosis or amebiasis within the first year after admission, and shigellosis and amebiasis rates were computed for all combinations of these variables. By identifying the combination of variables that characterize a patient, a prediction of the likelihood of disease contraction was made.

The initial reaction of the medical staff was not to utilize the typology but, rather, to mass treat *all* hospital patients in an attempt to eradicate the diseases totally. Over the long run, however, the expense and possible dangers of such drug use led to more selective drug use, based on information supplied by the typology.

The examples given illustrate some uses of typological schemes. In addition, it is possible to perform experiments, utilizing such schemes, for verification of their utility or modification of the typologies themselves. Pattern techniques, such as those illustrated by the examples, are not the only means of characterizing patients. Factor analysis may be similarly used to characterize the individual patient. An illustration of such use grew out of a study of the anthropometric characteristics of the mentally retarded (Dingman *et al.,* 1966). Seven measures of growth were reduced to three factors: Body breadth, body length, and head size. Utilizing head size, in particular, it was comparatively simple to isolate microcephalic and hydrocephalic patients on the basis of computed factor scores. The use of factor scores provides a profile of the patients which can be utilized in various ways, such as isolating patients with unusual profiles of measurements.

Classification of institutionalized retardates has always been an administrative and medical tool for treatment and prognosis. The application of advanced statistical methods can help improve the classification process, thereby improving treatment and prognosis.

Definition of Mental Retardation as a Part of a Community Study

Data from institutions for the mentally retarded give an incomplete picture of retardation, because it does not include information about functioning in the community. Consequently, specific knowledge about the characteristics of mental retardation cannot be generalized beyond the institution. Any investigator of mental retardation in the community faces the problems associated with the definition of mental retardation which his institutional colleague can ignore. If individuals are formally diagnosed by the medical profession as mentally retarded they are very likely to represent the more obvious cases which have required institutionalization through the courts or other legal proceedings. In the total community it is frequently found that, although persons may not be formally identified as retarded in connection with a particular agency, they are informally identified and are given help without the necessity of stigmatizing them as being different from others in the community (Edgerton, 1967).

One functional approach to identifying the retarded in the community has been to identify those individuals who are on the rolls of social agencies in the community. These agencies usually have information that suggests whether a person is retarded. Often, they definitely designate individuals as retarded for the purpose of obtaining financial reimbursement. A study of a community of 100,000 people revealed that it had approximately 240 community agencies that could provide some kind of service for an individual who is regarded as mentally retarded (Mercer *et al.,* 1964; Dingman, 1967; Mercer and Butler, 1967; Robbins *et al.,* 1967). A survey of those 240 agencies revealed the usual pattern found in studies of this nature; namely, that a substantial number of persons were listed and receiving service from at least three agencies. The agencies' records revealed a pattern of movement that is similar to movement in and out of the institution; namely, agencies have boundaries. They, too, are surrounded by a semi-permeable membrane so that when individuals apply, some are taken in and some are not. The length of time that individuals are served by the agency depends, to some extent, on how seriously they need that agency's care. The person with a great need for the services of a specific community agency is likely to appear on the agency's rolls early, stay on their records for a long period of time, and only be deleted from the rolls when and if he is transferred to another social agency.

Mental Retardation Agencies Serve as Models in Microcosm

There exists in the community a macrocosm of the same kind of interchange as in the institution. Persons are identified, treated, and then exchanged between agencies. Frequently, the structure of agencies enters into the transfer process just as it did in the programs in institutions; for example, if a community agency has a budget cut, then retardates may be redistributed so that they are served by other agencies. Among agencies, there appears to be some competition for retardates who are likely to be helped by the services they offer.

There also seems to be some avoidance of individuals who, while eligible for service, appear to have little potential for being helped. For example Crippled Children Services seem to have been given primarily to those who could be completely rehabilitated by medical treatment. If a patient has had the additional handicap of being mentally retarded, he has been relegated to a lower place on the waiting list because it is apparent that although the physical handicap of the child might be successfully treated, the mental handicap would remain. Similar situations occur with the deaf and the blind. Also, there is some evidence that mental hygiene agencies give preference to the bright, mentally ill patients on agency files because they can be "cured," whereas the mentally retarded are likely to be served only if they have obviously acute emotional distress.

Finally, in the community, retardates are known to be served in a particular program because of their personal relationship with a staff member. It is not unusual for patients to be transferred from agency to agency as their responsible case workers are transferred from agency to agency. Continuous supervision of a case is sometimes regarded as more important than the formal definition of the clientele of an agency as given in its official documents.

Understanding the movement of a retardate from agency to agency in the community is complex. The institution can be visualized as one of the many community agencies which serve a retarded individual at some point in his life. The models and statistics discussed in connection with an institution have general applicability for characterizing movement of retardates within the institution, admission to, and release from the institution, as well as living in a community, irrespective of service received by community organizations.

References

Baumeister, A. A. (ed.). *Mental Retardation.* Chicago: Aldine Publishing Company, 1967.

Bereiter, C. Some Persisting Dilemmas in Measurement. In C. W. Harris (Ed.) *Problems in Measuring Change.* Madison: The University of Wisconsin Press, 1963, pp. 3–20.

Brison, D. W. Definition, Diagnosis, and Classification. In A. A. Baumeister (Ed.) *Mental Retardation.* Chicago: Aldine Publishing Company, 1967, pp. 1–19.

Butterfield, E. C. The Characteristics, Selections, and Training of Institution Personnel. In A. A. Baumeister (Ed.) *Mental Retardation.* Chicago: Aldine Publishing Company, 1967, pp. 305–328.

Campbell, D. T. and J. C. Stanley, Experimental and Quasi-Experimental Designs for Research on Teaching. In N. L. Gage (Ed.) *Handbook of Research on Teaching.* Chicago: Rand McNally and Co., 1963, pp. 171–246.

Chiang, C. L. An Index of Health: Mathematical Models. *Vital and Health Statistics,* Center for Health Statistics, Series 2, No. 5, May, 1965.

Dingman, H. F. Adjustment of the Mentally Retarded in the Community Today. *Proceedings of the Joseph P. Kennedy, Jr. Foundation Symposium,* 1967.

————. An Automated Research Program. *Medical Record News,* 1962, 33, 2, 58–61, 88.

————. Some Uses of Descriptive Statistics in Population Analysis. *American Journal of Mental Deficiency,* 64, 2, 1959, 291–295.

Dingman, H. F., R. K. Eyman, and G. Tarjan. A Statistical Model for an Institution for the Mentally Retarded. *American Journal of Mental Deficiency,* 68, 5, 1964b, 580–585.

————. Mathematical Analyses of Hospital Release Data. *American Journal of Mental Deficiency,* 70, 2, 1965, 223–231.

Dingman, H. F., H. D. Mosier, and H. J. Grossman. Deviation in Somatic Growth; A Factor Analysis. *Child Development,* 37, 4, 1966, 949–957.

Dingman, H. F., G. Tarjan, R. K. Eyman, and C. R. Miller. Epidemiology in Hospitals: Some Uses of Data Processing in Chronic Disease Institutions. *American Journal of Mental Deficiency,* 68, 5, 1964a, 586–592.

Edgerton, R. B. A Patient Elite: Ethnography in a Hospital for the Mentally Retarded. *American Journal of Mental Deficiency,* 68, 3, 1963, 372–385.

————. *The Cloak of Competence.* University of California Press, 1967.

Edgerton, R. B. and H. F. Dingman. Good Reasons for Bad Supervision: "Dating" in a Hospital for the Mentally Retarded. *The Psychiatric Quarterly Supplement,* Part 2, 1964, 1–13.

Edgerton, R. B. G. Tarjan, and H. F. Dingman. Free Enterprise in a Captive Society. *American Journal of Mental Deficiency,* 66, 1, 1961, 35–41.

Eyman, R. K. The Effect of Sophistication on Ratio and Discriminative Scales. *American Journal of Psychology,* 1967, LXXX, 520–540.

Eyman, R. K., H. F. Dingman, and G. Sabagh. Association of Characteristics of Retarded Patients and Their Families with Speed of Institutionalization. *American Journal of Mental Deficiency,* 71, 1, 1966, 93–99.

Eyman, R. K., G. Tarjan, and D. McGunigle. The Markov Chain as a Method of Evaluating Schools for the Mentally Retarded. *American Journal of Mental Deficiency,* 72, 3, 1967, 435–444.

Goldstein, H. Population Trends in U.S. Public Institutions for the Mentally Deficient. *American Journal of Mental Deficiency,* 63, 1959, 599–604.

Kim, P. J. Pattern Study in Life Characteristics: Stochastic and Other Models I. *Biometrics,* 1968.

Kirk, S. A. Research in Education. In H. A. Stevens (Ed.) *Mental Retardation.* Chicago: The University of Chicago Press, 1964, pp. 57–99.

Kramer, M., P. H. Person, Jr., G. Tarjan, R. Morgan, and S. W. Wright. A Method for Determination of Probabilities of Stay, Release, and Death, for Patients Admitted to a Hospital for the Mentally Deficient: The Experience of Pacific State Hospital During the Period 1948–1952. *American Journal of Mental Deficiency,* 62, 3, 1957, 481–495.

Kullback, S., M. Kupperman, and H. H. Ku. Tests for Contingency Tables and Markov Chains. *Technometrics,* 4, 1962, 573–608.

Lazersfeld, P. The Logical and Mathematical Foundation of Latent Structure Analysis. In Samuel Stouffer, et al. *Measurement and Prediction,* Chapter 10. Princeton: Princeton University Press, 1950.

Levy, J. and R. M. Hunter (Eds.) *Data Collection and Utilization in Institutions for the Mentally Retarded,* WICHE, University East Campus, Boulder, Colorado, 1964.

Lohmann, W., R. K. Eyman, and E. Lask. Tiolet Training. *American Journal of Mental Deficiency,* 71, 4, 1967, 551–557.

Lord, F. M. Elementary Models for Measuring Change. In C. W. Harris (Ed.) *Problems in Measuring Change.* Madison: The University of Wisconsin Press, 1963, pp. 21–38.

Mercer, J. R. Social System Perspective and Clinical Perspective: Frames of Reference for Understanding Career Patterns of Persons Labelled as Mentally Retarded. *Social Problems,* 13, 1, 1965.

Mercer, J. R. and E. W. Butler. Disengagement of the Aged Population and Response Differentials in Survey Research. *Social Forces,* 46, 1, 1967, 89–96.

Mercer, J. R., H. F. Dingman, and G. Tarjan. Involvement, Feedback, and Mutuality: Principles of Conducting Mental Health Research in the Community. *American Journal of Psychiatry,* 121, 3, 1964, 228–237.

Miller, C. R., G. Sabagh, and H. F. Dingman. Latent Class Analysis and Differential Mortality. *Journal of American Statistical Association,* 57, 1962, 430–438.

Muench, H. *Catalytic Models in Epidemiology.* Cambridge: Harvard University Press, 1959.

O'Connor, G. and R. Hunter. Regional Data Collection as an Aid to Institutional Administration and Program Planning—1964–1965. *Mental Retardation,* 5, 4, 1967, 3–6.

O'Connor, G. and D. Payne. Statistical Expectations of Physical Handicaps in Institutionalized Retardates. (Unpublished), 1968.

Robbins, R. C., J. R. Mercer, and C. E. Meyers. The School as a Selecting Labelling System: A Study of One Year's Referrals to the Central Office. *Journal of School Psychology,* 5, 4, 1967, 270–279.

Robinson, H. B. and N. M. Robinson. *The Mentally Retarded Child: A Psychological Approach.* New York: McGraw-Hill, 1965.

Sabagh, G., H. F. Dingman, C. R. Miller, and G. Tarjan. Differential Mortality in a Hospital for the Mentally Retarded: A Study of Mortality Among Patients Admitted to Pacific State Hospital, 1948–1956. *Proceedings of International Population Conference,* Vienna, 1959, 460–468.

Sabagh, G., R. K. Eyman, and D. G. Cogburn. The Speed of Hospitalization: A Study of a Preadmission Waiting List Cohort in an Institution for the Retarded. *Social Problems,* 14, 2, 1966, 119–128.

Shafter, A. and R. M. Coe. Administrative Planning and Population Forecasting. *American Journal of Mental Deficiency,* 61, 1956.

Smith, H. L. and D. J. Levinson. The Major Aims and Organizational Characteristics of Mental Hospitals. In M. Greenblatt, D. J. Levinson and R. H. Williams (Eds.) *The Patient and the Mental Hospital.* New York: Free Press, 1957, pp. 3–8.

Stevens, H. A. and R. Heber. *Mental Retardation.* Chicago: The University of Chicago Press, 1964.

Tarjan, G. The Role of Residential Care—Past, Present, and Future. *Mental Retardation,* 4, 6, 1966, 4–8.

Tarjan, G., H. F. Dingman, R. K. Eyman, and S. J. Brown. Effectiveness of Hospital Release Programs. *American Journal of Mental Deficiency,* 64, 4, 1959b, 609–617.

Tarjan, G., H. F. Dingman, R. K. Eyman, and G. O'Connor. Evaluation of Management and Therapy of the Mentally Retarded. In J. Zubin and G. Jervis (Eds.) *Psychopathology of Mental Development,* 1967, 603–622.

Tarjan, G., H. F. Dingman, and C. R. Miller. Statistical Expectations of Selected Handicaps in the Mentally Retarded. *American Journal of Mental Deficiency,* 63, 3, 1960, 335–341.

Tarjan, G., R. K. Eyman, and H. F. Dingman. Changes in the Patient Population of a Hospital for the Mentally Retarded. *American Journal of Mental Deficiency,* 70, 4, 1966, 529–541.

Tarjan, G., S. W. Wright, H. F. Dingman, and R. K. Eyman. The Natural History of Mental Deficiency in a State Hospital. III. Selected Characteristics of First Admissions and Their Environment. *American Journal of Diseases of Children,* 101, 1961, 195–205.

Tarjan, G., S. W. Wright, H. F. Dingman, and G. Sabagh. The Natural History of Mental Deficiency in a State Hospital. II. Mentally Deficient Children Admitted to a State Hospital Prior to Their Sixth Birthday. *American Journal of Diseases of Children,* 98, 1959a, 370–378.

Tarjan, G., S. W. Wright, M. Kramer, P. H. Person, Jr., and R. Morgan. The Natural History of Mental Deficiency in a State Hospital. I. Probabilities of Release and Death by Age, Intelligence Quotient, and Diagnosis. *American Journal of Diseases of Children,* 96, 1958, 64–70.

Windle, C. Prognosis of Mental Subnormals. *American Journal of Mental Deficiency,* monogr., 66, 1962, Whole No. 5.

Zipf, G. K. *Human Behavior and the Principles of Least Effort.* Cambridge, Massachusetts: Addison-Wesley Press, 1949.

Zubin, J., and G. A. Jervis (Eds.). *Psychopathology of Mental Development.* New York: Grune and Stratton, 1967.

Dimensions of Institutional Life:
Social Organization, Possessions,
Time and Space

Institutions for the retarded, at the level of the popular or conventional knowledge, are straightforward and uncomplicated social organizations. The mass media in its various forms has given wide expression to the conventional and lay wisdom and there are many "facts" about institutions that nearly everyone who reads, "knows." It is "known," for example, that institutions are a poor substitute for home and family. It is "known" that institutions are not so progressive as other social organizations. It is "known" that institutions are resistant to change. All of these "knowns" that go to make up the conventional wisdom are being reinforced in many ways by well meaning but relatively unsophisticated interpreters whose writings *reach* the general public. By and large, the employees of institutions are not given to writing, especially those who form the tenured or experienced nucleus of the institutional work force.

Institutions for the retarded continue, like their retarded residents, to be stigmatized as being "slow to change" (retardates too have been popularly characterized as slow to change, rigid, and so on), "employing people who couldn't get a job elsewhere," (retardates have long held this stigma). Rather than the "sins of the fathers. . . .," what occurs in the case of institutional employees is more accurately translated, "sins of the 'sons.' " The employees and their "children" reciprocally and mutually share a variety of stigmas and the interdependency of this relationship subtly alters *both* employee and resident over the course of time. Articulate spokesmen for institutions have been few in number and efforts to translate accurately the complexities inherent in such social organizations may, relative to the growing number of institutions, become even rarer. As current rehabilitation philosophy gains momentum, and it has many visible spokesmen writing and speaking persuasively on its behalf, it becomes correspondingly less popular or possible for students of institutional social organization to reach the audience, academic or otherwise. Nevertheless, institutions long ago innovated in rehabilitation and the professional literature on mental deficiency (largely unread by the masses) over 50 years ago addressed the subject under the term *extra-mural placement*. Despite concensus that habilitation of retardates is desirable, it is exceedingly unlikely that institutional placement or various forms of milieu therapy closely approximating institutional placement will disappear in the future. For those employees who may work for a significant part of their lives in the institution and for those retardates who will be in their care, it is essential then that as many of the complexities of institutional operations, therapeutic or otherwise, be isolated and described to assist in making institutions more desirable places in which to work or live. This effort necessarily requires attention to the research on both retardates and institutional employees.

Research on mentally retarded individuals entails studying a variety of characteristics of individuals at various chronological ages (Mercer, 1965; Chandler, Shafter, and Coe, 1958). These mentally retarded are frequently clustered together in an institution or they are brought into laboratories from clinics or special schools. This study of individuals away from their total life situation gives a biased and one-sided view of the rich life of the persons with limited intelligence (Edgerton, 1963). There has been a substantial amount of research on the characteristics of the life of the retarded, particularly of those discharged into the community (Windle, 1962). But all too often even that research is confined to a study of demographic variables, functional intelligence measures, or other characteristics which do not round out our understanding of the total social matrix in which the mentally retarded live and work.

In any discussion attempting to convey findings of research on the characteristics of the life of retardates, it is essential, if such results arise from investigations on institutionalized retardates, that the sociocultural milieu of the institution be described to provide a perspective to the reader. The role of the employees and staff of institutions requires attention because in numerous ways, formal and informal, these individuals structure the lives of the retarded. Belknap (1956) in discussing the sociocultural aspects of an institution, has contributed from his knowledge of the formal social structure of the state mental hospital in a significant way. Cleland and Peck (1967) have discussed to a considerable extent the hierarchy of the hero constraints on an individual. These behavioral constraints consist of the institution manager, the employees in an institution, those volunteers who come into the institution to work under the guidance of the employees, the patient workers who work in the institution keeping the rules and structuring the culture according to the desires of the people in the hierarchy above him, and finally the patients themselves. The patient culture is shaped substantially by the attitudes of the managers, the employees, the volunteers as well as the perception by the patients of the culture that they hope to move into when they leave the institution.

How do the staff and the managers, given space and the volunteer helpers and the patient workers, structure the culture for the best benefits for the patients? Not too much has been written on the dynamic use of the structural aspects of the situation although the article by Henry (1964) on space and power in a psychiatric ward does open this topic of functioning in this kind of environment. Most of the literature on the structuring of life does not deal with institutions of the mentally retarded nor surveys of the life of the mentally retarded outside of the institutions. Attempts will be made to bring this literature to bear on the problems in mental deficiency and give some indications on what kinds of research within these institutions needs to be started. As the authors view research in mental deficiency, it seems evident that research should arise from the point of view of knowledge of the full life of the retarded insofar as it can be made explicit.

Social Organization

There is a social organization which exists in institutions for the mentally retarded (Edgerton, 1963). Depending on the level of activity of the persons in the institution, this organization does take some different shapes. If there are large numbers of delinquent, mildly retarded individuals in the institutions, the social organization of the dominant culture of the patients will be organized around the ideas and values of the delinquent society with which the patients are familiar (Edgerton, 1963; Edgerton and Dingman, 1964). That is, the patients will model themselves after the society to which they would like to belong, even though they were never themselves members of that society (Edgerton and Dingman, 1963). The more severely retarded patients have a social organization (MacAndrew and Edgerton, 1964), but it is not so formally integrated as the organization of the mildly retarded persons. Nevertheless, it has its own value system and its own rules of conduct. Even the very severely retarded patients have a kind of social organization in the sense that by exhibiting deviant behavior they can control factors in their environment such as who feeds them, what kinds of elementary privileges they are given, and to what extent the staff can spend time with themselves rather than coping directly with the demands of the patients (MacAndrew and Edgerton, 1964). It is most instructive to watch a helpless patient with an IQ of less than 20 lying in a crib completely without speech manipulating the movement of staff on the ward by her cries and her periods of silence and smiling contentment when she gets those things in the environment that she wants.

As patients become more sophisticated, the study of their control of the environment becomes much more complex (Edgerton, *et al.,* 1961). Investigation of several delinquent mildly retarded subcultures reveals, however, that the retarded institutionalized person was not a part of a delinquent gang, but that they are modeling their behavior after what they think a delinquent group of their agemates would be doing in the appropriate circumstances (Edgerton and Dingman, 1963). It is interesting to note, as Edgerton (1963) has done, that formal norms and sanctions are organized in and are enforced by the delinquent retarded culture on a set of behaviors they feel to be appropriate to the situation in which they find themselves. This nowhere became more evident than in the study of "dating" practices among the retarded where it was seen that the brighter patients usually selected a person to serve as a lookout and as a go-between for the couple who wanted to get together in some privacy (Edgerton and Dingman, 1964). The presence of the third party and of the go-between clearly gives evidence for a culture that can sanction such behavior and can impose sanctions when the behavioral norm is violated. The rules of social conduct, while not written down, are easy to follow for the alert observer because of the elaborate symbolism involved in keeping the role behaviors of the patients in correct perspective (MacAndrew, 1966). The existence of taboos to signify the dating relationships between members of the opposite sex and the use of gifts and ornaments to call attention to the role relationships between persons signify clearly and provide evidence of the statuses and functional capacities impugned on different persons in this system. In a recent paper (Philips and Dingman, 1968), it became apparent that these mentally retarded individuals can function according to the traits attributed to them instead of being limited to their functioning level within an austere and unguided environment. The guidance and the evaluation of patients needs to be specified in terms of the individual's integration into the social organization and into his capabilities in specified environments rather than trying to isolate measures of his capacity in a laboratory situation.

Possessions[1]

The possessions of the mentally retarded are clear and important indications of the capacity of the individual. The fact that an individual has many objects that are regarded as his own implies that the individual has some personality, some force, and some character with which the social organization must cope. If an individual could not express himself through his belongings, then the person would not have belongings. The objects might be stolen from an individual if he could not defend them in some way.

At first it may seem that the number of belongings of persons would be correlated with their functional intelligence. It would seem that the severely retarded would have few, if any, personal belongings over which they exerted control.

The severely retarded have many possessions, not physical ones necessarily that one could regard as objects that would be owned; but the retardate is quite definite for the most part about his relationship towards the place his bed belongs, the kinds of clothing he prefers wearing, the persons he wants to feed him, and the schedule on which he is fed, bathed, and clothed. The severely retarded are quite capable of making their wishes known and trying to work ways of getting their interests satisfied. They are not, on intimate acquaintance, passive and devoid of social stimulus power.

The mildly retarded are the ones who have large collections of objects that to them signify status. A mildly retarded person can frequently be seen with a transistor radio to his ear even if the battery does not work. It is the mildly retarded individual who has a collection of keys that do not unlock any door. It is the mildly retarded person who pulls together large collections of clothing so that they can dress in bizarre and unusual costumes for different kinds of social events.

The very mildly retarded delinquents are different. They have fewer belongings because they correctly regard the institution as only a temporary home. They try to choose belongings and garments that will not stigmatize them as belonging to an institutional culture. They are constantly trying to utilize the language and the implements of the society to which they hope to return. Given an opportunity, they frequently do escape into this society to which they aspire; and if they are sufficiently alert and have acquired skills, they, with the assistance of their "non-institutional" objects may adjust satisfactorily. Sometimes only the most bizarre kinds of occurrences will serve to point up the shortcomings of the retarded in the community. An

---

1. These observations came from a series of studies conducted with various students from several universities. None of them has yet been published, but they cover many different kinds of possessions owned by many patients of different intelligence and functional levels.

escapee for example, dressed appropriately can often get a service occupation as a bellhop in a large hotel or motel only to be discovered because he does not consider it ethical to take tips when he is getting a salary. This probably stems from the institutional culture where people in the institution are paid salaries and are prohibited from taking any gifts or emoluments from parents or relatives of the retarded in the institution. This entire range of behavior might be socially approved, practically, but when due to ignorance of the larger society's norms deviations are noticed, they serve to stigmatize the individuals as belonging to a group or sub-culture that is different from the modal society.

The Importance of Temporal and Spatial Boundaries

At the interface of the patient and employee culture there are two relatively fixed variables which serve in subtle ways to shape the behaviors of both groups. These variables, time and space, to a large extent effectively define the range *and* depth of human interactions within institutions and persuasively and subtly alter the institution itself.

All institutions for the retarded have boundaries. Physical time and physical space constitute two structural determinants of the institution and, within the fixed limits of both, the attainment of the institutional objectives of service, research, production and training must be attempted. Although it is obvious that any institution is located in space (e.g., 40 to 50 to 1,000 acres) and that any institution possesses 365 days per year, it is the manner in which these variables are utilized that provides both challenge and opportunity to institutions.

With time and space as guides, attention initially focuses on the administrative-professional employee category and the temporal changes occurring at this level. Alterations or redistribution of time within other employee, patient, and volunteer categories are subsequently discussed in any effort to reveal the dynamic interplay between all institutional participants and how time and space, in concert, act to slowly but inexorably, shape the patient-employee culture. Although discussion purposefully overdraws the negative aspects of informal time and space in institutions, it should be indicated that informality may also be adaptive. Edgerton and Dingman (1964) have illustrated that absence of formal structure or direction may, under certain conditions, be therapeutic.

Time as a Determinant of Institutional Social Interactions

One of the most pressing and persistent problems of institutions (Cleland & Peck, 1959; O'Gorman, 1958; Seitz & Cleland, 1967) and the helping professions in general (Margolin, 1966; Rosenthal, 1967) is the manpower shortage. So severe is this problem that an entire section of *National Action to Combat Mental Retardation* was devoted to exploration of ameliorative approaches to overcome serious manpower shortages at every level from attendants through scientists (President's Panel, 1962). A great many causes of such serious shortages have been isolated, described, and at least partially corrected. Low wages, poor working conditions, and long working hours are among the more obvious and, in times of relative affluence, easily remedied causes of manpower shortages. Other measures (e.g., scholarships and appeals through various mass media) have complemented the broad-scale effort to supply the manpower needs of institutions and other helping agencies. Yet the shortage continues. Perhaps some hidden sources can be isolated that may indirectly yield increments to the existing manpower pool. A partial solution lies in improved management of the time of top echelon administrators and professionals, a reduction of their own absenteeism.

The consequences of high absenteeism have long been a focus of management concern, with production, morale, and economic losses representing only a few of the consequences. Oddly, the importance of absenteeism as reflected in the industrial literature appears unidirectional—attention is focused almost singly on rank-and-file employees, with concensus that absenteeism is costly in psychological, social, and economic ways and represents a covert sign of hostility and withdrawal (Kerr, 1964).

Absenteeism can reflect legitimate causes. It can also reflect a type of avoidance behavior (Bass, 1965; Kerr, 1964; Knowles, 1952; Stagner, 1956). De Grazia (1962), in discussing worker protests, indicates that absences, disciplinary layoffs, resignations, and transfer requests are referred to by "students of industrial relations . . . as acts of 'job resistance,' and, in turn, their incidence is taken to indicate a low state of work morale." While most such studies focus on absenteeism among lower-ranked employees, it seems likely that similar or identical hypotheses may account for "managerial absences." From the viewpoint of attendants and other subprofessional institutional employees, it is easy to rationalize, "If the boss or doctor is gone so much, why should I stick around?" This somewhat heretical way of viewing absenteeism is logically important. Even if, as Wilensky (1961) suggests, "There is a general tendency for higher occupational strata . . . to work long hours," the focus of rank-and-file employees is on the *visible* aspects of work. It is quite possible that institutional (as well as other helping agencies) professional and administrative personnel are working *more* but showing less! This constitutes a phenomenon of importance in the manpower crisis of the helping fields—absentee management.

Insofar as the manifestations of absentee management in institutional settings are concerned, both economic and historical forces permit analysis.

What does the institutional employee perceive? The standard work week in institutions has been reduced eight or more hours per week during the past decade. In number of hours alone, there is simply less opportunity for an attendant to see the superintendent, physician, psychologist, or other professional staff member than was formerly true. The generally documented avoidance of patients and attendants by professional staff (Kahne, 1959; Scheff, 1961; Sullivan, 1962; Taylor, 1964) compounds the "absence" effect. The "absenteeism" of the managerial staff is increased by the multiple-reference groups, professional and civic, to which institutional leaders differentially belong and devote time (Cleland & Peck, 1967). Historically, the most recent deterrent to the manager or professionals' presence in the institution is the advent of federal grants which, ironically, call for a rather substantial outlay of extra-institutional attention (time) from responsible officials. As research and demonstration grant monies are received, meetings proliferate and gravitate to settings conducive to deliberation but out of sight of the majority of institutional employees. A recent addition to this array of forces tending to divert institutional leaders from the workers' view is another pressure, i.e., the call to establish community-based services or, in industrial terms, to diversify. Again, the institution loses the presence of top administrative and professional staff members as planning and implementation meetings proliferate. Inspection of the calendars and travel authorizations of those occupying the top ranks of institutional organizations leaves little doubt about the expenditure of management time away from the primary goal of the institution—the patients. Disregarding value judgments relative to such absences, it seems unquestionable that the phenomenon exists and that it is accelerating.

Assuming absentee management or legitimatized truancy is increasing among institutional administrators and professionals, what are the forseeable consequences? One of the important worker needs may be neglected, i.e., the ego needs. If managerial responsibility includes bestowal of attention as numerous authorities suggest (Barnard, 1964; Roethslisberger & Dickson, 1947; Scott, Clothier & Spriegel, 1954), managerial absenteeism, for whatever reason, will undoubtedly lessen the likelihood of meeting this primary need. Where such needs are not met clique formation increases (Kretch, *et al.,* 1962) and although this can be a positive force, all too often cliques are at odds with organizational objectives and are generally believed to reflect deficiencies within the formal organization.

During less affluent times in institutional history, when personnel shortages were chronically critical and capital expenditures for plant or equipment were utopian dreams, the responsibility for the maintenance of employee psychological needs (as well as recruitment and training) were often activities personally conducted by the superintendent. Such activities were, in real measure, "non-delegable" because only the absolute essentials for custodial treatment were budgetarily possible. In effect, the treatment team consisted of attendants, physicians, and a few nurses or teachers on the staffs of the more fortunate institutions. Such budgetary adversity forced institutional management into a paternalistic mold, and its parallels to the patriarchal family have been isolated and described by Cleland and Peck (1959).

Although paternalistic management is outmoded and generally decried, its strengths (and there were some) paralleled those of American industry a century ago: In the period of transition from old-style industry with employer, master workman, and apprentices forming more-or-less one large family, to new-style industry with the employment by one employer of workers in large numbers, the personal relationship of employer and employee disappeared to a large extent. This development not only deprived the employee of the expert supervision of his employer, but also tended to weaken the employer's feelings of personal responsibility for the welfare of individual workers (Health Bulletin, 1942). The reduction of management and professional encounters with personnel cannot be entirely attributed to the growth in size of institutions. For example, one particular institution had a resident population in 1952 of 2,000 and an employee complement of 400. By 1967, the same institution had a resident population of 2,300 and over 1,200 employees. Such examples are not isolated cases and many institutions have witnessed similar growth patterns as efforts are made to attain staff-patient ratios recommended by the American Association on Mental Deficiency and as research and demonstration projects swell employee ranks. The disproportionate growth of employees relative to residents, while largely encouraging, dramatically underscores the enigmatic nature of absentee management. There are now *more* employees to see the administrative and professional staff *less!* Personnel increases may not mean more time spent with patients *nor* any change in the way things are done. For example, Bensberg (1964) cites a study by Kong-Ming wherein nursing staff in an institution was greatly increased only to find the "patient-nursing hours changed very little. . . ." Drucker (1966) suggests overstaffing is a prime time waster and when "senior people in the group spend more than about one-tenth of their time on problems of 'human relations,' then the work force is almost certainly too large."

This growth phenomenon has serious implications for a major management responsibility, i.e., coordination. As Terry (1956) indicates, absenteeism seriously influences production and "when an employee is not punctual or does not appear for work the task of coordinating the group's efforts is made more difficult. . . ." Although Terry's remarks were directed primarily toward the rank-and-file employee, they are even more significant when the concern is the executive. Managerial absenteeism also reduces speed of decision and may seriously influence decision quality. For supervisory employees occupying a middle-management position, pressures from top and bottom impinge and if policy changes are delayed, frustration for the supervisor may be the inevitable result. In extreme absenteeism information on which executive decision-making is based can be biased beyond recognition or simply unavailable. For example, promising employees, capable of promotion, require identification, and most progressive organizations usually attempt to maintain a roster with long-range organizational needs focused on key positions while these, in turn, are aligned with probable retirements, deaths, and other forms of turnover. Because institutions are in a period of rapid expansion (Scheerenberger, 1965), personnel needs parallel those of industry and "In an expanding business. . . . there is not only the problem of keeping the present positions adequately manned but the necessity of training for the new positions to be created by the new plants" (Scott *et al.,* 1954). Training individuals to fill top administrative positions is a responsibility of leadership and requires the physical presence of those in leadership positions. All of these possible consequences of administrative-professional absenteeism represent the easily isolated aspects of the problem.

If precept or example is as important as commonly believed, absenteeism of administrators and professionals in institutional settings, legitimatized or not, is unlikely to elicit the best in production, morale, and punctuality from sub-professional employees. In 1966, American industry lost $10 billion in paid-for but absent labor, and institutions enjoy no special immunity. The multiple activities currently demanding a greater share of the institutional administrators' or professionals' time are being expanded rapidly. Undoubtedly, many new programs will prove to be valuable, but external pressures should not obscure the obvious, though often overlooked, fact that direction of most institutions for the retarded is not a part-time job.

In an admittedly speculative vein, Hicks (1966) suggests a more complex consideration—namely, the "jet-age syndrome." This author indicates that certain research reveals "it may take a traveller who jets across time zones up to a week to return to normal and to perform at his best level. . . ." Other studies cited by Hicks show "that the problem of the jet age is not the time in the air but rather where one lands in relation to where one started." As travel in pursuit of grants, professional meetings, invited addresses, and other accompaniments of affluence increases, one can only speculate as to consequences at the level of institutional operations.

It has been suggested that absentee management derived its impetus from the recent affluence in the helping professions. This phenomenon, although discussed in relation to institutions, is probably evident in other helping agencies and universities as well. It has been suggested that certain consequences of this absenteeism appear to violate basic managerial principles and may importantly influence morale, turn-over, absenteeism, and production among the employees comprising the institutional majority, i.e., attendants and other subprofessionals. For the sincere administrator and professional employee (and most are) this obvious erosion of time can cause divided loyalties and occasion serious guilt feelings. If any, or all of these consequences of the phenomenon are valid, what corrective measures seem indicated?

A study of turnover and absenteeism among institutional non-professional ranks and a similar study of administrative and professional institutional personnel could be easily accomplished from existent records and comparisons of turnover, and absenteeism rates between sub-professional and professional levels could be made on both intra- and inter-institutional bases. Authentication of marked absenteeism at the highest ranks should suggest corrective measures.

What correctives appear necessary would depend, of course, on the magnitude and nature of executive absenteeism. One possible corrective relates to absences that appear to arise on the basis of individual differences among administrators and professional staff. Illustrative of this are those external programs relative to community-based extensions of the institution in which the superintendent or his staff fill an advisory role. Superintendents and other institutional executives occupy a line position ordinarily requiring somewhat different talents or skills than does a staff advisory role. However, some administrators prefer and enjoy a staff advisory role, and for them meetings outside the institution wherein a staff rather than line role is indicated, are more rewarding. Formerly, individuals in institutional line positions but prefering the advisory function had no choice, but the current diversification underway in institutions admits of a sufficient outlet for staff type preferences. Such a study may provide some index of occupational satisfactions among top-echelon people, and subsequent reassignment may be indicated.

Another method for reduction of absenteeism at any level is afforded by environmental modification. Professional and administrative avoidance of patients (and attendants) is sometimes, as Sullivan (1962) suggested, due to one-way status conferral. Much attention is currently devoted to the systematic bestowal of social reinforcement at the patient level; institutions could profit by a similar focus on employees. Rewards, systematically geared to employee needs could include staged participant observation through appropriate building design, unique utilization of consultant personnel, and role-rotation—all designed to foster closer relationships and mutual rewards between sub-professional and professional level staff (Cleland & Peck, 1967).

Other alternatives might include conducting community meetings in the institution, introducing some rewarding feedback to institutional administrators and devoting greater attention to existing promotional practices. Administrative feedback to institutional-based executives often leaves much to be desired. Institutional administrators and staffs in undesirable locations, isolated from the hub of a given state's relevant professional activities, might, of necessity, absent themselves more frequently than their counterparts in institutions with a more favorable location. Whether evidence would support such an hypothesis, or whether circumstances would dictate less absence might suggest alternative approaches to the issue of absenteeism, but some attention to systematic visitation from the central administration and some reassurance that higher authority values attention to the job should be made explicit because "the value that the manager places on the elimination of tardiness or absenteeism will be reflected to a great degree by the employees" (Terry, 1956).

In summary, the problem of executive absenteeism and time erosion in institutions appears to represent one hidden cause of the current manpower shortage. Further, it differs somewhat from its manifestation in industry because absenteeism in competitive industry is subject to economic correctives, i.e., survival of the organization is not automatic as it is (perhaps unfortunately) in the public-supported institution. As external activities and monies chip away at the time of institutional leaders and rank-and-file employees' awareness of this behavior mounts, it appears reasonable to assume that "following the leader" will seriously affect institutional operations. Absenteeism and its correctives are discussed in detail in the standard industrial literature (Kerr, 1964; Scott, *et al.*, 1954; Stagner, 1956).

The manner in which time is distributed in institutions is of considerable importance. Manpower management has been described as "activity concerned with servicing and maintaining the work force by conserving and effectively utilizing it so that its power is not wasted and maximum effectiveness is obtained" (Benn, 1952). Before such management can be established, the distribution of time must be thoroughly understood. Of all the complexities of institutions, time as distributed among employees and patients has undergone the most dramatic, albeit subtle change over the past several decades. The reduction from the 48-hour work week for attendants in most institutions in 1948 to a nearly universal standard 40-hour week in 1968 should illustrate the importance of this variable. Quantitatively, this change based upon a 50-week work year would mean 2,400 hours for the 1948 attendant as contrasted to 2,000 hours for the 1968 attendant. Obviously, the issue is not to return to earlier working hours but to understand the *qualitative* aspects of such a dramatic change. Some approximation of the importance of the qualitative change occurring subsequent to such a time change is afforded by examples from the patient level. A great amount of study has been given to the effects of long-term institutionalization of retardates' performance on both cognitive and noncognitive tasks. Badt (1958), Sarason and Gladwin (1958), Hobbs (1964), and others have associated length of institutionalization to performance decrements while others (Clarke & Clarke, 1954; Zigler & Williams, 1963) have suggested that factors other than length of institutionalization *per se* are required to account for such changes. Two studies (Cleland & Patton, 1968; Cleland, Patton, & Dickerson, 1968) utilized matched groups of retardates on a furlough or no furlough basis during the summer academic recess and found in both studies that subjects having longer (actual time in residence) tenure reflect generally better overall adjustment. Such studies reflect on an important methodological point, i.e., time *actually* in residence rather than length of institutionalization based upon admission date, yields qualitatively different behaviors and might provide alternative interpretations to studies failing to take furloughs into account. In like manner, appraisal of the distribution of time worked by attendants (and other institutional employees) currently in the work force would yield vastly different degrees of actual experience with retardates. Qualitatively, one might expect in institutions having experienced the greatest work week modification over a 20-year period, marked attitudinal differences between attendants of 5 years' tenure and those of 20 or beyond.

The latter group, for example, may have acculturated to the patient culture to such an extent that any change is strongly resisted. For the more limited institutional objectives of a decade or more ago, this time burden (by today's standards) may have yielded a set of attendant behaviors that were quite adaptive, but maladaptive insofar as the current and broadened mission of institutions is concerned. Training is today more formalized and in many cases is offered new employees in regularly scheduled classes on "company time." What was formerly learned through direct, face-to-face experience at the attendant level is currently "learned away from the ward" and often, away from the retardate.

Other temporal modifications have occurred to alter the institution in subtle but important ways. As affluence and technological advances intersect, patterns of living at the ward level are modified. Television, now commonplace on most wards, has permitted striking changes in attendant control of patients. Twenty years ago, bedtime came early except, perhaps, for retardates occupying statuses of privilege gained through work. More patients, therefore, are awake longer than formerly—a phenomenon literally forcing the night shift to observe their charges in at least a quasi-alert state.

This broadens shift exposure and stretches the knowledge of attendants to include the patients' night behaviors.

A concomitant modifier of temporal relations (experience) within institutions is the volunteer movement. As recreation programs were extended through volunteer efforts, the need to enlarge the volunteers' role subtly produced both temporal and spatial modifications. Volunteers entered the ward and retardates received more varied stimulation for extended periods of time. Social activities sponsored by volunteers required longer periods for completion, and night activities have served to keep the retardate "out of bed" and awake. The retardates' awake time has expanded and serves to promote greater exposure to significant adults. In place of prolonged exposure to a few attendants, retardates today experience more attendants *and* others as their awake time increases. Attendants and other institutional employees, are, in fact, in some cases moving toward an "experience-exposure" to retardates that may actually not exceed that of some volunteers. In one institution, four volunteers average over 6,000 hours or more than three years' experience, while another institution boasts one volunteer with over 15,000 hours *or* seven and one-half years' experience on the basis of a 40-hour, 50-work week year! The consequences for institutional operations of these temporal alterations are important ones.

Some institutions are currently engaged in "work out-live in" rehabilitation efforts as a trial or prelude to ultimate discharge. Often retardates under such work arrangements return to the institution an hour or so after administrative and professional staff have gone off-duty. In such cases, occasional crises arising outside the institution are relegated to employees having little, if any, authority for decision. Postponement of decisions pending the next duty period of the administrative-professional staff may seriously influence relations with employers of retardates and frustrate the entire rehabilitation effort. An example relevant to manpower management is seen in institutions having clerical-administrative-professional staff on an eight to five schedule and whose attendant personnel are on shifts of seven to three; three to eleven; eleven to seven. The time distribution afforded attendants from top staff under this schedule would be seven, two, and zero hours for the first, second, and third shifts. However, a shift from eight to five to nine to six for the administrative and professional staff and an attendant shift change from the present schedule to six to two; two to ten; and ten to six would give five hours administrative-professional coverage to the first shift, four to the second, and no charge for the third shift.

Effective utilization of *existing* manpower could benefit from attention to those subtle but important changes that have occurred in institutions over the years. Shorter working hours are generally welcomed by every employee level, but to challenge the sacred cow of traditional schedules amounts to a radical innovation. Nevertheless, "employers can increase output in two principal ways: by hiring more workers and by using workers more efficiently. . . ." and the later case can arise only if management "identifies its new problems correctly and responds to them intelligently and creatively." (Silberman, 1966). Although alterations in schedules typically bring resistances from employees, there are methods for introducing shift changes that may increase acceptance.

Institutions, in the process of change, should not ignore changes occurring in the community. Typical of the changes or problems facing the urban community are traffic congestion, noise, air pollution, police protection, and a host of other issues. An example of how community-institutional problems can be simultaneously attacked is afforded by a large, multi-purpose institution located in a community of over 240,000. Adjacent to the institution are two other large employers, all having identical shifts for office personnel. The scene at 8:00 a.m. and 5:00 p.m. is one of marked congestion wherein all three empty their parking lots into a major thoroughfare in a manner resembling "a free-for-all." Not only are employees frustrated, but as employee expansion continues in these facilities, city traffic control people are faced with a serious safety problem. Simply going into a nine to six office worker schedule for any of the three facilities would largely resolve the problem, and if it were the institution, improved supervisory coverage would result. Were the attendant shifts changed to a six to two, etc., basis, supervisory coverage for the second shift would double, and the morning crises attending patient awakening would benefit from a more favorable attendant-patient ratio. While the prospect of schedule alterations may seem burdensome much can be gained that may aid employee, patients, and community alike. Clearly, manpower management and the mental health manpower shortage could be furthered without exclusive reliance on the classical "we need more employees" theme.

By the end of 1959 the practice of moonlighting was occupying the divided attention of fully five per cent of the United States' labor force and is on the rise (de Grazia, 1964). Even among retarded, institutionalized, "patient helpers" moonlighting or multiple job-holding has been observed (Cleland & Swartz, 1968). Obviously, moonlighting exists among institutional employees and perhaps differentially so among those occupying the lowest salary bracket. The consequent divided loyalties, differential advancement rates, fatigue, and so on are detrimental to the institution and probably to the employee as well. What can be done to utilize this knowledge to improve the institution's position in recruitment, turnover reduction, and improvement of patient care? Current rigidity of state policy is defeating of efforts of institutional administrators to alter pay plans to meet existing competition in certain labor pools and represents a major roadblock to improved manpower management. Silberman (1966), discussing the current "labor shortage" in business and industry indicates, "As the labor market continues to tighten, employers' ability to hire additional workers will depend more and more on the speed and imagination with which they adjust to the new conditions of supply. . . ." One such adjustment might utilize the tendency to moonlighting. Because moonlighters' average time on their second job is 12 hours per week (de Grazia, 1964) the moonlighters' problem would be simplified if institutions offered a five-day, nine-hour shift in lieu of the typical five-day, eight-hour shift, with the inducement of overtime rates for the extra hours' work. Currently, such alterations are difficult because most publically supported institutions are on a straight time pay basis. But such policy changes to permit overtime pay for longer shifts might assist not only the moonlighters in reducing travel time and lessening fatigue, but would also put an additional hour of experience *and* trained help at the institution's disposal. Such a plan to "recapture the moonlighter" would probably have greatest effect if introduced at the mid-line supervisory level. Experience and depth of supervision in this employee group could be employed to advantage in assisting the growing numbers of "entry-level" attendants in orientation to their new jobs. Redistribution and recapturing time lost at both administrative and mid-line supervisory ranks thus allows organizational experience to be arrayed in phalanx style to meet and cope with institutional problems.

If the alleviation of value discrepancies as a source of conflict among attendants and professional-administrative staff (Barnett & Bensberg, 1964; Shotwell, Dingman, & Tarjan, 1960) is possible, temporal organization must improve to encourage greater face-to-face contact. The institutional manpower shortage is not unlike that of industry. Silberman (1966) puts it squarely: Again and again in the past, United States business has shown a remarkable capacity to use whatever supply of labor happened to be available, changing the people to fit the job requirements and changing the job requirements to fit the people. Business did it in World War II, when sharecroppers were turned into shipbuilders, domestics into riveters, overnight. . . . From farmer, domestic, or housewife *to* attendant—the re-training and recruiting problems of institutions do not seem more difficult than industry's during World War II; what does appear different is the institution's continuing reliance on organization and manpower management methods that have scant relevance to minor crises, let alone all-out "war on mental retardation."

Despite the obvious differences among institutional professional and sub-professional personnel such as educational and socioeconomic backgrounds (Bensberg & Barnett, 1966) it is of interest that little attention is given toward individualizing institutional pay plans. Unlike private industry which adapts frequency of pay to varied worker needs, publically-supported institutions are often tied to a policy of 12 monthly checks per year. That ability to delay gratification, especially financial rewards, differs widely along developmental and socioeducational dimensions (Mischel, 1962) is well known and is directly acknowledged in industries' numerous pay-plans. Here, as earlier noted, timing deserves consideration. To allow for employee differences in regard to frequency of payment necessitates change and policy flexibility. Bi-weekly payment for sub-professional workers may well be worth the effort.

Any conceivable schedule modification here, as with other institutional changes, should be preceded by thorough analyses of the community's modal payment schedules, especially in those sectors of business-industry or service that constitute the major competition for labor supply. Occasionally the institution may dramatically improve their competitive posture for labor in the surrounding labor pool through such modifications. There may also be additional benefits of improved morale or productivity. In any event, timing of one of the most powerful material incentives, payday, presents an opportunity for institutions to examine their current position relative to broader social change. Changes and their relevance to intra- and extra-institutional circumstances in any of the areas mentioned may directly or indirectly reflect on the evolutionary or developmental position of the institution itself.

Space as a Determinant of Institutional Social Interactions

In many ways the institution can be viewed as a microcosm of the surrounding community. Illustrative of the broader problems facing institutions *and* communities is the issue of urban planning and population density (Chinitz, 1966). Chinitz, discussing New York as a metropolitan region, suggests that "The density of the New York area is not likely ever to be duplicated in the U. S. . . . the overall density of the Region is 2,337 per square mile. . . ." Two particular institutions dramatically indicate that population densities (space per person) are a legitimate concern of institutions as well as urban planners. Institution A has a resident population of 2,300 and a campus of 80 acres (⅛ square mile). On this basis, population density per square mile exceeds 18,000! Institution B, having an identical resident population but possessing 640 acres (one square mile), has a density of 2,300. On the surface, institution A with a density exceeding the New York area as a whole, is subject to severe overcrowding. This is not the whole story, however. The manner in which space is distributed and organized— in brief, space utilization—makes a difference. Institution B throughout much of its history maintained a large dairy and farm operation which usurped 600 acres. Today, farming operations have ceased and campus *per se* occupies 70 instead of the former 40 acres. Hence, institution A devotes more space to serve an identical population. For the future, B possesses much greater flexibility in design and spatial grouping in any projected physical plant expansion, while A can only turn to high-rise construction. Clearly, space utilization within the institutional milieu is a multifaceted problem and although opinions abound relative to limiting the size (space distribution) of institutions, the issue is a highly equivocal matter (Cleland, 1965; Ullmann, 1967).

Geo-politicians have directed our attention toward space through their analyses of the history of welfare. Origins and outcomes of nearly every major conflict have, in some manner, related to spatial acquisition. Initiation of conflict has often been justified on grounds of needed living space and reparations extracted from the vanquished nation typically involve territorial concessions. At the institutional level, as at the international level, political ideologies dichotomize into isolationistic versus interventionist. Spykman (1942) has indicated that the rationale for United States' isolationists on the international scene rests principally on the issue of space, i.e., protective oceans on both coastlines. Due to transportation and other technological advances, this rationale is today largely untenable. So too, at the institutional level has the isolationist rationale been destroyed where based on distance from an urban center. Institutional locational considerations (Cleland, 1963), expansion of once "distant" community boundaries, and transportation and technological advances have effectively reduced this keystone of isolationistic views. Institutional sites are no longer chosen on the basis of the once powerful motivation of separating the deviant from the larger society. Today, the absence of a spatial barrier is generally seen by both institution and community as a good thing; although in times of crisis, i.e., a spectacular mass escape or a heinous crime by a patient, the old defenses of "separation by distance" are easily mobilized within the community. Space and its management or distribution remains as a potential source of conflict or peaceful co-existence between the institution and the community.

Space, like time, is constantly undergoing subtle transformation in the institution as volunteers, visitors, employees systematically require additional parking lots, offices, or waiting space. This space erosion occurs so slowly that effects may go unnoticed until a crisis arises. Additions of employees, volunteers, and visitors are viewed almost universally in a positive manner by administrative and professional staff during the acquisition phase. Increments should be viewed in relation to both rate of growth and available space and should not, naively, be accepted as an unmixed blessing (Cleland, 1965). Awaiting pronounced reverberations from the patient or employee cultures for application of corrective measures is hardly judicious administration and often results in decisions under crisis and thus is often grossly distorted.

In addition to space losses or redistributions arising from generally positive ways such as staff increments, other less desirable spatial alterations are often externally imposed upon institutions. Political intervention through either elected representatives or quasi-political pressure groups may be motivated by a desire to improve patient welfare, but pressures to admit patients out of turn or to admit those who are ineligible (on grounds of professional judgment) may cause repercussions within the institution that overextends capabilities of both staff and facility. Admission of one patient having a marked character disorder and who is not truly retarded can disrupt established *and controllable* balances of power at the interface of the attendant-patient cultures.

Adopting methods of geo-politics and examining the institution in this relation is merely another molar-level approach to further our understanding of how space influences and shapes the employee-patient culture.

In institutions space may conveniently be ordered into three categories: patient space, employee space, and mutual space. A relevant approach to understanding the manner in which culture is shaped by spatial boundaries or distribution is provided by ethologists. This discipline, devoted to the study of innate behavior patterns, also emphasizes the importance of space. Ardey (1966) views territory as "an area of space . . . which an animal or group of animals defends as an exclusive preserve . . . (and) possession of a territory lends enhanced energy to the proprietor." Patient space too is compromised of a variety of "territories." The restrooms, beds, and night stands represent a few of the more common areas ordinarily reserved for patient use, but none, ordinarily, are inviolable private areas. In practice, patients at any level of retardation seek out areas of relative privacy. For the profoundly retarded whose capacity for mobility through space is limited, one finds a not infrequent positioning in spots of relative privacy, i.e., under their bed, in the same chair or corner day after day, or similar unoccupied spots where "squatter's rights" are open. Higher-grade retardates, being generally more mobile, often make rather sophisticated and extended use of space. Working patients "take-over" storage space in their work places. Over the years, employees yield informal "ownership" or "title" to this space and possessiveness on the "owner's" part is speedily conveyed to any and all intruders.

Patient space is often extended in more subtle ways. The higher-level retardates have earned favor by gradually becoming an indispensable "assistant" to ward attendants through the performance of various routine ward duties or by helping control, feed, or dress less capable retardates.

The more able may receive as pay, more space. With truly private space at a premium, bestowal of an additional square foot by the attendants constitutes a potent reinforcer. The retardate, once possessing additional space, may work feverishly to ward off any threatened takeover by an ambitious newly admitted patient. Such spatial acquisitions may be in the attendant's office under a medicine cabinet, in a supply closet, or clothing room, almost always under the benevolent protection of the attendant. A major factor in "legalizing" such a "property title" is that supervisory attendants on *all shifts* reach consensus that the "owner" has earned this right. Such informal practices may have their origin when poverty budgets yielded very poor staff-patient ratios. In such origins then, these rewards could be considered quite adaptive, although in institutions today they may run counter to rehabilitation objectives and other institutional programs. Regardless of the relative therapeutic efficacy of this practice, this informal technique of space management undoubtedly still operates as a powerful reinforcer in a setting where space is a primary possession. For the recipient of this persuasive motivator, behavior may be modified in a direction judged favorable by attendants but judged otherwise by professionals and less-favored peers. Clearly, ability to predict staff and patient behaviors presupposes, as Moos and Daniels (1967) rightly suggest, some knowledge of the staff and ward setting as well. Spatial acquisition and its practice constitutes yet another shaping force for students of institutions to explore. Others, notably Henry (1964), have discussed space and power in the context of the mental hospital and his observation that attendants selectively reward the more reality-oriented patients, i.e., those least in need of help may suggest further approaches that could enhance understanding of patient and employee culture.

Employee as well as patient space commands attention. At the lower employee ranks, space specifically allocated to a given employee is often understandably less than that allocated patients. Many service-industry employees of the institution (e.g., laundry workers, food service workers) have no private space other than that briefly owned during rest breaks. Obviously, informally bestowed space obtains at this level as well as the patient level and the acquisition mechanisms are quite similar. Supervisors may grant space on the basis of "good worker" or out of fear of reprisal. Although the process is similar to that of patients' spatial acquisition, a more threatening problem appears, i.e., precedents established at this level are more liable to result in organizational conflict because *employees,* unlike patients, are accountable for their actions. Tenure accumulates differentially in a relatively small employee minority (Belknap, 1956)—an element tending to increase the likelihood of territorial acquisition or power but *only* in the hands of a few.

Although the tendency for space to gravitate toward long-tenure employees appears congruent with the concept of "reward for long service," the informal nature of this process may foster conflict when naive professional or sub-professionals inadvertently violate these boundaries which the "owner" has assumed to have the stature of legal property. Notwithstanding recent improvements in employee work conditions and salary, the continuation of "informal rewards" once established, is difficult to extinguish. At higher staff levels, personnel have an equally strong interest in space and here too, territorial rights are stoutly defended. Generally, the range of space follows rank, and top administrative-professional staff theoretically have free access to nearly all space in the institution although, in practice, exercise of this "right" may be quite limited. Higher ranking officials' "spatial holdings" are customarily more extensive and private, and even in instances of "my door is always open" one finds an array of buffer zones that rather effectively forewarn of an intruder's approach. In summary, space comprises a powerful aspect of the institutional value system. It enters importantly into the daily lives of patients and employees at nearly every rank and carries such weight that any reduction amounts literally to diminished status for the person who loses "ground."

For institutions being called upon to diversify—to extend services to include outpatient diagnosis, operate halfway houses, and additional services, new challenges and threats to the territorial integrity of institutions arise. Time sharing of professionals between the institutions and community agencies represents only one instance in which "dual hats" may often require "dual desks" or space. As newer services develop, as cities expand and surround once isolated institutions, and as technological change widens the base of the institutional professional staff, a more intelligent approach to space management will be required. Additional parking lots to accommodate staff increments not only influence costs, they diminish the institutional recreational areas appreciably. New approaches for dual use of parking space during slack periods are required and time management will dictate introduction of new schedules to meet changing community labor practices. Isolationism appears to be an untenable and outdated philosophy and institutions of the future, sensitively attuned to internal and external change, will be required to meet demands for diversified services and research in a lawful and orderly fashion. When time and space as elements determining and shaping the employee-patient culture are brought under more rational control and their informal and often contratherapeutic workings give way to rewards of a more therapeutic and controllable nature, patients and employees alike should mutually benefit and discover more constructive outlets than have heretofore appeared possible.

Summary

Behavior shaping through strategies and techniques of classical or operant variety has received considerable emphasis in institutions over the past decade (Bailer, 1967). The present effort has addressed several of the relatively subtle and molar-level behavior shapers which, as certain evidence suggests, are nonetheless influential in modifying the retardate-employee social organization. This dynamic interplay of time, space, possessions can be seriously considered to influence the overall milieu and may be therapeutic for either the retardate or the employees upon whom good programs depend (Cleland & Swartz, in-press).

Institutions for the retarded, like retardates themselves, are subject to wide individual differences and for this reason, discussion focused on elements shared in common—time, space, possessions. Additional attention should be given these parameters that appear to occupy a strategic role in shaping and determining the institution's place in the future. It appears that the success of behavior modification techniques at the molecular or individual level will be seriously impaired unless complementary efforts are directed toward organizational (social system) modification. While control of the subtle and molar shaping forces may be considerably more difficult to schedule, efforts to do so should enhance the effectiveness of all who live or work in institutions and to ignore these appears administratively hazardous.

References

Ardey, R. *The territorial imperative*. New York: Atheneum, 1966.
Badt, M. I. Levels of abstraction in vocabulary definitions of mentally retarded school children. *American Journal of Mental Deficiency*, 1958, 63, 241–246.
Bialer, I. Psychotherapy and other adjustment techniques with the mentally retarded. In A. A. Baumeister, (Ed.), *Mental retardation*, Chicago: Aldine Publishing Co., 1967.
Barnard, C. I. *The functions of the executive*. Cambridge: Harvard University Press, 1964.
Barnett, C. C. and G. J. Bensberg. Evaluation: A basic tool in training of attendant personnel. *Mental Retardation*, 1964, 2, 224–230.
Bass, B. M. *Organizational psychology*. Boston: Allyn & Bacon, Inc., 1965.
Belknap, I. *Human problems of a state mental hospital*. New York: Blakiston Division, McGraw-Hill Book Co., 1956.
Benn, A. E. *The management dictionary*. New York: Exposition Press, 1952.
Bennis, W. G. and E. H. Schein (Eds.) *Leadership and motivation—Essays of Douglas McGregor*. Cambridge: The M. I. T. Press, 1966.

Bensberg, G. J. and C. D. Barnett. *Attendant training in Southern residential facilities for the mentally retarded: Report of the SREB Attendant Training Project.* Atlanta: Southern Regional Education Board, 1966.

Bensberg, G. J., C. D. Barnett, and W. P. Hurder. Training of attendant personnel in residential facilities for the retarded. *Mental Retardation,* 1964, 2, 144–151.

Chandler, C. S., A. J. Shafter, and R. M. Coe. Arraignment, examination, and confinement of the mentally defective delinquent. Presented at the 82nd Annual Convention, Dallas, Texas, May 1958.

Chinitz, B. New York: A Metropolitan region. In *Cities: A scientific American book.* New York: Alfred A. Knopf, 1966.

Clarke, A. D. B. and A. M. Clarke. Cognitive changes in the feebleminded. *British Journal of Psychology,* 1954, 45, 173–179.

Cleland, C. C. Locational variables in the establishment of institutions. *Training School Bulletin,* 1963, 60, 123–129.

————. Evidence on the relationship between size and institutional effectiveness: A review and analysis. *American Journal of Mental Deficiency,* 1965, 70, 423–431.

Cleland, C. C. and W. F. Patton. Sustained versus interrupted institutionalization. In Jervis, G. A. (Ed.), *Expanding concepts in mental retardation.* Springfield: Charles C. Thomas, 1968.

Cleland, C. C., W. F. Patton, and W. L. Dickerson. Sustained versus interrupted institutionalization: II. *American Journal of Mental Deficiency,* 1968, 72, 815–827.

Cleland, C. C. and R. F. Peck. Intra-institutional administrative problems: A paradigm for employee stimulation. *Mental Retardation,* 1967, 5, 2–8.

Cleland, C. C. and J. D. Swartz. Deprivation, reinforcement and peer support as work motivators: A paradigm for habilitation of older retardates. *Commuity Mental Health Journal,* 1968, 4, 120–128.

————. *Mental retardation: Approaches to institutional change.* New York: Grune & Stratton, Inc., 1969.

de Grazia, S. *Of time, work, and leisure.* New York: Doubleday & Co., 1962.

Drucker, P. F. How to manage your time. *Harpers,* 1966, 233, 56–60.

Edgerton, R. B. A patient elite: Ethnography in a hospital for the mentally retarded. *American Journal of Mental Deficiency,* 1963, 68, 3.

Edgerton, R. B. and H. F. Dingman. Good reasons for bad supervision: "Dating" in a hospital for the mentally retarded. *Psychiatric Quarterly Supplement,* Utica: State Hospitals Press, 1964, 1–13.

————. Tatooing and identity. *International Journal of Social Psychiatry.* IX, 2, 1963.

————. Tatooing. *Abottempo,* 1964, 2, 4.

Edgerton, R. B. and G. Sabagh. From mortification to aggrandizement changing self-concepts in the careers of the mentally retarded. *Psychiatry,* 1962, 25, 263–272.

Edgerton, R. B., G. Tarjan, and H. F. Dingman. Free enterprise in a captive society. *American Journal of Mental Deficiency,* 1961, 66, 35–41.

Health Bulletin for Teachers. The health and safety of the worker. New York: Metropolitan Life Insurance Company Press, 1942, 13, 29–32.

Henry, J. Space and power on a psychiatric unit. In A. F. Wessen (Ed.), *The psychiatric hospital as a social system.* Springfield: Charles C. Thomas, 1964.

Hicks, C. B. Jet-age blues. *Today's Health,* 1966, 44, 66–68.

Hobbs, M. T. A comparison of institutionalized and non-institutionalized mentally retarded. *American Journal of Mental Deficiency,* 1964, 69, 206–210.

Kahne, M. C. Bureaucratic structure and impersonal experience in mental hospitals. *Psychiatry: Journal of Studies of Interpersonal Processes,* 1959, 22, 363–375.

Kerr, C. *Labor and management in industrial society.* New York: Doubleday & Co., Inc., 1964.

Knowles, K. G. J. C. *Strikes—A study in industrial conflict.* Oxford: Basil Blackwell, 1952.

Kretch, D., R. S. Crutchfield and E. L. Ballachey. *Individual in society.* New York: McGraw-Hill, 1962.

MacAndrew, C. and R. B. Edgerton. I.Q. and the social competence of the profoundly retarded. *American Journal of Mental Deficiency,* 1964, 69, 385–390.

————. Procedure for interogating non-professional ward employees. *American Journal of Mental Deficiency,* 1964, 69, 347–353.

————. On the possibility of friendship. *American Journal of Mental Deficiency,* 1966, 70, 612–621.

————. The everyday life of the institutionalized "idiots." *Human Organization.* 1964, 23, 312–318.

Margolin, J. B. News and notes. *Community Mental Health Journal,* 1966, 2, 186.

Mercer, J. R. Social system perspective and clinical perspective: Frames of reference for understanding career patterns of persons labeled as mentally retarded. *Social Problems,* 1965, 13, 18–34.

Mischel, W. Preference for delayed reward as a function of age, intelligence, and length of delay interval. *Journal of Abnormal and Social Psychology,* 1962, 64, 425–431.

Moos, R. H. and D. N. Daniels. Differential effects of ward settings on psychiatric staff. *Archives General Psychiatry,* 1967, 17, 75–81.

O'Gorman, G. A hospital for the psychotic defective child. *Lancet,* 1958, (Nov.) 951–953.

Philips, S. U. and H. F. Dingman. On the construction of persons. *Mental Retardation,* 1968, 6, 20–22.

President's Panel on Mental Retardation. *A proposed program for National action to combat mental retardation.* Washington, D.C.: U.S. Gov't. Printing Office, 1962.

Roethslisberger, F. J. and W. J. Dickson. *Management and the worker.* Cambridge: Harvard University Press, 1947.

Rosenthal, N. H. The health manpower gap: A high hurdle. *Occupational Outlook Quarterly,* 1967, 2, 1–8.

Sarason, S. B. and T. Gladwin. Psychological and cultural problems in mental subnormality: A review of research. *American Journal of Mental Deficiency,* 1958, 62, 1115–1307.

Scheerenberger, R. C. A current census of state institutions for the mentally retarded. *Mental Retardation,* 1965, 3, 4–6.

Scheff, T. J. Control over policy by attendants in a mental hospital. *Journal of Health and Human Behavior,* 1961, 2, 93–105.

Scott, W. D., R. C. Clothier, and W. R. Spriegel, *Personnel management.* New York: McGraw-Hill, 1954.

Seitz, S. and C. C. Cleland, Changing existing attitudes—A dissonance approach. *Psychological Reports,* 1967, 20, 51–54.

Shotwell, A., H. F. Dingman, and G. Tarjan. Need for improved criteria in evaluating job performance of state hospital employees. *American Journal of Mental Deficiency,* 1960, 65, 208–213.

Silberman, C. E. *The myths of automation.* New York: Harper & Row, Inc., 1966.

Spykman, N. J. *America's strategy in world politics.* New York: Harcourt, Brace, & Co., 1942.

Stagner, R. *Psychology of industrial conflict.* New York: John Wiley & Sons, Inc., 1956.

Sullivan, H. S. *Schizophrenia as a human process.* New York: W. W. Norton & Co., 1962.

Taylor, H. G. Attendants: Assessment and application. *Mental Retardation,* 1964, 2, 83–88.

Terry, G. R. *Principles of management.* Homewood, Ill.: Richard D. Irwin, Inc., 1956.

Ullman, L. P. *Institution and outcome.* Oxford: Pergamon Press, 1967.

Wilensky, H. L. The uneven distribution of leisure: The impact of economic growth on "Free time." *Social Problems,* 1961, 9, 32–56.

Windle, C. Prognosis of mentally subnormals. *American Journal of Mental Deficiency,* 1962, 66, 5.

Zigler, E. and J. Williams. Institutionalization and the effectiveness of social reinforcement: A three-year follow-up study. *Journal of Abnormal and Social Psychology,* 1963, 66, 197–205.

Institutional Programming and Research: A Vital Partnership in Action

During the past century Western man has developed a special system for dealing with the mentally retarded: The residential institution. He did so not as a result of scientific study, but out of humanitarian impulses. The development of residential facilities for the retarded coincided with the growth of institutions for other chronic disabilities, notably mental illness and tuberculosis. The professional humanitarians, physicians or educators, who were placed in charge of these residential care centers, had little to guide them but their own good intentions and the prevailing climate of public opinion, the *Zeitgeist*. Residential institutions multiplied helter-skelter, without specific planning and guided by no body of scientific knowledge.

By the 1920's new residential facilities for the retarded were springing up all over the country. A stratified corps of institutional directors, attendant supervisors, and other administrative personnel had arisen. While individual members of this corps occasionally moved from one institution to another, most of them remained as apparently self-perpetuating administrations of their particular institutions or state systems. Because most institutional personnel, the attendants, remained in their positions relatively

1. This chapter was prepared with the assistance of grant number RD–1816–P of the Vocational Rehabilitation Administration, U.S. Dept. of Health, Education and Welfare.

short times, it fell to this administrative corps to provide continuity to programs and philosophies. Moreover, the lack of any objective body of knowledge about how best to design institutional practices resulted in considerable diversity between institutions, and the quality of institutional programs came to depend largely on the humane dispositions of their particular administrative officers. As these dispositions varied, so did the quality of residential programs for the retarded. In the United States today, more than 200,000 retarded persons reside in more than 150 institutions whose programs vary with the humaneness and competence of their various administrative officers.

Concurrent with the growth of residential programs for the retarded, but entirely independent of it, the social and behavioral sciences developed rapidly. These disciplines concerned themselves with human growth and development from infancy to adulthood and with the effects of wide-range environmental conditions on cognitive and emotional growth. But until very recently the impact of the behavioral sciences upon institutional management has been limited primarily to the clinical use of instruments designed to measure functioning in intellectual and self-care areas.

The Intelligence Quotient was adopted as the criterion for admission to residential facilities for the retarded almost as rapidly as intelligence tests and psychometricians became available. There the matter rested. After admission, which in most cases resulted in life-long institutional residence for the retardate, repeated psychometric evaluations were made, but their results seldom influenced decisions concerning the management of the individual. An even more serious neglect of the potential contribution of the social sciences was the failure to attend to the accumulating evidence that a child's total milieu contributed greatly to his growth and development. The I. Q. of the institutionalized retardate, once assigned, became immutable.

The Effects of Institutionalization

During the 1940's and 50's the research evidence continued to accumulate, and it indicated almost unanimously that institutional rearing created serious lags in children's emotional, behavioral, and intellectual growth. Bowlby's (1951) influential monograph summarized the studies on the effects of maternal deprivation, and it dramatically highlighted the dangers inherent in removing a child from his home. The consensus of this massive evidence, summarized later by Yarrow (1961) and Butterfield (1967) was that, in general, children should be reared at home. However, certain exceptions were noted: Some institutions appeared to have less detrimental effects than others, and some manifested no negative effects at all. For example Klackenburg (1956) found no ill effects in children raised in Scandinavian nursing houses, and Freud and Burlingham (1944) noted that among displaced English children during World War II no ill effects were exhibited. Children reared in communal nursing homes in Israeli Kibbutzim showed even "better emotional control and greater overall maturity . . . than control children living with their own parents" (Rabin, 1958). It became evident from the available research that *some* institutions have a seriously deleterious effect on child development, while others do not. The studies cited above dealt with so-called normal children (i.e., not labeled retarded), but similar evidence had begun to accumulate (e.g., Lyle, 1960) which clearly showed that institutionalized retardates were developing at a slower rate than non-institutionalized controls.

The apparent conclusions which can be drawn from the research on institutional rearing are:

1. Institutional child rearing is generally less conducive to child growth and development than normal home care.
2. Some institutional environments are less harmful to child growth and development than others.

The Residential Institution as a Research Subject

The supposed need of the retarded, the force of tradition, and sometimes financial considerations, lead to the establishment of many large (1,000 or more residents) residential institutions in the United States. A very large number of studies about the nature of mental retardation was carried out in these facilities. Partially because of convenience (availability of subjects and personnel) and partially because of the implicit assumption that retardates would behave in similar fashions regardless of their environment, no efforts were made to cross-validate these studies in other institutional environments. Until recently virtually no studies had been available about the institution itself.

The dearth of descriptive information about institutions for the retarded is unfortunately not unique. A similar absence of data exists in other areas. For example, only one researcher (Rheingold, 1960) working with normal children in an "at home study" described the homes in other than anecdotal or clinical terms. Attempts to focus on causative aspects of the milieu's effects on the retardate's behavior have been undertaken only recently. Nevertheless, attempts to modify the retarding effects of institutional rearing upon the retarded are not new.

Perhaps the most rigorous, most careful, and certainly the most influential series of longitudinal studies was conducted in Iowa under the direction of Skeels (1939). Skeels arranged for 13 orphaned or abandoned children to be reared as "house guests" in an institution for the retarded, to be cared for by attendants and older retardates and thus to receive intensive "mothering" and individual attention. After about two years eleven of these specially handled children were placed in adoptive homes. During even the brief interval before adoptive placement, marked gains in intelligence were noted in the group reared in the institution for the retarded. A similar group who remained to be reared in the orphanage showed no such gains. Recently a 30-year follow-up of these "children" has become available (Skeels, 1966), and most impressive differences between the experimental-institutional and control-orphanage groups were revealed. All of the persons with the special early experience in the institution for the retarded had become productive citizens; one had graduated from a state university and eight others had graduated from high school. Most of those originally reared in the orphanage, however, were now residing in institutions for the retarded as adults, and only one had completed high school. Skeels' studies clearly suggest that institutions for the retarded need not have the detrimental effects upon their residents that are so frequently ascribed to them.

If public residential care *per se* is not retarding child growth and development, it is necessary to explore the specific factors which make up the extremely complex human system termed *institution for the retarded,* to isolate specific influential factors, and then to implement these research findings in practical ways.

Although many of us have been impressed with the paucity of stimulation and the inadequacy of care in large institutions, these conditions have rarely been described objectively. Perhaps the sole exception is a study of one West coast institution (Thormahlen, 1966). Thormahlen found that less than 2 per cent of the attendant's time was spent training children and that 36 per cent of the time attendants encouraged dependent behavior among the residents. One third of the time of the personnel of this facility was spent actively preventing the retarded under their supervision from developing self-care skills. Thormahlen also found that ward practices were designed to make the acquisition of self-care most difficult. For example, girls were required to wear dresses which buttoned in the back; the least capable children wore high topped tennis shoes which required complicated lacing and tying skills; there was no toilet paper in the toilets, no forks and knives on the tables, and virtually no toys in the "playrooms."

Thormahlen also reported that the staff-resident ratio had little effect on the quality of care actually received by the retarded children. Instead "an increase in personnel tended to produce a more dependent child since there were then enough staff members to assume more responsibilities and more tasks for the children. In addition, increased staffing tended to accentuate role stratification . . . and resulted in the employees remaining in the kitchen, clothing room, etc., rather than being in a position to interact with children (Thormahlen, 1966, p. 57)." It seems clear that this institution is not performing as adequately as most persons concerned with caring for the retarded would hope. Still, it would be an error to assume that all residential facilities are equally depriving. For example, Butterfield and Zigler (1965) were able to demonstrate experimentally that children in two institutions within the same state manifested substantially different degrees of "social hunger," i.e., a need to be in the physical proximity to non-retarded persons. This finding suggests that the two institutions provide their residents with different amounts of social interaction.

Implementation of Research Findings

Research findings imply that typical, traditional institutions have substantial shortcomings, that in most cases a retarded child should remain at home as long as possible to maximize his development, and that increased interpersonal contacts (such as in the Skeels' study) help to turn an otherwise detrimental milieu into a beneficial one.

It might be added here that developmental retardation is directly proportional to the time spent in an institution. Grissey (1937) and Kephart and Strauss (1940) demonstrated 30 years ago that retardates institutionalized at earlier ages showed greater I.Q. losses than those institutionalized at later ages. Butterfield (1967) in summarizing the accumulated research evidence concluded that the younger the retardate placed in an institution the more susceptible he is to the detrimental effects of this kind of placement.

These findings seem to demand that traditional institutional programs be revamped and a new approach to residential care be developed. Numerous efforts in this area are now in operation and one state, Connecticut, is attempting to change its entire institutional system in line with the research data and conclusions cited above. Connecticut's current contribution to residential care is known as the "regional center." Without suggesting that the Connecticut approach is the best or the only solution to the problems posed by institutional deprivation, it is described here merely as one example of how research findings have been acted upon in an effort to improve residential care for the retarded. More and different efforts must be made if we are to meet our professional and ethical responsibilities to those retarded who are placed in residential institutions.

The Regional Center

It seemed to the Connecticut Office of Mental Retardation that research findings clearly required a basic change in their conceptualization of how to meet the needs of Connecticut's mentally retarded. The term *service* had to be expanded to include services rendered to retardates residing at home, especially younger ones. Merely upgrading residential programs was not enough, although that too was needed. The regional center in the Connecticut program is first and foremost an attempt to assist parents and communities to retain their retarded.

The task of the regional director is to supply all necessary assistance to the parent so that he will be able to maintain his child at home and thus to permit as many retardates as possible to remain in the community. Also, those retarded persons who are admitted to the regional center for residential care should be integrated into the community at large as much as possible.

The basic services which the regional centers try to provide are:

SERVICES TO RETARDATES AND THEIR FAMILIES
LIVING IN THE COMMUNITY

Day-care Services for young, severely handicapped, or otherwise impaired children who are ineligible for public school special education classes. These services are rendered directly by the center, or by parent groups who receive guidance from the center and financial support through the Office of Mental Retardation.

This kind of service relieves the parent of the need for continuous supervision of the retarded youngerster, and has thus permitted the return of women to the (tax paying) labor force. It also helps prepare the child for public school. Many of these youngsters are "graduating" to the special education classes within their communities.

Sheltered Workshops for older retardates who have reached the maximum age of school attendance and can lead a productive, though non-competive existence. The problem of programming for the adult retardate is especially important. Because medical advances have increased the life-span of retardates to near-normal length, most persons designated as being retarded are chronological adults. These retarded men and women can be an asset rather than a burden to their communities. To make this possible the regional center and Office of Mental Retardation provide supervision, guidance, and financial aid to community-based sheltered workshops. Also such workshops are frequently maintained on the grounds of the center.

Professional Services to Parents, Children, and Agencies. Parents and social agencies frequently need guidance and information about services which are available to the retarded. The regional center tries to serve as a central clearinghouse for information about all activities suitable for retardates and to make its knowledge available to all. Having such knowledge is also frequently helpful to the regional center. They have found that diagnostic services can often be obtained at community clinics and hospitals. Connecticut is a small enough state to permit relatively easy access to such community facilities, thereby reducing the diagnostic capabilities which must be provided by the regional center itself.

Recreational Facilities for the retarded, especially for adolescents and adults, though vitally necessary, are usually scarce. The regional center provides such facilities in the evenings and on weekends. The mere presence of a place where a retardate is welcome often makes the difference between a successful and unsuccessful community adjustment for him. Those retardates who live nearby take frequent advantage of this opportunity.

During the summer months, regional centers conduct special recreational programs for all retardates, including those whose programs are provided by other agencies during the rest of the year. Many school children enroll in this regional program.

A major task for recreation directors is the opening of general community recreational resources to the retarded. Community centers, "Y's," youth organizations (Boy Scouts, Campfire Girls, etc.) have been alerted to the needs of retarded children and have responded well.

Educating the Community is an intangible, though clearly basic necessity for the initiation of a successful regional program. The centers can succeed only if retarded persons are seen by the population at large as potentially productive and intrinsically worthy individuals. Such attitudes are not established merely by lectures and talks to selected groups (PTA's, church groups), though these are also important, but primarily through demonstration in one's own agency. Thus, the task of alerting the professional community to modern treatment philosophies in retardation is especially acute.

Medical practitioners are frequently unaware of educational and rehabilitative methods which have been developed for the retarded. Psychiatric clinics for children and adults have traditionally not given their services to the retarded and their families and are in need of guidance about how they can serve this population. This educational task of the center is carried out by persistent and frequent joint case-conferences in which the professionals in the centers involve themselves with the professionals in the community. Potentially the community possesses all the resources for working with the retarded, but many decades of neglect have brought about persisting attitudes of hopelessness, which have led to the neglect of retardates and their families. Many years of patient education efforts through daily contacts with key professionals will be needed before a meaningful change in attitude will take place, but the regional centers are a beginning.

Services to Retardates in Residence

In spite of all the efforts made to enable parents and communities to retain retardates at home, it sometimes becomes necessary to place a child in a residential facility. Such placement is most often not necessary for the welfare of the retardate. Rather, it arises out of social or psychological needs of parents, or is due to the absence of parents and other relatives (Klaber, in press). Admission to an institution to the retarded has traditionally been considered an "all or none" affair: a child's admission constituted a significant break from his previous existence. Placement was considered to be a permanent solution to whatever problems had been presented by the youngster.

The regional center instituted a new system of admissions designed to meet immediate, short-term needs of children and parents. Instead of the permanent Probate Commitment which had been in effect hitherto, provisions for "voluntary" or "informal" admissions were made. This procedure permits short-term residence in state facilities for the retarded and allows guardianship to remain with the parent. Parents are now able to secure residence for reasons of acute family stress (e.g., birth or death of a family member), short-term residential evaluation of a retardate (e.g., to determine accurately his suitability for semi-independent living), or even for family vacation. Length of such short-term admissions ranges from 24 hours to six months.

Special care is taken that residents of a regional center do not lose their ties with the community at large. As many services as possible are secured from the community, and the desirability of return to a child's own home, foster home, or hostel is stressed.

Educational Services to the retarded residents of the center is rendered by the town in which the center is located. School-age children designated as being "educable" or "trainable" are sent to the local schools. The program is funded through a tuition plan in which the state reimburses the host-town in full. Naturally, such an arrangement can operate only if the number of such students is kept within reasonable boundaries. The small capacity of regional centers ensures the manageable size of these groups. If a child is excluded from public school, he is served by educational facilities maintained at the regional center.

This service is also open to retarded in the community who have been excluded from public school. Whenever a retarded child is excluded from a school system, the Office of Mental Retardation is notified by the State Department of Education. The Office relays this information to the appropriate regional center who must investigate the case. This investigation alone has reduced the number of school exclusions. However, when a child cannot be retained in school the center will work out a plan for him which utilizes community or regional center resources.

Vocational Habilitation for mildly and moderately retarded adolescents and adults is incorporated in the training department of the center. Attempts are made to place as many retardates in productive jobs as possible. The mildly retarded adults at the regional centers who assist in the maintenance of the institution and care of younger residents receive wages (at present, $10 per week). They are then assisted in spending their earnings judiciously.

To facilitate return to community living some retardates are given the opportunity to reside in the center and to work at a job outside the center. They are gradually encouraged to take up supervised, semi-independent residence at a carefully selected home. Those adults who are unlikely to achieve a level of functioning which would permit competitive employment are placed in sheltered workshop situations which will permit them to produce useful work according to their ability. They, too, receive remuneration according to their ability.

Residential Care represents the institution counterpart of parental care. In a family, however, two individuals expend considerable time and effort not only on the physical care of their offspring, but also on their children's psychological and emotional development. To permit residents of regional centers to achieve reasonable development, they, too, must receive stimulation and support. To achieve this aim, regional centers use a variety of means: small unit size (12 to 20 children per child-care unit) is conducive to individual interaction of aides and their charges; hence, buildings are designed to have very small day-rooms which can be attended to by one worker. Special efforts are made to bring people from the community into contact with individual residents. Federally financed programs have been particularly helpful in this area; foster grandparent programs, for example, permit the utilization of poor, elderly citizens for this kind of work.

Every effort is made to maintain contact with the child's family. Visiting hours are therefore completely open, with parents and friends being welcomed in the actual residential units.

Health Services are not handled by a house staff, but are obtained through clinics and hospitals in the community. Medical practitioners are retained on a consulting basis. Typically, one physician comes regularly to the center once a week (though he is on call at all times), as does a local dentist. Whenever the need arises, medical specialists are consulted. Seriously ill residents are taken to a community hospital.

Such an arrangement has the dual advantage of using the best available medical personnel, while at the same time educating these professionals in the area of mental retardation. Many of these physicians return to their private practices with a changed outlook towards the problem of institutionalization.

Other Services which require professional consultants (speech pathology, clinical psychology, physical and occupational therapy, etc.) may be rendered directly by the house staff, or typically a sub-professional, full-time staff member would be used. He would consult with a fully trained professional who is primarily affiliated with another community agency. For example, a speech teacher with a bachelor's degree may be on the full-time staff and consult with a speech pathologist who holds a Ph.D. degree and is affiliated with a local university.

The Service List

All the identified retarded persons in the region are known to the center whether or not they need service at a given time. The purpose of this list is to permit effective life-time planning for the individual and his family. Thus, parents are urged to use the center's resources for crisis counseling (e.g., in case of parental illness, the retarded who has lost a job). The knowledge that a giver agency, a known quantity, is interested in the retarded and his parents lends a sense of security to the family.

The service list aids in forestalling the sudden emergencies which have confronted the admission committees of the traditional facilities so frequently. The follow-up of the entire case load permits methodological, life-time help when needed, and thus strengthens the home in its ability to retain the retarded person.

Research and Programming

The Connecticut Program shows that institutional programs can be designed to be not only humane but also to be consistent with conclusions based on research. Conversely, it is also possible to design research programs which meet the needs of institution administrators. The administrator needs to know how to make his facility benefit its residents. The administrator can do this if he knows the actual events taking place in his facility and their effects on child behavior.

In the field of mental retardation the situation is no different than in any other area of habilitation. All states maintain facilities, usually called "schools" where retarded children and adults reside. Ostensibly, retardates are sent there to learn and be trained in personal, academic, and vocational skills. The effectiveness of these facilities has traditionally been "assessed" through impressions and subjective reports. These reports suggested that there were indeed significant differences between institutions, but these differences were expressed either in abstract terms (e.g., good atmosphere, nice attitudes) or in terms of architectural, financial, and personel ratios (e.g., cu. ft. of air per bed, daily per capita costs, attendant to client ratio). With the assistance of a VRA grant we set ourselves the task of assessing institutions more objectively in both human and actuarial terms. The following is a brief report of our findings.

The Aims of Institutions for the Retarded

To assess the effectiveness of an organization its goal must be explicitly understood. Institutions for the retarded typically lack clearly stated objectives. Brochures, pamphlets, or other publications usually express a general view to the effect that "X Training School effectively maximizes the potential of each individual in residence." Such statements are gratifying, unassailable, but unfortunately, also meaningless. However, it is possible to formulate a number of criteria which are explicit, simple, and observable. We do not content that these goals encompass the entire range of institutional effectiveness, but no institution can be judged effective unless it achieves at least these three things:

1. Increases in the residents' ability to care for themselves (self-sufficiency).
2. Improvements in the residents' cognition (intellegence).
3. A state of general well-being of the residents (adjustment or happiness).

Methodology

In behavioral science three methods of scientific investigation are usually employed: experimental manipulation under laboratory conditions, measurement of abilities of attitudes through validated instruments, and behavior observations under natural conditions. We employed all three methods to assess institutions.

Because the ultimate subject of our research was the institutional system, rather than behavior of retarded children, it was imperative to investigate a variety of institutions, rather than children in only one residential facility. Such investigations are, unfortunately, very rare in the field of retardation. King and Raynes (1968) have demonstrated that institutional "wards" regiment their residents much more than "hostels" do, despite similar residential populations and staff ratios. King and Raynes did not describe, however, the detailed functioning of their institutional settings. Thormahlen

(1966) described repeated observations in one institution in great detail, but did not choose another kind of facility for comparative purposes. It was our intent to both describe and contrast institutions for the retarded.

Our basic approach was to approximate the hypothetical ideal case of admitting the same child to different institutions. We did this by matching mentally retarded residents of different institutions as closely as possible on several variables. We assumed that differences among such matched groups of retardates would reflect their differential institutional experiences.

Table 6–1. Matching Data On Subjects In Six Institutions For The Retarded

Institution		Series I			Series II		
		A	B	C	D	E	F
MA	MEAN	3.12	2.92	3.19	1.77	1.75	2.02
	SD	1.62	1.84	1.33	1.04	1.04	1.24
IQ	MEAN	28.88	27.15	29.31	21.10	23.10	23.48
	SD	14.00	10.48	7.96	8.79	8.85	8.55
Age at Admission	MEAN	6.41	6.64	6.25	7.05	6.90	6.11
	SD	2.14	2.03	1.66	3.19	3.17	2.97
CA	MEAN	10.96	10.52	10.52	15.48	15.40	15.48
	SD	1.88	1.99	2.22	3.91	3.84	3.83

The Institutions and the Matching Process

We studied six state-supported institutions for the retarded. Three of these facilities were in one state, two in another, and one in a third state. We divided our study into two series of subject samples. Series I consisted of three matched samples of 17 children from each of three of the six institutions, and Series II of three samples of 44 children from each of the other three residential facilities. By matching every child with two other children, we are, in theory at least, studying the same child in three separate settings.

The matching itself was performed on a purely actuarial basis, from records supplied by the institutions. We matched the children as closely as possible on the following variables: age, age-at-admission, sex, race, IQ, and MA. We eliminated from our study children diagnosed as mentally ill, and persons with disabling sensory handicaps (hearing and vision, Table

6–1). We also attempted to match gross diagnostic categories, and thus always matched mongoloids with other Down's Syndrome cases, seizure patients with other epileptics, and so on. A close match of parental socio-economic status was not feasible, but a sample of 20 parent-pairs clearly demonstrated the comparability of the matched groups. Our groups seem to contain a representative sample of parental backgrounds.

The first series of matched triads consisted of 51 children, 17 from each of three institutions, A, B, and C.

Institution A is a medium-sized facility which is divided administratively into three separate and distinct areas of service: a boy's village, a girl's village, and a compound for the severely retarded. The institution was originally designed to serve the mildly retarded, and efforts were made to simulate home environments by building relatively small living units with "house parents" who lived in. As admission pressures eventually resulted in the construction of larger living units, the admission of youngsters and more severely retarded and a greater emphasis on nursing type care. The official philosophy, however still emphasized the ideal of small units, educational approaches and an atmosphere of homelike care.

Institution B is a large facility (population more than 4,000) which is divided into two strictly separated administrative units: male and female. These two segments are substantially autonomous with respect to child-care procedures and are geographically distinct. Apparently the founders of the facility felt that their population would consist of ambulatory reasonably self-sufficient individuals whose major needs are shelter and food. Large dormitories and centrally located eating facilities suggest as much. The relatively new influx of more severely retarded, younger, and less self-sufficient residents prompted a building program stressing full-service edifices. These buildings are designed to meet all the needs of its residents, including food services and a variety of therapies. The philosophy is essentially medical, and stresses physical habilitation.

Institution C is also a large facility whose original design stressed efficiency and low-cost services for severely handicapped individuals. Buildings are very large, several of them have more than one story, and space is designed primarily for the placement of beds. Recreational facilities and educational and recreational programs are minimal. This institution is the only one in our survey which did not have some playground area for each building. The institution is not divided into separate services; rather, it is administered centrally.

The second example series consisted of 132 children, 44 each from Institutions D, E, and F.

Institution D is a medium-sized facility whose original plant was composed almost entirely of multi-storied buildings. It was apparently originally believed that ambulatory, self-sufficient individuals would reside there Originally, there had been total segregation of sexes but, more recently, there have been administrative changes permitting personnel and residents to move from one dormitory to another depending on need. Newer buildings are designed for full service and include day rooms and dining halls. Educational activities are carried out in a relatively new school building which is located at the outskirts of the grounds.

Institution E is a new retardation facility. It is located in older buildings which were originally designed to serve chronically ill children and adults, but the physical plant is not indicative of the facility's philosophy of care. The number of residents is very small (fewer than 300), and a heavy emphasis is placed on supplying the needs of the retardates through outside community resources. Schooling, medical care, and so on are provided by town or private resources. The per capita expenditure for residents in Institution E was more than double the average of the other institutions in our sample. Volunteers, a variety of specialists, and other personnel abound creating an unusually high caretaker to retardate ratio.

Institution F is a medium-sized (close to 2,000 residents) facility. It had the most neglected physical plant of all institutions studied, with old, multistoried buildings and unpaved roads. The original philosophy probably was essentially similar to that of Institution D, but a much older school building testifies to a much earlier interest in educational activities. Many of the old buildings have been modified to include school or education rooms. The institution is centrally administered without a sharp division between male and female services.

Residents of Institution A were matched with Institutions B and C, but a unique opportunity presented itself in Institution E. A number of its residents had been transferred five years earlier from Institution D for purely administrative reasons. It was possible to match these persons retrospectively on measurements obtained at D with youngsters who had remained at D. The second group is thus an attempt to obtain longitudinal measures, albeit retrospectively.

Measuring Institutional Experience of Residents

To obtain a behavioral description of our subjects and, more importantly to determine how their institutional environments impinged upon them we constructed an observation schedule consisting of both subject and environmental variables. Included in our observations were: the behavior of the child and the behavior of the individual interacting with the child. When observing the child's behavior we recorded self-directed behavior (crying rocking, finger posturing, other stereotypes, inactivity, etc.) and outer-directed behavior (smiling, laughing, dancing, destructive and aggressive acts, playing with people and with objects, talking, listening, watching, and other items).

The "other person," the individual who was observed to interact with a subject, was classified according to whether he was an attendant, or any non-retarded adult other than an aide. We recorded whether he responded to a demand on the child's part, or whether he initiated the interaction. We then described the interaction (taking care of the child's physical need, conversing or playing with the child, punishing him, showing physical affection, etc.).

Four research assistants, two men and two women, were employed in all the observations. This staff was comprised of recent college graduates in psychology and education who had neither educational background nor experience in research or in the field of mental retardation. Their lack of preparation in scientific areas was more than compensated for by their freedom from established attitudes to mental retardation and total naivete with respect to our hypotheses.

The research assistants underwent an intensive eight-week training program in the use of the observation scale. At the end of training the inter-rater reliabilities were all .85 or greater. The fact that this highly satisfactory level could be achieved after only two months of training suggests that observational assessment of the behavior of mentally retarded individuals is both feasible and practical.

While it is highly desirable to learn about the behavior of institutional retardates through such observations, they are insufficient in yielding the data necessary for the evaluation of adjustment. Fortunately, a number of experimental procedures have recently been developed and perfected in psychological laboratories. These techniques have yielded reliable results in special situations, but have not been attempted in "field conditions." For example, rocking behavior among severely retarded has been described as dependent on external events (Klaber & Butterfield, 1968). Such behavior can be measured with relative ease and might be used to assess quickly the impact of external events (i.e., ward activities) upon the retarded. We used this method to describe some of the inter-institutional differences.

Social deprivation measures have rarely been used to measure inter-institutional differences. Butterfield and Zigler (1965) and Klaber, Butterfield, and Gould (1969) however have demonstrated that two institutions for the retarded within the same state-system may act in distinctly different ways upon mildly retarded children, one institution apparently satisfying the social needs of its residents much better than another. Through extending social reinforcement techniques to tasks relevant to more severely retarded children and adults, we were able to assess the social reinforcement value of other institutions. We have adapted a special technique to this end and have demonstrated its usefulness in inter-institutional comparison (Klaber, Butterfield & Gould, 1969).

Child behavior was also assessed with traditional scales and psychometric tests. These measures are especially useful in serving as guideposts of functional levels.

Our three approaches to the assessment of behavior of the institutional retardate were thus:

1. Detailed behavior observations.
2. Laboratory techniques adapted to the life-span on the retardate, and to inter-institutional comparisons.
3. Psychometric tests and rating scales.

We believe that this three-pronged approach yields a substantial fund of data about the "output" of the institutional system or the "product" of the organization. As yet we have said little about the system itself, its workers (aides), managers (professional staff and administration), and some of the consumers—the parents.

While a substantial number of studies dealing with the expressed attitudes of institutional aides is available in the literature (Butterfield, 1967), only one has been concerned with direct observation of aide behavior (Thormahlen, 1965). We have substantial data on how aides express themselves on paper and pencil inventories, but only scant information on their actual behavior. The evidence we *do* have suggested little relationship between these two assessment methods.

To overcome the inherent rigidity of a pre-formulated inventory, we supplemented our evaluation with a Sentence Completion Test. Such a projective device requires the respondent to supply his own answers, and thus overcome the social desirability effect which tends to be more powerful in conventional inventories. Carefully devised scoring categories permitted us to achieve 87 per cent or better agreement between two raters. This instrument was used with parents and with aides. We also administered a revised version of the Parent Attitude Research Instrument to these groups in the hope of using the projective and the objective instruments jointly.

Results

Perhaps the most vital aim of institutional management is to develop greater self-sufficiency among its severely retarded residents. The published purpose of the so-called training programs in institutions stress the fostering of greater independence among their charges. The ability to care for one's own needs, to dress, feed, and toilet oneself, to communicate and make one's needs known are surely among the most important aspects of self-care.

To assess these vital aspects of self-care we constructed a special scale. This instrument was more detailed at the dependent end of the scale than the Vineland Social Maturity Scale and simpler than the Cain-Levine Social Competency Scale. It consisted simply of nine areas of self-sufficiency arranged in order of ascending independence (drinks from bottle; is spoon fed; feeds self with spoon, but is very messy; feeds self with spoon neatly; feeds self with fork; feeds self independently, but has meat cut; uses knife for cutting and spreading). We were not interested in what the child might do under ideal circumstances, but what he actually *does* under the daily living conditions of institutional life.

Because completing our self-care scale required mere observation, we obtained extremely high inter-rater reliability. Scores obtained by our own workers correlated .98; attendants' scores correlated .94. Average scores of two attendants and two of our observers correlated .92. In practice we relied upon the average of scores reported independently by this highly reliable instrument.

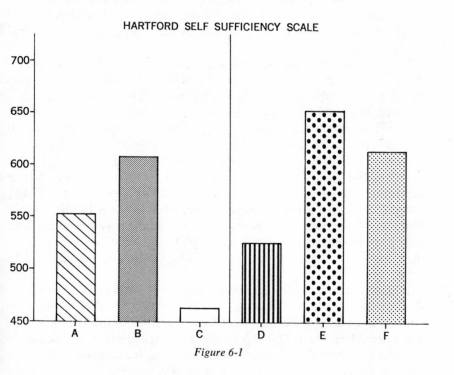

Figure 6-1

Because the children were matched according to measured intellectual ability, differences in self-sufficiency must, of necessity, reflect the effects of institutional programming. Figure 6–1 presents graphically the results of a comparison of self-sufficiency between the institutions.

It is clear that in both Series I and II one institution produces much less self-sufficient children than the other two. In Institution C and Institution D, the residents do less for themselves in areas such as feeding themselves, toileting and dressing themselves.

It may be argued, however, that these residents do less by themselves because they are being properly cared for. The over-riding question then remains whether children in various institutions experience similar degrees of happiness. We have attempted to assess the elusive quality of "happiness" or "adjustment" in behavioral terms. By sampling the behavior of mentally retarded individuals over substantial periods of time and throughout their waking day, it was possible to rerecord their responses reliably. Certain behavior patterns are likely to reflect good adjustment (e.g., smiling, playing with toys, talking and interacting with others), while others are clearly symptoms of poor adjustment (e.g., autistic behavior, aggression, withdrawl). By combining the frequencies with which these two classifications of behavior were observed, it was possible to construct an objective and reliable assessment of behavioral adjustment and apply them to our matched triads.

We employed an adjustment index calculated by summing arithmetically the incidence of clearly adjustive behavior and clearly maladaptive behavior. By assigning positive scores to the former, and negative scores to the latter, the predominance of adjustive over maladjustive behavior (or *vice versa*) can thus be readily ascertained. These data were obtained from almost 10,000 independent time samples, and are highly representative of behavioral observations the layman would term happiness.

Figure 6–2 clearly demonstrates that institutions differ in the state of adjustment ("happiness") they confer upon their charges. In Series I Institution C is predominantly an unhappy one, while in Series II Institution D bears this distinction. The same facilities showed the lowest degree of self-sufficiency among its charges. The ability of retarded children to care for their own needs is apparently correlated with the happiness manifested by them.

A third measure of institutional effectiveness is intellectual development. Because our sample was matched for IQ we could not demonstrate such differences on a cross-sectional basis for Series I, but Series II yielded data which could be evaluated retrospectively on a longitudinal basis. The matching data were based on tests administered by the institutional staffs to the samples six years or more in the past. It was possible to reexamine the

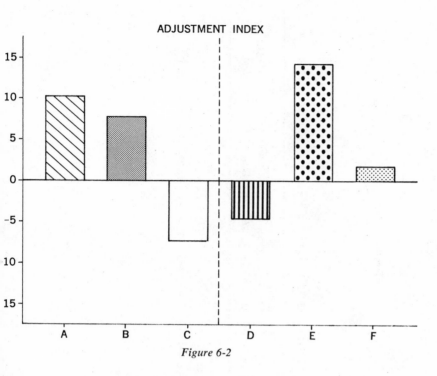

Figure 6-2

children for the purposes of our research. These examinations were undertaken by the institutional staff at C, F, and by totally naive psychologists at D and E. The results of this assessment are summarized in Table 6-2.

Table 6-2 shows that Institution D manifests the greatest relative decline in IQ because of a failure to show any mental growth in the children; Institution E, however, shows a substantial increase in Mental Age (by as much as one third from the original baseline), whereas Institution F shows a moderate increment in MA, and consequently a moderate decline in IQ.

Examining the data on happiness, self-sufficiency and intellectual growth to each other, we can discern a similar pattern for each of these three variables. Institutions in which retarded children are happy are also ones in which the children have grown more intellectually and achieved greater independence.

The Effective Institution

Assessing institutional effectiveness is made possible through the use of the methods described above. An institution in which children are happy, self-

Table 6–2. Changes in IQ and MA Over Six Years

| | Institution D | | | | Institution E | | | | Institution F | | | |
| | IQ | | MA | | IQ | | MA | | IQ | | MA | |
	Mean	SD	Mean	SD	Mean	SD	Mean	SD	Mean	SD	Mean	SD
1960 or before	21.1	8.8	1.77	1.04	22.8	8.6	1.75	1.04	23.5	8.6	2.02	1.24
1966	10.8	8.7	1.75	1.22	16.6	11.3	2.33	1.58	16.2	10.3	2.35	1.54
Per cent change	−49%		−1%		−27%		+33%		−31%		+16%	

sufficient, show intellectual growth, manifest minimal stereotype (such as rocking), and manifest no excessive need for social reinforcement can be described as being an *effective institution.* A facility in which most of these factors are present to a small degree is *ineffective* in terms of its therapeutic milieu.

In our sample of six state institutions, Institutions C and D are ineffective institutions. These two agencies stand out because of the consistent low rank they obtained on all measures. These completely independently gathered assessments are so consistent as to allay any doubts about the validity of this conclusion. Institution E emerges as clearly effective, while F appears to be moderately effective.

Establishing the effectiveness of an institution is an important step in and of itself. It may have vital bearing on the question of institutionalizing a mentally retarded child (Klaber, in press). Yet such a designation merely enables us to label a facility—it does not explain the variables and causes which make for effectiveness.

It is reasonable to assume that effectiveness is dependent on many variables: per capita cost, physical plant, as well as the behavior of the professional and ward personnel. We were unable to investigate all these factors fully. We have, instead, concentrated on the human element, especially the ward personnel.

Aides and Their Charges

Because it is likely that it is the behavior of those persons who come in contact with the children that will be most influential in modifying child behavior, we observed this behavior on the part of the attendants as they interacted with our matched triads of retardates.

For example, we recorded the percentage of the incidents in which we observed conversations between aide and child. We rerecorded the percentage of observed incidents when one of "our children" was ministered to physically. Table 6–3 shows some of the results obtained from three institutions. It clearly emerges from this table that our children received greater attention from aides in Institution E, than either Institution D or F. They had more conversations with aides, they received more physical care, and received responses to their demands more frequently. As we have already seen in Institution D, unhappy behavior predominates over happy behavior, intellectual growth is slower than other facilities, and the residents do not act as independently as in the other two agencies. A strong relationship between the actions of the attendants and the capabilities of the children is clearly suggested. Moreover, the evidence of the social deprivation experiment is also fully consistent with the same variables.

Table 6–3. *Incidence of Attendant-Child Interactions*
(Per cent of Total Interactions)

	Institution		
	D	E	F
Shows physical affection	.44	.80	.37
Converses with individual child	2.20	4.36	1.96
Takes care of physical need	2.85	4.24	2.50
Responds to child	1.93	2.72	1.39

The Retardate and his Interpersonal Environment

We do not mean to imply that the retardate in an institution receives all of his interpersonal stimulation from attendants. Quite to the contrary, by far most of his experiences are with other retardates and with older less handicapped persons called "working patients," "working boys," "trainees." A surprisingly large number of interactions comes from other, non-retarded persons on the ward. These individuals are volunteers, professionals (e.g., physical therapists), and individuals employed specifically to interact with children.

Table 6–4 delineates the sources of interpersonal contacts of the children in our sample. In five out of six institutions peer contacts (i.e., other ward residents of similar degree of retardation) constitute the most prevalent source of interpersonal relations. Significantly, however, in Institution E, our most effective facility, this is not the case: Attendants and other non-retarded adults interact as frequently with the residents of the residents interact with each other. Institution E is our most effective facility in which the children were observed to be happiest. The often heard statement to the effect that "retarded children are happiest among their own kind" has therefore no basis in fact.

Table 6–4. *Sources of Interpersonal Contacts (Per cent)*

Sources of Inter- personal Contact	Institution					
	Series I			Series II		
	A	B	C	D	E	F
Aides	22.0	11.3	23.7	25.9	30.8	23.4
Trainees	2.1	7.9	3.0	10.8	3.2	7.7
Peers	63.4	60.9	67.4	48.9	31.7	57.0
Nonretarded adults	12.5	19.8	5.9	14.4	34.3	11.9

Another finding which was surprising to us is shown in Table 6–5. In the institutions which we observed the contribution of non-attendant appeared to be much greater than we had anticipated. This observation led us to compute the expected rate of interpersonal interaction of this personnel and compare it with the observed rates. We may assume, for example, that if three attendants and one volunteer are present in a ward, the volunteer's contribution is 25 per cent of the total observed interpersonal interactions.

Table 6–5. Expected vs. Actual Interpersonal Contacts of Nonattendant Personnel

	Institution					
	A	B	C	D	E	F
Expected	.23	.51	.12	.36	.83	.37
Actual	.57	1.75	.25	.56	1.12	.51

A glance at Table 6–5 will dispel this notion rapidly: Most non-attendant personnel interact much more with the residents than expected on a purely statistical basis. This finding is potentially highly significant, demonstrating the need for specialized personnel, free of housekeeping and administrative duties, whose duties, whose job, is the human relationship between child and adult. Our data also suggest that reliance on "working patients" or "trainees" is inadequate and, on the whole, not satisfactory. Our data suggest, therefore, that programs using such older and more capable retardates are probably of limited utility.

An interesting side light of our findings was the fact that one of the most potent indicators of satisfaction we identified was the amount of non-nutritive sucking the retardates engaged in. The incidents of oral self-stimulation (thumb-sucking, licking of objects, strings, rags, dolls) manifested a perfect negative rank order correlation with self-sufficiency and adjustment. It appears that this very simple behavior pattern which is so easily observed can serve as an excellent indicator of institutional effectiveness.

The Typical Routine

Although there are certain similarities in the observed institutional routines, there are also some glaring differences. For example, all six institutions claim that schooling is available to all those who are eligible (i.e., educable and/or trainable), yet the percentage of matched children *actually* attending school varies greatly.

School Attendance

Series I

	A		B		C
No.	Per cent	No.	Per cent	No.	Per cent
13	76	12	71	3	18

Series II

	D		E		F
No.	Per cent	No.	Per cent	No.	Per cent
6	14	15	35	12	27

As in all our previous measures, C and D have significantly fewer children attending school programs than the other two facilities in their respective series. Because it is reasonable to assume that teachers interact more with individual children than aides, this fact contributes even further to the social deprivation of the residents. Moreover, it is concluded that a given child may have a two to three times better chance to attend formal school classes in one institution than in another.

On the ward the most typical "activity" was simple idleness (i.e., sitting down or doing absolutely nothing). In both series this factor appeared to be related to the amount of interactions available with aides and the other adults.

Inactivity (percent of observations)

	Series I			Series II	
A	B	C	D	E	F
33.16	27.94	49.74	44.40	26.70	36.20

It is clear that the residents of E are much more active than the matched residents of D and F, and those in C are less stimulated than their matches in A and B.

Between roughly one-third and one-half of the time of the severely retarded resident of a typical institution is spent in doing nothing (not even television watching). A substantial amount of time (between 15 and 20 per cent) is spent in autistic behavior, such as uncontrollable jumping, head banging. It is necessary to mention here that we have found no effect of the institutional environment on this behavior pattern. Evidently none of the institutions we studied have developed effective methods in treating such extreme withdrawl symptoms.

To understand the task of the aide better we observed attendants in Institutions C, D, and E while on the ward.

Here we did not observe matched residents, but attendants while they were in the immediate vicinity of the retarded children. We used a time-

Table 6–6. In-Room Activities of Aides
in Three Institutions
(Per cent of Observations)

	Institution		
	C	D	E
Child care (active)	28.40	25.40	30.64
Talks to child	22.53	23.07	28.59
Plays	5.10	1.90	7.57
Punishment	2.82	5.12	4.38
Ward routine	11.77	15.00	11.65
Supervision (passive)	24.71	17.08	15.60
Self-directed	11.66	23.75	13.69

sample method of two-minute intervals (two minutes of observation followed by a two-minute rest period, in blocks of 30 minutes each).

Table 6–6 shows the summed times of attendants engaged in given activities. Child care activities include feeding, bathing, and the like, while passive supervision indicates that the attendant is merely standing by to see that no harm comes to the children. "Ward routine" refers to physical activities directed to the maintenance of the ward, while "self-oriented" describes activities unrelated to the aides' work-assignment. Institution D's aides are more likely to idle, watch TV or engage in their own hobby than attendants at either C or E. However, workers at C must spend much more time in supervising residents than the personnel at E.

It is clear that aides in different institutions are maintaining significantly different work assignments. Each institution has created its own typical work distribution, but the reasons for this phenomenon are not evident. Curiously, Institution D which has emerged as the worst facility on all our measures has maintained the most active in-service training program over the years, while E (our most effective facility) has instituted such a service only recently. The superintendents of all institutions claim to encourage interactions with children and seemingly attempt to do all in their power to implement their ideas. So far we have found little evidence that effective modification of aide behavior results from the administrative measures instituted by the directors of the facilities, or that in-service training changes attendants' interactions with children.

Attitudes of Attendants

Attendant behavior is undoubtedly related to the attitudes which they hold with respect to the mentally retarded; unfortunately, we have been unable to find any studies which compare different institutions, nor are there any studies available which relate attendants' manifest verbalizations to observed behavior (Butterfield, 1967).

In evaluating training programs for attendants such an approach seems crucial, for administrators are less interested in producing socially approved verbal responses than in proper, or desirable child-rearing activities. We attempted to measure verbal attitudes through the use of two instruments: a modification of Schaefer and Bell's PARI (Schaefer & Bell, 1958) and a sentence completion test constructed by our own task.

The modification of the PARI was a very simple one: We inserted the word "retarded" before any mention of child in the test, and substituted "retarded infant" for the word baby. We thus arrived at a new scale we called R-PARI (*R* standing for Retarded). We had hoped to be able to demonstrate the different attitudes of workers in different institutions and perhaps even to correlate these with attendant behavior. Our results, however, were quite disappointing. The relative agreement and disagreement of attendants in Institutions D, E, and F was almost complete. Only one sub-scale of a total of 23 yielded a difference beyond the .01 level of probability. This sub-scale was entitled "Suppression of Sexuality." It contains such items as "Retarded children who take part in sex play become sex criminals when they grow up." Attendants at D agree much more frequently that suppression of sexual behavior is of importance in caring for retarded children. We wondered whether this attitude was related to the fact that complete segregation of the sexes was the rule at D until recently, whereas E and F were relatively more relaxed in this respect.

In spite of this one interesting difference we were much more impressed by the apparent general homogeneity of attitudes as expressed on the R-PARI. Although the attendants differ markedly in their behavior, they do not express verbally divergent opinions.

To maximize the possibility of self-expression on the part of the aides we constructed a Sentence Completion Task consisting of 20 sentence stems, all relating to mental retardation. The completed sentences were scored according to specific instructions for each sentence. We were able to achieve 87 per cent agreement among raters, the remaining 13 per cent were resolved by majority score (agreement of two out of three raters). Selected sentence stems relating to certain issues are discussed below.

DIFFERENCES BETWEEN INSTITUTIONS

Although institutions differ in so many respects from each other, the attitudes of attendants show remarkable consistency. The differences which we found were, curiously, unrelated to job performance. We had expected, for example, the morale of the "bad" institution in a sample to be worse than in the other two facilities; such was not the case. We attempted to measure this factor through responses to the sentence stem "as a rule state institutions for the retarded." By assigning positive or negative values to such responses it is possible to gauge the attitude of the respondents to state institutions. In this case about one half of all responses received a positive rating in Institutions D and E (48 and 57 per cent respectively) but only 8 per cent in Institution F felt kindly toward their place of employment and similar agencies. We were so surprised at this result (both the failure to differentiate between "good" Institution E and "bad" Institution D as well as the extremely low rating of Institution F) that we investigated relevant literature in industrial areas. We found that a review of studies affecting employee-management relationships concluded that "there is no simple relationship between job satisfaction and job performance" (Vroom, 1964). Our findings are evidently consistent with similar research in other areas.

The only other significant differences between institutions (at the .01 level or smaller) was in the general feeling of aides toward the retarded. The sentence stem "mentally retarded children are often" was completed in purely negative terms by 71 per cent of the attendants in Institution D, by 48 per cent of the aides in Institution F, and by a mere 33 per cent of the personnel at E. Clearly, the attendants at E perceive retardates less as possessing a multiplicity of bad qualities (such as being hyperactive, difficult to manage) than personnel in other institutions. We might even say that they like them better.

COMMONALITY OF AIDES' ATTITUDES

Most attitudes we measured show typical response patterns among aides regardless of the institution which employs them, and regardless of the in-service training they received. Below are some of the highlights of our findings.

PARENTS

Aides have virtually nothing positive to say about parents of retarded children. They manifest negative attitudes towards "fathers of retarded children," "mothers of retarded children," and, therefore, not surprisingly towards "parents of retarded children."

EDUCATION

Attendants are clearly in favor of "schooling for the retarded child" and 83 per cent are for encouraging this activity. However, when the concept of "schooling" is made more concrete and their attitude toward teachers is tapped, fully two-thirds (66 per cent) respond negatively by criticizing the professional educators. Apparently it is easier to be for "education" than to like the teachers personally.

INSTITUTIONAL PROBLEMS

To elicit a critique of institutional practices the sentence stem "The trouble with institutions for the retarded . . ." was used. Responses were scored in terms of administrative and physical difficulties; thus the response "are understaffed" would be an example of the former, while "having poor bathing facilities" would be an example of the latter. Attendants are overwhelmingly of the opinion that administrative practices are the root of the major problems (76 per cent) with only (24 per cent) indicating physical shortcomings as being particularly vexing.

THE MENTALLY RETARDED AND THE ENVIRONMENT

Mental retardation is viewed on several items in relation to society at large, rather than as an isolated phenomenon (78 per cent); the greatest danger to a retarded child is seen in psychological rather than physical injury (62 per cent); the greatest problem with a retarded child is seen in terms of external forces dealing with the child, rather than as an integral part of his being retarded (67 per cent). The aides thus clearly view mental retardation as a social problem.

Professional Personnel

Attendants and ward personnel are not the only people concerned with the welfare of the residents. The professional staff has certainly a major impact on the lives of the retardates residing in an institution. Observational methods are not suited for assessment of these persons, and we had to restrict ourselves to purely descriptive methods in dealing with this group. We surveyed the professional cadres of the institutions, somewhat informally, gathered some information about their qualifications, and interviewed the institutional directors.

PROFESSIONAL QUALIFICATIONS

It is extremely difficult to judge the efficiency and competence of professionals. We have come therefore to rely on the standards, rules, and degrees bestowed on such workers by their professional peers. We were impressed by the relative dearth of fully qualified persons in positions which permit their coming in contact with residents.

MEDICINE

All six of the institutions in the sample offered medical services to the retardates. Five had a medical staff in residence. Only one institution, however, employed physicians who held non-administrative, full-time positions with a specialty diploma from a recognized specialty board. This institution employed four such well-qualified physicians all of whom were pediatricians (it must be noted that less than 50 per cent of the institution's residents were 16 years old or younger). Two facilities employed diplomates in psychiatry and neurology as superintendents, but neither of these people had time for individual treatment.

All institutions claimed to use medical consultants, but it was impossible to determine how frequently they actually made use of them. Our impression was that they were used most sparingly. None of the facilities used a Board Diplomate in Psychiatry in a strictly clinical capacity, i.e., in working directly in the treatment of residents on a sustained basis.

CLINICAL PSYCHOLOGY

While all six facilities had full-time personnel in psychology, only two had a Ph.D. on its psychology staff. Two additional facilities employed psychologists with doctorates in other than clinical positions, one in research and one in administration. A number of Ph.D.'s were used in part-time positions in five institutions for a variety of services, including clinical supervision, in-service training, and research. None of the psychologists were diplomates in clinical psychology or in any other psychological specialty.

SOCIAL WORK

Only one of the six social service departments we visited was directed by a person holding a Master's Degree in the field of social work. Most other persons serving in the capacity of "social worker" were either completely untrained college graduates or had an incomplete social work education.

NURSING

Our survey of nursing personnel is very incomplete because institution administrators did not know the academic background of persons working as nurses on their staff. They were more concerned with meeting minimal state specifications than with hiring outstanding or unusual professional excellence. As far as we could establish there were no nurses holding a Master's Degree employed in any of the institutions, and we guess that a high percentage of the nursing positions designed to be staffed by Registered Nurses were in reality filled by Licensed Practical Nurses.

EDUCATION

Comparatively speaking, the professional training of educators was more adequate than in any other professional discipline. All institutions had individuals with Master's Degrees in charge of educational programs. Most of the teachers were licensed to teach in public schools in their respective states, though a relatively large number would not qualify for certification in the field of mental retardation in the community programs.

Some Reasons for the Personnel Shortage

Almost all administrators queried realized the shortages of their professional staffs, and attributed it to two specific factors: low salaries and national shortage of personnel. They were united in claiming that properly trained professionals were not attracted to their facilities for these reasons.

An informal survey, however, revealed that the reasons most often given for professional shortages are open to question. It was possible to ascertain that a number of well qualified persons had served in the six institutions but had left them. It appears that the problem lies not in attracting, but in retaining professional personnel.

During the past five years two persons with doctorates in education had left the institutions; five psychologists with doctorates, two social workers with MSW degrees, and one RN with an MA were identified as having "passed through" the employ of the six facilities. We were unable to ascertain any Board of Diplomates among physicians who left the agencies.

We were able to interview informally three of the psychologists, one social worker, the nurse, and one board-eligible physician who had left the six institutions. We also interviewed the superintendents. These interviews strongly suggested that the former employees viewed their reasons for leaving the institutions very differently from their employers. The tenor of complaints of the former employees was best described by one psychologist who said simply, "I wasn't appreciated," whereas, the typical response of the administrators was the answer "he simply didn't fit in." All professionals complained that their superior was not acquainted with their own specialty, but insisted that he was qualified to pass on the competence of their job performance. All felt harassed and required to conform to a general institutional pattern which was ill designed to meet the needs of professional personnel. They felt that their graduate education had prepared them for independent action, not for conformity.

Among the specific examples the workers gave as particularly upsetting were opening of official mail addressed to them, lack of cooperation and interest in research activities (this area has been documented by Baumeister, 1967 and Wolfensberger, 1965), lack of professional associates, and—most frequently of all—lack of respect for their professional skills. In a way, then, the superintendents who said that they "didn't fit in" was right. The question remains whether it is the institution or the professional worker who should accommodate the other.

The high degree of competence of the individuals who had left the institutions is attested to by the fact that two of the psychologists and both educators are currently on the faculties of universities and the other professionals hold positions at least comparable to the ones they had left. They were unanimous in stating they were not earning substantially more money, but that their work assignments were much more pleasurable.

Parents

The institutional system can easily be likened to any organization; its input is the newly admitted retarded children; its output is the development of these youngsters. The output varies from facility to facility. The process (behavior of personnel) is specific for each institution. One area is still unexplored—the consumers of the output.

In theory, all the citizens of the state are the consumers of state services. It is they or their elective representatives who decide upon the continuation, expansion, or contraction of the system. In fact, however, the average citizen knows little and cares less about the effectiveness of institutions for the retarded. The real consumers are the parents of the mentally retarded children.

Parents of children in institutions and those whose youngsters might be admitted to such facilities are the citizen-consumers of the institutional output. They are the only group of persons outside the system directly concerned with its operation.

It is surprising how little research has been done with groups of parents of institutionalized children. Two recent comprehensive research surveys in retardation fail to mention the word "parent" in their index. Most of the research has been conducted among those who have retained their children at home, not among those who have placed their offspring in an institution. We felt that our approach to the entire institutional system would be incomplete without the inclusion of the parents in our investigation.

We investigated both expressed attitudes and observable behavior among the aides and we intended to use a similar approach with parents. Verbal attitudes were tapped by using the same instruments we used with aides (the R-PARI and our Sentence Completion Task), while the parental behavior we selected for our study was the number of visits they paid to their institutionalized children in the course of a year. We complemented our study by administering the verbal instruments to parents who had retained their children at home.

PARENTAL ATTITUDES

Having established significant behavioral differences of parents in different institutions (Klaber, in press) we proceeded to search for possible variations of parents who have children in different facilities. To this end we administered the Sentence Completion Task to 14 parents with children at E and to 30 parents with children at D. These admittedly very small samples were obtained during parents meetings. The parents who were visiting their children thus do not constitute a random sample. We have attempted to collect such data also from the parents of our sample, but were able to obtain a response-rate of only 30 per cent. The fragmentary material, which was extremely expensive to collect, seemed to reflect the trends of the larger sample.

The most interesting finding of an analysis of the Sentence Completion Task was the lack of differences between the two groups. It seems that the verbal attitudes of parents with children in different institutions is homogeneous, while parental behavior is not.

The self-image of the parents was a poor one. Parents saw themselves overprotective or neglectful, feeling sorry for themselves, guilt-ridden, and ineffectual. It is evident from their responses that they are in need of psychological assistance which few of them had. Although several of the facilities studied claimed in the brochures and interviews that therapeutic counseling was available to parents, we were unable to substantiate a single case of a sustained relationship of a qualified professional in the employ of an institution (psychologist, psychiatrist, psychiatric social worker) and a parent. The presence of the severe damage to the parental self-image points up the need for such a service.

The parents of children in both effective and ineffective institutions perceived the attendants in unrealistically favorable terms. The sentence stem, "Attendants in institutions for the retarded are . . ." was frequently completed in quasi religious terms, e.g., "to receive a special reward in heaven," "angels of mercy." Frequently, they were described as "better than the real father and mother" or as "wonderfully trained and well qualified for the job." Fully 91 per cent of the parents had favorable comments about the aides. The distortion of reality testing in this area was highlighted by the total inability to distinguish between effective and ineffective institutional practices.

The same perceptual distortion with respect to the adequacy of institutional care was evident on answers to the sentence stems, "As a rule state institutions for the retarded . . ." "The trouble with institutions for the retarded . . ." The latter sentence was, of course, deliberately slanted to elicit negative attitudes; yet it failed to do so in the majority of cases. Parents would admit problems in states or institutions other than their own, e.g., "I find no trouble at D," or "In X State I know of no trouble; I hear the other states are terrible." The institutions were seen as "making their lives more pleasant," "as a rule not as good as E," "are ideal and most essential for the children." A small minority state there was some overcrowding and "lack of home atmosphere."

The sentence stem, "I often wonder why the mentally retarded . . ."

yielded the greatest number of unanswered records. About one half (49.6 per cent) of the parents left this item blank. Our puzzlement about this phenomenon was dispelled when we persued and analyzed those records which did have an answer; it became abundantly clear that the parents suppressed or perhaps repressed their wish that the retarded child did not exist. Typical sentence completions were "are allowed to live often long lives by a loving God, especially severely retarded living on and on to a life of nothingness," "were put on this world by God," "are born," "are the way they are."

These responses and lack of responses serve as an additional indicator of need for professional help for parents. Reliance or denial and repression in defending against the psychological trauma of retardation constitutes by definition a maladaptive response to environmental stress.

PARENTS WITH CHILDREN AT HOME

After we analyzed the responses of parents who had placed their children in residential state-supported facilities, the question of whether their responses were the result of retardation in the family *per se* or whether they are applicable to a special reference group arose. In the hope that such a comparison group would enable us to determine psychological facets associated with institutionalization we attempted to collect data from parents who had elected to retain their retarded child at home.

We obtained our sample from a local parent group and from a parochial school with a religious program for retarded children. The two groups of parents were comparable in education and income, but the home group was younger and their children were primarily moderately retarded; the institution group was older and their children were mostly severely and profoundly retarded. Such differences are in line with expectations; yet they impose certain limitations on the interpretation of the results.

There are some significant differences between the groups of parents who have elected to retain their retarded children at home and those who institutionalized their retarded offspring.

Mentally retarded children are seen in a more positive light by the home group, but mentally retarded adults are not. Almost half (40 per cent) of the home group gave positive responses to the sentence stem, "Mentally retarded children are often . . ." but only 15 per cent of the same group had a positive completion to the stem, "Retarded adults tend to . . ." The institution group remained consistent with 19 per cent and 16 per cent positive responses respectively.

INSTITUTIONS FOR THE RETARDED

There was a clear-cut difference in parental attitude toward institutions and attendants. The institution group was convinced of the excellence of the facilities in which their children are placed, while the home group was convinced of the opposite. The praise lavished on the institutions was so extravagant as to suggest severe distortions in reality in this area. For example, attendants were described as "angels," "much better than any parent could hope to be," "the most wonderful people I have ever met," etc. The item designed to elicit complaints about these facilities ("The trouble with institutions for the retarded . . .") was frequently answered in terms of complete denial, and even more frequently in terms of "no trouble in X State, but bad in others." The home group was much less favorably impressed by the attendants, frequently referring to their lack of training.

Perhaps the most interesting difference found between the two groups was in relation to the realism of expectation expressed by them. The sentence stem, "I often wish that retarded children . . ." was scored in terms of specific desires (e.g., "had more school programs available") and magical fantasies (e.g., "could all be cured"). On this item parents with children at home showed a high degree of realistic specificity, while almost half (46 per cent) of the institution group expressed totally magical and frequently extremely rejecting attitudes (e.g., "I often wish that retarded children didn't exist.").

The differences between parental groups suggest a significant breakdown in reality testing of parents who place their children in institutions. We do not know, of course, whether this difference occurred before or after the placement of the child. We suspect, however, that this impairment of judgment occurs *before* the decision to institutionalize a child is made and is symptomatic of it.

As "consumers" the parents lack the objectivity and critical facility to serve as the regulatory agent which is inherent in a free-market economy. Supervisory agencies within the state system are too involved in the power-politics of the larger state machinery. It appears, therefore, that an independently financed agency (perhaps at a university or a charitable foundation) will have to be given the authority and the necessary access to numbers of residential institutions. The most promising strategy involves inter-institutional comparison. No parent organization and no single state system has the necessary resources to undertake such studies. Regional and national authorities seem, therefore, to be a necessary part of a system of ongoing and permanent evaluation of institutional effectiveness.
tiveness.

The Researcher and the Administrator

It is incumbent upon the administrator to follow research evidence in his practices and not to rely on his own "common sense" or humane impulses solely. It is the researcher's duty to search for meaningful answers to administrative questions rather than to work on problems which only interest other researchers.

While it is assumed, albeit too optimistically, that administrators read the research literature, there exists little opportunity for the researcher to learn of the needs of the administrator. It is obvious, therefore, that research activities must be developed at the state administration level in a way to permit research personnel to be *in* the state facilities but not *of* them.

Below is a list of some questions asked by administrators, which have been partially answered through research. This list is sadly short, and probably not complete, yet it demonstrates the kind of problem frequently asked and answered to some extent with the aid of research methodology.

1. *Is a retarded child better off at home rather than in our institution?* On the whole, yes (Butterfield, 1967).

2. *Is this true with respect to all homes?* Probably not. Zigler (1961; 1966) suggested that pre-institutional experiences have an effect on intellectual and motivational development. The greater the retardates' deprivation at home the less damaging the institutional effect.

3. *Is this true with respect to all institutions?* No. Institutions differ from each other; some are less detrimental to growth than others (Klaber, 1969).

4. *Can special programs within an institution ameliorate the usually detrimental effects?* Yes. Many experiments and programs have shown this. Most impressive among them is Skeels' (1966) work in which he showed that short-term institutionalization under special care conditions in childhood may lead to fully productive adult living.

5. *Do such programs constitute a good measure of the effectiveness of our institution?* No. Many institutions have special programs for a very limited number of children, but the average resident receives little attention (Klaber, 1969; Thormahlen, 1965).

6. *Does the effectiveness of an institution depend on the interpersonal interactions of residents and staff?* Probably yes. Residents in institutions with a high amount of human interactions reduce need for dependency (Zigler, 1966) and are correlated with smaller intellectual deficits (Klaber, 1969).

7. *If that is the case, is the staff-to-resident ratio the sole determining factor in creating a favorable environment?* Surprisingly, no. More attendants mean greater role stratification (Thormahlen, 1965), but not necessarily a better atmosphere of treatment (King and Raynes, 1968), professionals and volunteers contribute more in interaction terms than attendants, and unit-size seems more important than the attendant-resident ratio (Klaber, 1969).

8. *Is the small institution clearly superior to the large one?* Evidence is still very inconclusive. King and Raynes (1968) have found that similar-sized facilities may have very different child care programs, depending on their

respective designations as wards or hostels. Klaber (1969) describes a small institution as being more effective than several large ones, yet it seems much too early to generalize about institutional size.

9. *Does in-service training of attendants make the crucial difference between effective and ineffective programming?* Unfortunately there is no evidence to support this contention. While it sometimes is possible to train attendants to answer questionnaires correctly (Butterfield, 1967), child care practices under actual observations seem unaffected by training programs (Thormahlen, 1965; Klaber, 1969).

10. *Would parents visit in institutions more often if they were residing in closer proximity to them?* Probably not. Klaber (in press) found that, at least within a radius of one hundred miles, parental visits are not determined by distance. Parents do visit children in institutions where the residents are better adjusted more frequently.

11. *Since institution size, attendant training, distance from home, or staff ratio seem not to be crucial in determining institutional effectiveness, is not then the administration, supervision, and management responsible for conditions?* Unfortunately we do not know. No research results concerning the role of the superintendant, the activties of the professional staff, supervisory methods, etc., are yet available. Clearly, much work is needed in this area.

The entire area of human systems, as related to mental retardation, is unexplored. The complex interactions of attendants, supervisors, administrators, and professionals have yet to be described. Most difficult of all is the question of intervention in a service system: the procedures involved in changing programs to maximize their efficiency. The difficulty in accomplishing this task is exemplified by the history of a technique which is currently termed *Behavior Modification*. This approach to changing behavior had its origin in the 1930's. With Skinner's (1938) publication of the characteristics of operant conditioning the foundations of all the principles of modifying the behavior of organisms had been established. This early work, however, concerned itself primarily with the behavior of animals. It took many decades before researchers used these relatively simple techniques with people. Today it is recognized that operant conditioning may be used to eliminate maladjustive patterns among the retarded (e.g., head banging) and to promote socially desirable actions (e.g., table manners). Yet, in spite of more than 30 years of experience, no institution had adopted a facility-wide program for all its residents using this approach. Sometimes psychologists are permitted the use of one ward to demonstrate this technique, sometimes a number of attendants are assigned to them, but nowhere has this technique changed the behavior of the entire system. Why then has the system failed to respond to a technique with demonstrated advantages? Evidently because the researchers saw as their client (or subject) the retarded child rather than the administrative structure, and the administrators viewed the researchers as remote from the everyday problems of programming. Until these two groups of professionals came to rapproachment which would permit cooperative attack on problems of common interest, the impact of research on institutional management will remain marginal. It is incumbent on both groups to find common ground for action. The failure of a technique with demonstrated results to penetrate the system must not be permitted to recur. The channels of two-way communication must be opened lest advances be stifled in self-defeating reverberating circuits.

References

Baumeister, A. A. A survey of the role of psychologists in public institutions for the mentally retarded. *Mental Retardation,* 1967, 5, 2–5.

Bowlby, J. *Maternal care and mental health.* Monograph Series No. 2, Geneva: World Health Organization, 1951.

Butterfield, E. C. The characteristics, selections, and training of institution personnel. In A. Baumeister (Ed.). *Mental retardation: Appraisal, education and rehabilitation.* Chicago: Aldine Publishing Co., 1967a.

—————. The role of environment factors in treatment. In A. Baumeister (Ed.). *Mental retardation: Appraisal, education, and rehabilitation.* Chicago: Aldine Publishing Company, 1967b.

Butterfield, E. C. and E. Zigler. The influence of differing institutional social climates on the effectiveness of social reinforcement in the mentally retarded. *American Journal of Mental Deficiency,* 1965, 78, 48–56.

Freud, A. and D. T. Burlingham. *Infants without families.* New York: International University Press, 1944.

Grissey, O. L. The mental development of children of the same IQ in differing institutional environments. *Child Development,* 1937, 8, 217–220.

Kephart, N. C. and A. A. Strauss. A clinical factor influencing variations in IQ. *American Journal of Orthopsychiatry,* 1940, 10, 343–350.

King, R. D. and N. V. Raynes. Patterns of institutional care for the severely subnormal. *American Journal of Mental Deficiency,* 1968, 72, 700–709.

Klaber, M. M. Parental visits to institutionalized children. *Mental Retardation,* 1968, 6, No. 6, 39–41.

—————. The retarded and institutions for the retarded—a preliminary research report. In S. B. Sarason and J. Doris (Eds.). *Psychological problems in mental deficiency.* New York: Harper and Row, 1969.

—————. Should a retarded child be institutionalized?—a question of ethics for the consultant psychologist. *Community Mental Health Journal,* in press.

Klaber, M. M. and E. C. Butterfield. Stereotyped rocking—a measure of ward effectiveness. *American Journal of Mental Deficiency,* 1968, 73, 13–20.

Klaber, M. M., E. C. Butterfield and L. J. Gould. Responsiveness to social reinforcement among institutionalized retarded children. *American Journal of Mental Deficiency,* 1969, 73, 890–895.

Klackenburg, G. Studies of maternal deprivation in infant homes. *Acta Paediatricia,* Stockholm, 1956, 45, 1–12.

Lyle, J. G. The effect of an institutional environment upon the verbal development of imbecile children: I Verbal intelligence. *Journal of Mental Deficiency Research,* 1960, 4, 1–13.

Rabin, A. I. Some psychosexual differences between kibbutz and non-kibbutz Israeli boys. *Journal of Projective Techniques,* 1958, 22, 328–332.

Rheingold, H. L. The measurement of maternal care. *Child Development,* 1960, 31, 565–573.

Skeels, H. M. Adult status of children with contrasting early life experiences. Monographs of the *Society for Research in Child Development,* 1966, 31, No. 3.

Skeels, H. M. and H. B. Dye. A study of the effects of differential stimulations on mentally retarded children. *Proceedings and Addresses of the American Association on Mental Deficiency,* 1939, 44, 114–136.

Skinner, B. F. *The behavior of organism: An experimental analysis.* New York: Appleton Century Crofts, 1938.

Thormahlen, P. W. A study of on-the-ward training of trainable mentally retarded children in a state institution. *California Mental Health Research Monograph,* 1965, No. 4.

Vroom, V. H. *Work and motivation.* New York: Wiley, 1964.

Wolfensberger, W. Administrative obstacles to behavioral research as perceived by administrators and research psychologists. *Mental Retardation,* 1965, 3, 7–12.

Yarrow, L. J. Maternal deprivation: Toward an empirical and conceptual reevaluation. *Psychological Bulletin,* 1961, 58, 459–490.

Zigler, E. Research on personality structure in the retardate. In Ellis, N. R. (Ed.), *International Review of Research in Mental Retardation,* New York, Academic Press, 1966.

————. Social deprivation and rigidity in the performance of feeble minded children. *Journal of Abnormal and Social Psychology,* 1961, 62, 413–421.

Behavior Modification of Residents and Personnel in Institutions for the Mentally Retarded

Operant conditioning techniques are being used more and more widely to teach severely and profoundly retarded institutionalized persons. These techniques can be used successfully with individuals who have limited behavioral repertoires and who lack language skills, and they seem highly appropriate for those retarded persons who usually have little or no language, often are not toilet trained, frequently cannot use utinsels to feed themselves, and so on.

Ellis (1963) was the first to suggest that procedures based on operant principles be used to train severely and profoundly retarded institutional residents. Dayan (1964) followed this suggestion and developed a toilet training program which was carried out by attendants under the supervision of psychologists. Incontinent retardates were placed on the toilet every two hours and were rewarded for eliminating in it. By the end of the six-month training period the incidence of soiling and wetting was markedly less than at the beginning of the program.

Similar projects have been conducted at other institutions. A self-help and social skill training project was executed at Pinecrest State School (Bensberg, Colwell, and Cassel, 1965). A group of profoundly retarded boys were toilet trained, taught to feed themselves, to dress themselves, and to carry out simple tasks. Operant conditioning procedures have also been used at Parsons State Hospital and Training Center to teach self-help and social skills to severely and moderately retarded girls (Girardeau and Spradlin, 1964; Gorton and Hollis, 1965). Other institutions have also adopted procedures to teach self-help and social skills to the severely and profoundly retarded.

The Operant Conditioning Method

The basic principle of the operant conditioning method is that voluntary behavior is influenced by its consequences. The most effective way to generate or modify behavior and maintain it is to make it contingent upon reinforcement. There are two classifications of reinforcement. One increases the probability of behavior recurring through its presentation, or accelerates behavior. This is called *positive reinforcement,* for example, food, or candy, or praise. The second classification of reinforcement indirectly decelerates behavior that produces an aversive consequence and directly accelerates behavior that either prevents, or avoids, or terminates the aversive consequence. This is called *negative reinforcement*—and includes electric shock, physical violence, withholding privileges, incarceration, or other forms of punishment.

Not only the presentation of reinforcement strengthens behavior, but the temporal characteristics or *schedule* with which it is presented also produces a profound effect upon responses. If a reinforcement is given only following a specific number of responses the behavioral pattern will differ markedly from that which occurs when reinforcement is presented only after a response occurs following a specified interval of time. In the first case, reinforcement is contingent upon a specified number of responses occurring. As a result of the contingency, responses occur frequently or at a high rate. In the second case reinforcement is contingent upon a response occurring following the passage of a specified time interval, and only the response which occurs after the interval has passed will produced reinforcement. As a result few responses will occur until just before the minimal interval is completed.

Continuous reinforcement is given after each response occurs. *Intermittent* reinforcement is given less than every time a response occurs. Reinforcement which is presented after a specified number of responses occur or for a response that occurs after a predetermined interval are examples of intermittent reinforcement. A continuous reinforcement schedule is typically used to develop new patterns of behavior, while intermittent reinforcement schedules are used to maintain behavior after it develops. Intermittent reinforcement schedules are more economical and produce forms and temporal patterns of behavior which cannot be generated with continuous reinforcement. They also produce greater resistance to extinction than continuous reinforcement.

The second principle, which makes it possible to teach complex behavior to severely and profoundly retarded persons, is *shaping.* Shaping is the basic behavior modification procedure used in operant conditioning, and it is this procedure which enables the trainer to teach these retardates complex behavior they probably would not learn otherwise. The term *shaping,* as it is used here, incorporates two other operant conditioning principles: *chaining* and *successive approximation.* Chaining refers to the process of teaching an entire behavioral unit by singly conditioning each behavioral component and then conditioning the components to one another. For example, the complex behavior, toiletting, can be broken down into ten behavioral components: 1. the person responds to bowel and bladder cues; i.e., he becomes aware that he is about to elminiate; 2. he inhibits the elimination; 3. he walks to the toilet; 4. he pulls down his pants and underclothing; 5. he sits on the toilet seat; 6. he eliminates; 7. he cleans himself; 8. he gets off the toilet; 9. he pulls up his pants and underclothing; and 10. he walks away from the toilet. These ten behavioral components can conveniently be thought of as the "links" that comprise the complex chain of behaviors called *toiletting.*

Individual behavioral components are conditioned by successive approximation, which consists of reinforcing closer and closer approximations to the desired behavior. For example, many retardates are "restless" and will sit on a toilet seat for only a few seconds before getting up. It is desirable that they sit for three or four minutes to increase the probability that they will eliminate in the toilet. Sitting time might be increased by first requiring the retardate to sit for five seconds before reinforcing him. If he would sit for five seconds with no difficulty, the sitting period could be increased to six seconds; after he would sit reliably for six seconds it could be extended to seven seconds, eight seconds, then ten seconds, then twelve seconds, then fifteen seconds, and so on. By gradually increasing the required interval that is reinforcement contingent, sitting time could be increased to three minutes.

As Reese (1966) has pointed out, reinforcement of successive approximations has two effects: it strengthens the response being reinforced, and it increases the likelihood that a closer approximation to the final behavior will occur. As new approximations are reached and reinforced, earlier ones extinguish. If the trainer moves too slowly the chance of other responses occurring will be decreased; if he progresses too rapidly, demanding an approximation that is, as yet, not likely to occur, the behavior that has been conditioned may extinguish, and the trainer will have to backtrack to an earlier approximation and repeat the procedure. Skillful use of the successive approximation procedure consists of selecting the right responses to reinforce and knowing how long to reinforce each approximation before moving to the next one.

Not only is it important to teach new behavior, it is also important for the behavior to occur under the appropriate circumstances. The new behavior (as well as old behavior) should occur at the right time and in the right place. That is, the behavior must be brought under *stimulus control*. Stimulus control refers to conditioning behavior to occur when a specific signal or cue is given. This is done by presenting the cue to an individual and reinforcing the appropriate behavior when it occurs in the presence of the cue and not reinforcing it, or even punishing it, when it occurs in the absence of the cue (or preventing the behavior from occurring in the absence of the cue). When the behavior will reliably occur in the presence of the cue it is said to be under the control of that cue, hence the term *stimulus control*. For example, if an institutionalized retarded child will walk to the toilet whenever the attendant says "go to the toilet," then the act of walking to the toilet is under the control of the attendant's vocal cue, "go to the toilet." Complete toilet training of such a child involves bringing defecation and urination under the control of the toilet itself, as well as bowel and bladder cues. The toilet becomes the central cue for defecation and urination. This is done by reinforcing him for eliminating in the toilet and not reinforcing or even punishing him for eliminating elsewhere.

In summary these three principles, reinforcement, shaping, and stimulus control, constitute the basis for applying the operant conditioning method. Through skillful application of the principles of shaping and reinforcment, severely and profoundly retarded persons can acquire new behaviors. Once the behavior has been acquired the principles of stimulus control and reinforcement make it possible to ensure that the behavior will occur appropriately.

Shaping and Maintaining Behavior: Mentally Retarded Residents

The procedure based on the principle of shaping incorporates the programming aspect of behavioral development or modification.

The first step in teaching self-help and social skills is to identify clearly the specific skills of interest and to isolate terminal behavior that identifies each skill. If, for example, one wants to toilet train a child, he should identify the terminal behavior that defines toilet training. This is usually defined as the child's being able to respond independently to his own bladder cues, walk to the toilet, and eliminate without assistance from an attendant or trainer.

The second step is to identify the component behaviors that comprise the terminal behavior. The complex behavior, toiletting, for example, can be broken down into ten steps, or behavioral components. This process is one of the most important steps in training. Success or failure of the training program is dependent upon a correct identification of all the crucial component behaviors. If some essential components are omitted, the complex behavior may not develop properly. If the complex behavior can be reduced to a series of simple component behaviors, particularly those essential to the complex behavior, the probability is greater that all retardates will learn the complex behavior.

The more deficient a retardate's relevant behavioral repertory, the more component behaviors will have to be shaped when teaching him any given skill. His level of sophistication should be determined first, i.e., whether he will pay attention, follow simple instructions, and so forth. If not, these basic behaviors should be shaped first.

The retardate's behavior must be brought under some degree of verbal control. He should be trained to follow certain basic instructions, such as "Come here! Sit down! Go to the toilet!" and "No!" This step facilitates controlling him during training. An important verbal cue, which can serve as a reinforcer, is "Good boy!"

The basic procedure of chaining is followed in shaping behavior. After the important behavioral components have been identified, the response directly preceding the presentation of reinforcement is usually shaped first. In the toilet training example the terminal response is defecation or urination in the toilet. If this behavioral component is dependent upon another (e.g., sitting on the toilet) then, of course, the second should be shaped first. The behavioral components are usually shaped, one at the time, in a backwards fashion. This "backwards" approach may be based more on tradition than necessity, but it is the conventional way to shape behavior. If the child will reliably sit on and eliminate in the toilet he may next be trained to pull down his pants, sit, and eliminate. Then he would probably be taught to locomote to the toilet, pull down his pants, sit, and eliminate.

Presentation of reinforcement is usually given following the terminal response (e.g., defecation). However, when behavioral components are being shaped initially, reinforcement may be given even when a small step or component is completed. For example, in training a child to put on boxer-type shorts the trainer first analyzes the complex act into small steps which the child can easily master. He begins by shaping the last step first, the one which completes the act and results in reinforcement from the trainer, i.e., pulling the shorts up to the waist. If the child has not acquired the three basic behavioral components upon which the training program depended—grasping his shorts by the waistband, understanding the verbal command, "Pull up your shorts!" and the relationship between following instructions and obtaining reinforcement, each would have to be conditioned first and reinforced independently before progressing to pulling up the shorts.

Assuming the child would follow simple instructions, he might first be trained to grasp his shorts by the waistband. Grasping the waistband would be reinforced. Then the trainer might pull the shorts down two inches below the normal position and say, "Pull up your shorts!" while at the same time placing the child's hands on the waistband and pulling his arms upward and then reinforcing him for this response. The act of the trainer's assisting the child in going through the motion is called a *prompt*. He is being provided additional information or cues. Such a pantomime procedure is probably superior to verbal cues alone when working with severely and profoundly retarded children. When the child can reliably pull up his pants with help the trainer begins to withdraw his assistance gradually until the child is pulling up his pants independently. The process of gradually removing cues is called *fading*. Next the trainer may pull the pants down four inches from the normal position and say, "Pull up your pants!" and reinforce him for pulling them up. After he reliably demonstrates he can complete this phase of training the trainer progressively pulls the pants down a little further, repeating the procedure, until the child can pick them up on command, put a foot through each leghole, and pull them up.

The process by which a retardate is taught to pull his pants up by first pulling them two inches down from the normal terminal position, getting him to pull them up, reinforcing him, then pulling them down four inches, and again getting him to pull them up, reinforcing him, etc.; until finally, he can pull them up all the way after he gets a foot in each leghole, is an example of *successive approximation*.

The child should clearly demonstrate he has mastered each step or link in the chain before he progresses to the next step. How long he will be kept at any step will depend on his individual rate of learning and the adequacy of the programming. If he is moved to the next step too soon his behavior may begin to deteriorate. If this should happen, it is necessary to back up to an earlier step he previously completed successfully, and if his performance at this point is satisfactory the shaping procedure can be resumed until all the steps or components in the chain have been completed. Considerable "backing up" may be required when training the severely and profoundly retarded.

REINFORCEMENT

Conditioning new behavior and bringing all behavior under stimulus control is accomplished through a reinforcement process. As additional components are added to a behavior chain the effectiveness of the reinforcement may become a crucial factor in the operant conditioning method. As more and more responses are required for a given reinforcement, the stability of the performance will be increasingly dependent upon the effectiveness of the reinforcement (Ferster and Skinner, 1957; and Lawson and Watson, 1963). The selection of a suitable reinforcement for a particular child is an important factor.

Specific consequences that have reinforcement properties vary from individual to individual. While one child may like candy; another will not eat it. The second child may like to play games with an attendant, while a third child may prefer playing with a toy either to eating candy or playing games with an attendant. The extent to which the reinforcement is effective for training will depend upon the value of the reinforcement for the individual. Reinforcements need to be selected specifically for each person, and some rule of thumb is needed to provide a basis for selecting them.

The *Premack hypothesis* provides a useful basis for selecting reinforcement (Premack, 1959). Reinforcement is defined in terms of the probability of occurrence of behavior. Reinforcements are high probability behaviors, i.e., behaviors which persons like to engage in, such as eating candy, playing games, playing with toys, eating meals, going to the playground, or listening to music. Premack proposes that the behavior to be shaped is usually a relatively low probability behavior, i.e., it normally does not occur often. To increase its rate of occurrence, he suggests that the occurrence of high probability behavior should be made contingent upon the occurrence of low probability behavior. For example, giving a retardate candy to eat could be made contingent upon eliminating in the toilet. If eating candy is a low probability behavior but playing tag with the attendant is a high probability behavior, then playing tag with the attendant could be made contingent upon eliminating in the toilet. Under these conditions the rate of eliminating in the toilet should increase. The rule of thumb suggested by the Premack hypothesis is to use high probability behaviors as positive reinforcers.

The effectiveness of a reinforcement also is influenced by *deprivation* states. If a retardate who like candy gets a lot of it independent of training, he will probably not crave it to the extent that he would if he were not receiving candy regularly. The more candy he eats the more he will be *satiated* by candy and the less he will crave it. So one way to increase the effectiveness of a reinforcement is to deprive the child of it under ordinary circumstances and use it only during training. Because satiation decreases the effectiveness of a reinforcement, edible type reinforcements should be given in small amounts. Candy should be given in small pieces, food of other kinds in small bits, and liquid reinforcement in small quantities. If a game is being used as a reinforcement, then each reinforcing event should be relatively brief because satiation may also occur with activities such as games (Cofer and Appley, 1964; Kish, 1966). However, the effectiveness of reinforcement is also determined by their *size* or quantity, so care should be taken to determine that the amount given each time is great enough to maintain the behavior although not so large that the retardate will become satiated after he obtains only a few reinforcements. The time interval between the occurrence of the behavior and dispensing the reinforcement also influences its effectiveness. The optimum way to administer reinforcement is to give it within a half second or less after the behavior occurs. When the interval between response and reinforcement increases, two things happen: the influence of the reinforcement on desired behavior decreases; the reinforcement accelerates the behavior occurring at the moment it is given—perhaps some behavior unrelated to that desired by the trainer. So, when the presentation of reinforcement is delayed, not only will the desired behavior be minimally affected, but other, perhaps undesired behavior, will be inadvertently conditioned.

The necessity of providing immediate reinforcement produces something of a dilemma. The act of presenting a child with reinforcement such as candy usually requires one or two seconds, even with an electromechanical reinforcement dispenser. Therefore, some cue is needed which can be given immediately to signal the reinforcement is forthcoming. This cue will become a conditioned reinforcement as a result of being associated with other reinforcements. A very convenient cue is saying "Good boy!" when the retardate makes a correct response and then presenting the unconditioned reinforcement as quickly as possible. The vocal conditioned reinforcement, "Good boy!" can be a relatively effective reinforcement in and of itself.

The training process consists of accelerating appropriate or desirable behavior with positive reinforcement and decelerating inappropriate or undesirable behavior with negative reinforcement.

Accelerating Behavior

Most positive reinforcements used with retardates can be conveniently classified as *edible, manipulatable,* and *social.* Edible reinforcements include food substances such as candy, cookies, and fruit juice; manipulatable reinforcements include toys, crayons, paints, playing games alone, watching television, or listening to music; social reinforcements are those that occur when the retardate interacts with people such as playing games with an attendant or peer, being hugged, patted, or praised. Some reinforcements are a combination of manipulatable and social such as an attendant playing a game of ball with a child.

Numerous kinds of edible substances have been employed as positive reinforcements and appear to be the most effective class of reinforcement (Watson, Orser, and Sanders, 1968; Watson and Sanders, 1968; and Ferster, 1961). Sweet food stuffs such as cookies, candy, ice cream, jello, grapes and coca cola are favorites among trainers as well as other substances like metracal, baby food, pop corn, and regular meals (Bensberg, Colwell, and Cassel, 1965; Giles and Wolf, 1966; Baumeister and Klosowski, 1965; Gorton and Hollis, 1965; Hollis, 1966). Some training programs have used deprivation conditions to make the reinforcement more effective (Fuller, 1949; Spradlin, Girardeau, and Corte, 1965; Whitney and Barnard, 1966). Watson and Sanders (1968) have compared reinforcement preferences of severely and profoundly retarded children over a period of months for candy, snacks, and manipulatable reinforcements. Candy was preferred to snacks by most children. Both candy and snacks were preferred to manipulatable reinforcements, such as watching live animals, watching electromechanical toys operate, viewing movies and listening to music.

Reinforcement preferences vary among retardates. Some show little preference for candy or sweets (Baumeister and Klosowski, 1965; Giles and Wolf, 1966; Watson, Orser, and Sanders, 1968; Watson and Sanders, 1968). Manipulatable and social reinforcements may be satisfactory for such children. Toys have been found to be effective manipulatable reinforcements. Children may perform tasks to watch electrical-mechanical toys operate (Baumeister and Klosowski, 1965; Watson, Orser, and Sanders, 1968; Watson and Sanders, 1968) or play with a ball or doll for a brief period (Giles and Wolf, 1966). One child was given an old shirt to tear (Baumeister and Klosowski, 1965). When manipulatable reinforcement is used the child is typically allowed to play with the toy for only a brief period to reduce possible satiation effects.

Social reinforcements consist of words of praise, hugs, playing games with the child, and attention in general (Bensberg *et al,* 1965; Giles and Wolf, 1966). Giles and Wolf gave retardates a ride in a wheelchair. "Good boy!" is a social reinforcement. Some children would probably prefer social reinforcement to any other class of positive reinforcement.

Reinforcement may also be classified in terms of reinforcement history —unconditioned and conditioned reinforcement. Unconditioned reinforcers are those which are not dependent upon a history of conditioning for their reinforcement properties. Conditioned reinforcements were originally relatively neutral and acquired reinforcement properties as a result of being associated with unconditioned and other conditioned reinforcements. Unconditioned reinforcements are generally more effective than conditioned reinforcements. One possible exception to this statement is the generalized conditioned reinforcement. However, conditioned reinforcement offers certain advantages over unconditioned reinforcement. It has a less disruptive effect upon ongoing behavior because it requires no consummatory response. By using conditioned reinforcement in conjunction with unconditioned reinforcement, a higher rate of behavior can be maintained and greater control can be exercised over its form and temporal pattern than by the use of conditioned reinforcement alone.

A generalized conditioned reinforcer is a stimulus that has been associated with a number of unconditioned or conditioned reinforcements and has acquired some of the reinforcement properties of each (Skinner, 1953). It has two major advantages over unconditioned reinforcement: generalized reinforcement is relatively independent of specific deprivation states, and it may take on greater incentive value than unconditioned reinforcement because the effects resulting from association with each primary reinforcement may summate (Ferster and DeMeyer, 1962). It should then ultimately be the most powerful type of reinforcement. Money and attention from other humans are the most common examples of generalized reinforcement. Social reinforcements are either single or generalized conditioned reinforcement.

Token or generalized reinforcements make it possible for the retardate to select edible, manipulatable, or social reinforcement (assuming all are available), allowing him to satisfy the particular deprivation state that is greatest at any given moment. Girardeau and Spradlin (1964) and Lent (1967) used a token reinforcement system with severely retarded adolescent girls. They performed specified tasks for tokens which could be exchanged for candy, gum, hair clips, perfume, lipstick, crayons, and paper. Watson, *et al* (1968) reinforced retarded children with poker chips. The poker chips could be used to operate four types of dispensing machines: one which contained candy, one which contained snacks, one which held live animals in different compartments, and one which showed movies or electrical-mechanical toys or played music. Birnbrauer (1967) and Sidman (1967) have also used a token reinforcement system with retardates.

Probably the potentially most effective use of a generalized reinforcement procedure is to use it to increase the conditioned reinforcement properties of attendants and others to make them more effective reinforcers. Attention from a "significant" person, i.e., one with whom the retardate has considerable contact and upon whom he is dependent for everyday nursing care, appears to be an effective reinforcement for most retardates. Bensberg *et al.,* and Colwell have all reported that attention or approval from such attendants appears to be sufficient for maintaining behavior once it is conditioned. By pairing the attendant with other reinforcing consequences she should become conditioned to be a more effective reinforcer, and approval and attention from her as well as physical contact—hugs, pats, and caresses—should be more reinforcing than otherwise. It might be possible to increase her reinforcement properties even more by having her use vocal reinforcement with considerable reinforcement properties in and of itself and pair it with other reinforcement. For example, one could take an automated token reinforcement system, such as the one used by

Watson, *et al.*, where there were a large number and variety of reinforcements. If a tape recorded voice said "Good boy!" each time the retardate spent a chip, then the conditioned reinforcement properties of the vocal reinforcement, "Good boy!" should increase. The same conditioning process could be carried out manually as well. An attendant or trainer could say "Good boy!" each time the child received reinforcements of different kinds as well as simultaneously reinforcing him in other ways.

A third source of reinforcement, in addition to the attendant and some tangible reinforcement such as candy, is the task itself. Some tasks should have greater reinforcement properties than others. Retardates would probably prefer playing musical games to simply pulling a lever if both tasks produced the same kind of extrinsic reinforcement. A task can be positively reinforcing, relatively neutral, or negatively reinforcing. A good example of a positively reinforcing task is the "fun and games" type of activity that is ingeniously applied by music therapists. In a demonstration of music therapy, Nicosia (1968) used a combination of imitation and music to shape the behavior of a small group of retardates. She served as the model and had these children imitate her to musical accompaniment. The "games" component of the activity appeared to have rather powerful reinforcement properties. In addition, music and songs also appeared to have important stimulus control properties by acting as mediators of behavior. Smaltz's (1968) behavior maintenance technique, which is based on teaching retardates to sing a song whose lyrics describe the activities that comprise a task, should have such stimulus properties. As they sing the song they carry out the activities described in the song. Singing the song appears to serve two functions: it reinforces their behavior, and the words of the song act as prompts to control the specific components of the behavioral chain.

A task, such as pulling a lever on a variable interval schedule, may be either relatively neutral or even have aversive properties, particularly as a function of time. Retardates at Columbus State School have shown decreased response rates over extended periods of time, and some even stop pulling a manipulandum after several weeks, although they are reinforced with tokens. If, after they stop pulling the lever, they are given tokens *gratis* they still go and spend them. Presumably this type of task can become aversive over time. Initially, lever pulling is probably a rather novel task. Novelty itself can be a source of reinforcement. Novelty may decrease as a function in time until the task becomes relatively neutral, and it may become monotonous or aversive.

Both unconditioned and conditioned reinforcements are given by the attendant or trainer to the retardate for emitting some specific behavior. Ferster (1966) calls these "arbitrary" reinforcers. Such reinforcers are controlled by the attendant and are dependent upon the attendant for their occurrence. The behavior being reinforced by the attendant is also under her control; she is one of the stimuli controlling the behavior. The occurrence of the behavior is highly dependent upon the presence of the attendant who provides both some of the stimulus control for the desired behavior and reinforcement. Behavior may be so dependent upon the presence of the attendant it may not occur in her absence. This factor places a rather drastic restriction on the stability and durability of the behavior. There appear to be at least two solutions to this problem. One is the use of automation (Watson, 1968) and the other is the use of "natural" reinforcers (Ferster, 1966). Watson has argued that automation can be used to supplement the attendant and to make the retardate's behavior partially independent of the attendant. Two examples should clarify this point.

One common problem at Columbus State School with retardates is regurgitating food and then reingesting it. Although such behavior may have no adverse effect on the health of the retardate it disturbs and disrupts the normal daily activities of attendants, ward matrons, and other institutional staff members. Initial attempts to eliminate this behavior were carried out directly by an attendant who punished regurgitation. The retardates soon discriminated between regurgitating when the attendant was within 10 or 15 feet and regurgitating when she was 20 or more feet away or out of sight. Her presence had apparently become a discriminative stimulus for *not* regurgitating and her absence or minimal distance was a discriminative stimulus for regurgitating, if other necessary conditions were satisfied. The problem was to punish regurgitation independently of the attendant so the effects would extend beyond her physical presence. An attempted solution was to use a portable electric shocking device sewn in a vest worn by the child. A radio receiver, connected to the shocking device, supplied shock whenever a transmitter was operated. Thus the source of punishment was made independent of the attendant as far as her descriminative stimulus properties were concerned. Unfortunately, someone had to be available to operate the transmitter, and the shock level was insufficient to suppress the behavior.

Another more complete approximation to the use of automation to replace the attendant as a source of reinforcement and stimulus control is the automated toilet training procedure described by Watson (1967, 1968). The two most important behaviors to shape in toilet training are: elimination in the toilet, and independently responding to bowel and bladder cues that signal elimination is eminent. The first problem was solved be developing a photoelectric cell switch which was activated whenever the retardate eliminated in the toilet. This switch then operated a reinforcement dispenser which produced candy. The operation of the reinforcement device was completely independent of the attendant. With respect to the second problem, an automated signalling device is being developed to cue retardates to walk to the toilet when elimination begins to occur. The retardate wears training pants equipped with a moisture sensitive switch which is connected to a small tape recorder located in a vest worn by him. Whenever he begins to urinate or defecate the resulting moisture activates the switch which activates the tape recorder which says, "No, Johnny!" (or whatever his name is) "Go to the toilet!" Assuming "No!" has been made a conditioned aversive stimulus and locomoting to the toilet is under control of the verbal cue "Go to the toilet!" the retardate should go to the toilet. The purpose of the device is to condition physiological bowel and bladder cues as discriminative stimuli which control locomoting to the toilet. After conditioning is completed the device will be faded and eliminated. "No!" presumabily serves as punishment for premature elimination. If not, it can be conditioned.

Automation can be viewed as either an intermediate step or a final step in behavior control of retardates. In the two examples above it was intended to be an intermediate step. From a "prosthetic" environment point of view it could be considered a permanent source of reinforcement and control (Lindsley, 1964). If it is considered to be an intermediate step, then other forms of reinforcement must be substituted.

Baer and Wolf (1967) have suggested the use of "natural" reinforcers. Such reinforcers are already in the retardate's environment. An example is a hot object such as a stove or soldering iron. Once the child touches such an object and is burned, *not* touching it becomes a positive reinforcement. Another example is operating a water fountain. Turning the valve controlling water is reinforced by the presence of water. These kinds of reinforcement occur relatively independently of other humans, and therefore the behavior will be maintained even in the absence of others. By shaping the retardate's behavior so that it will be maintained by natural reinforcers, the behavior has become independent of the attendant herself and the behavior should be both more stable and more duarble. If the ultimate goal in training retardates is to develop durable behavior, then natural reinforcers are a necessity and should constitute the final step in any training program. In essence, employing natural reinforcers is simply a matter of identifying high probability behaviors already present in the retardate's environment and making their occurrences contingent upon low probability behaviors *a la* Premack.

DECELERATING BEHAVIOR

Positive reinforcement is relatively ineffective for reliably eliminating undesirable behavior in the severely and profoundly retarded. The primary effect of positive reinforcement is to accelerate behavior (Morse, 1966).

There are four procedures which are commonly used to eliminate or decelerate behavior: *extinction, satiation, conditioning an incompatible response,* and *application of aversive events.*

Although extinction is a commonly used and sometimes effective procedure, it has two disadvantages: The trainer or controlling authority does not always have complete control over all reinforcements, and therefore, he cannot effectively withhold all reinforcement. Masturbation is a classic example. Second, one of the effects of extinction is to increase the response rate before it decreases it. If one is attempting to eliminate self-destructive behavior, e.g., head banging, the effects of the extinction procedure might produce severe and even irreversible physical damage to the retarded. Extinction is probably most effective when it is used in conjunction with reinforcement to produce an incompatible response. If a child cries to receive attention and has vocal skills, an effective way to eliminate attention-getting crying might be to ignore crying and give the child attention when he calls the attendant by name. As the attention-getting response of calling the attendant by name increases, crying to obtain attention will probably decrease. Goldiamond (1968) has suggested a way to condition an incompatible response that does not produce a rate increase of the undesirable behavior. He suggests that if one continues to reinforce the undesirable behavior, but gives greater reinforcement to the occurrence of the desirable behavior, the desirable behavior may predominate over the undesirable behavior which may finally disappear. Goldiamond used such a technique to eliminate stuttering. He instructed the parents of a child who appeared to stutter to obtain attention to continue to reinforce stuttering to keep the rate from increasing (which might have frustrated the parents further), but also to encourage him to speak fluently and reinforce him generously when he did. Goldiamond's reasoning was that stuttering produced aversive as well as positive consequences for the child, i.e., it was obvious deviant behavior, thus the final reinforcement value for fluency was greater than for stuttering.

Satiation can be used effectively to either decelerate or eliminate undesirable behavior. Ayllon (1963) has used this method to eliminate hoarding towels in a psychotic adult. She had persisted in keeping extra towels in her room. The hospital staff began to bring her towels intermittently throughout the day when she was in her room and continued to do so for a number of days. She stopped hoarding towels. To use a satiation technique, it is first necessary to identfy the source of reinforcement.

Probably the most effective way to eliminate specific behavior is to punish it with an aversive consequence. The term *punishment* refers to a deceleration of the future probability of a specific response as a result of an immediate consequence for that response (Azrin and Holz, 1966). The presentation of the aversive consequence is made contingent upon the occurrence of a specific response.

What are the characteristics of an ideal aversive consequence to be used to punish undesirable behavior? Azrin and Holz have considered this problem in detail. Such a stimulus should be one whose intensity can be varied along a broad range and whose value can be specified precisely. This is necessary because intensity of the aversive stimulus is an important factor influencing the effectiveness of the punishment procedure and because there are individual differences with respect to reaction to a specified value of the stimulus. Electric shock provides one of the best examples of such a stimulus. The intensity can be reduced to a point that is undetectable and can be increased to an intensity that is very painful and still not harmful.

The contingencies of punishment should be specified only by the trainer and not by the subject. If the trainer specifies that the retardate receive punishment each time he hits his head against the wall, it is important that the retardate does not develop tactics which allow him to beat his head against the wall without being punished. Similarly, if an aversive stimulus of a specific intensity is to be used, it is equally important that the subject does not control the intensity. Needless to say, the retardate often adds reinforcement contingencies to the ones set up by the controlling authority. The effectiveness of punishment will be reduced to the extent that he does develop procedures which allow him either to avoid or reduce the effect of the punishment stimulus.

There are three basic ways an aversive stimulus can be applied: *punishment, escape,* or *avoidance.* Punishment is the application of an aversive stimulus after a particular response occurs. The presentation of the stimulus is response contingent. For example, the retardate slaps his head and this act results in an electric shock. Escape is the termination of an aversive stimulus made contingent upon a response. A child touches a hot stove, his fingers are burned, and he terminates the painful stimulus by removing his fingers. An avoidance situation is one in which the organism can make a response which prevents or delays the occurrence of aversive consequence. One child gives a more aggressive child a toy when he demands it, and as a result, avoids being hit. The primary difference among these three situations is the specific condition that produces the aversive stimulus. In the case of punishment, a specific response *produces* the aversive stimulus; in escape, a specific response *terminates* the stimulus that is already present in avoidance, a specific response *prevents* the consequence from occurring or *prolongs* the presentation of it. If the person does not make the response within some interval in the avoidance situation, he receives the aversive stimulus. Punishment has been used more than escape or avoidance procedures in institutions for the retarded.

The effectiveness of punishment appears to be determined by the intensity of the aversive stimulus, the manner in which it is introduced, immediacy of punishment, the schedule of punishment, and whether some alternative response is available (Azrin and Holz). An aversive consequence presented at a high intensity is more effective for permanently suppressing behavior than one presented at a moderate or low intensity and then increased gradually. Sudden introduction of punishment at a substantial increase in intensity will further suppress responding even after the organism has been exposed to shock for several days. The permanency of the suppression effects of shock is reduced when the presentation of shock is delayed. Continuous punishment suppresses responding more effectively than intermittent punishment. Alternative responses may also have a significant influence on the effectiveness of punishment. Azrin and Holz report that time out from reinforcement suppresses a given response only when some alternative response that will provide the organism with reinforcement is available.

The term *time out* refers to removal of the opportunity to obtain reinforcement contingent upon the occurrence of a response. Removal of the opportunity to obtain reinforcement is accompanied by a cue that indicates to the child he cannot obtain reinforcement for some specified interval. If the response being suppressed is the only outlet for satisfying an important deprivation state it would seem that another means of responding should be made available to the child. For example, if a retardate is breaking windows or injuring other residents to obtain attention and this response is suppressed via punishment, it would be wise to shape a more sociably acceptable attention getting response pattern, rather than simply suppressing the destructive response. Otherwise, the important deprivation state would remain unsatisfied. This may be the type of situation that actually leads to "symptom substitution."

Some aversive consequences that have been investigated are electric shock, noise, an air blast, response cost, time out from reinforcement, conditioned aversive stimuli (Azrin and Holz), and novelty (Kish, 1966). Electric shock has been studied most extensively and appears to be the most effective and most conveniently applied form of punishment (Azrin and Holz). A wide range of intensities are available, and the intensity of the stimulus can be specified precisely. It is easy to administer shock. Grids can be mounted in floors; manipulanda can serve as electrodes; portable, miniaturized, remotely controlled devices can be attached to the subject; or "shock sticks" can be used. Shock has two basic disadvantages. Because of individual differences in skin resistance from moment to moment, it is not always clear just how much current the subject is receiving, and the retardates often learn to escape or minimize the effects of shock. Thus they establish contingencies in addition to those set up by the controlling authorities.

Noise is evidently not so effective as electric shock. It can be precisely specified and controlled, but even at high intensities it does not produce a complete reduction in responding. Above certain decibel values, noise can damage the hearing system.

Response cost is basically a "fine" system. The subject pays for making certain responses. If, for example, he is getting tokens for correct responding, he gives back tokens for incorrect responding. Response cost produces an immediate reduction in responding that is almost complete. Two conditions are necessary to use response cost as a reinforcer. The subject must accumulate some minimal number of reinforcement to pay the fine, and generalized conditioned reinforcement is usually the most convenient form of reinforcement because it is not always possible to recover unconditioned reinforcement such as candy or cookies.

Time out from reinforcement is probably the least effective of the aversive consequences. Azrin and Holz report that it does not, in and of itself, reduce the future probability of responding, the definition given for punishment. However, it has been found to be effective when an alternative response that would produce reinforcement was available. Conditioned aversive stimuli have been studied and used rather extensively with both animals and humans. Such stimuli appear to be effective for suppressing undesirable behavior and will continue to be effective if the conditioned aversive stimulus is occasionally associated with the unconditioned aversive stimulus.

Novelty can also serve as an aversive consequence. Kish cites a number of experiments in which novelty appeared to be aversive to organisms. This can be thought of as the "strangeness" or bizarre aspect of the environment producing fear in an organism.

Most of these factors of aversive consequences influencing the effectiveness of punishment are based on studies using infrahuman organisms as subjects.

Several studies have been reported recently that investigate the influence of punishment on elimination of undesirable behavior in severely and profoundly retarded persons. This research probably received its greatest impetus from the work of Lovaas and his coworkers (1964). He reported the use of painful electric shock to suppress self-injurious behaviors in autistic children. Since that time similar procedures have been used with the severely and profoundly retarded (White and Taylor, 1967; Tate and Baroff, 1966; Whaley, 1967).

Tate and Baroff used response contingent electric shock to eliminate self-injurious behavior in a severely retarded nine-year-old boy. White and Taylor used electric shock to punish ruminative behavior—regurgitating their food and rechewing it—in two severely and profoundly retarded children.

Hamilton and Standahl (1967) reported an impressive application of response-contingent electric shock to eliminate stereotyped screaming behavior in a 24-year-old profoundly retarded female in an institution ward. In addition to eliminating the response by using response contingent shock, they also evaluated the extent to which the effects of punishment generalized to other vocal behavior. The subject exhibited three types of stereotyped vocal sounds: screaming, "mooing," and "chattering." But only screaming was punished. Screaming was for all practical purposes eliminated, but chattering and mooing showed no systematic changes that could be related to electric shock. This study shows that the effects of shock were specific to shocked behavior as opposed to suppressing vocal behavior in general.

Whaley eliminated self-destructive behavior in a six-year-old Mongoloid whose IQ was 15 by using a combined punishment-avoidance procedure. The behavior in question was ear-pounding. The child would repeatedly strike his ears with his fists. A special pair of electroconductive mittens were constructed and placed on his hands. Whenever the mittens contacted the head or other parts of the body he received shock. Training progressed in two stages. First, the self-injurious behavior was suppressed with low intensity response contingent shock. As a result of response contingent shock, self-injurious behavior was completely suppressed. Second, an incompatible response was conditioned employing electric shock. The subject was required to make certain minimal contact with a toy to avoid shock—the avoidance phase of training. After the incompatible response was conditioned, the child would not strike himself as long as he held the toy. After conditioning, when the subject did not possess the toy in the experimental room where avoidance training had taken place, he engaged in self-restraining behavior that was incompatible with the previously punished self-injurious behavior. This study provides an excellent example of one of the most effective ways to eliminate a response. First the undesirable responding is suppressed; then it is replaced with an incompatible response—one, which because of its very presence, prevents the undesirable response from occurring.

Watson (1968) used a conditioned aversive stimulus procedure to eliminate undesirable behavior in severely and profoundly retarded children. The procedure employed a Pavlovian-type higher order conditioning technique. Three different stimuli were used, only one of which was an unconditioned aversive stimulus. Subjects received punishment in the following manner: the first undesirable response produced a low tone; the second and third undesirable responses produced a low tone plus a tape recorded vocal "No!"; the fourth undesirable response and each undesirable response thereafter produced a low tone, a "No!" and a brief, moderately intense electric shock. After several pairings of the three stimuli, both the tone and the "No!" acquired aversive stimulus properties. Once they became aversive, subjects usually stopped responding in the presence of "No!" before they received the electric shock. The performance data suggests that, following conditioning, tone alone was least aversive, tone plus "No!" was intermediate in degree of aversiveness, and low tone plus "No!" plus shock was most aversive.

Such a procedure should have at least two advantages over an unconditioned aversive stimulus alone. Because there seems to be a wide variation in individual differences in reacting to any given aversive stimulus, a single aversive stimulus of a given intensity level may be too weak for one subject to be effective, optimum for a second subject, and too intense for a third. One of the disadvantages to intense punishment is that it may drive the subject away from the cite of stimulation (Powell and Azrin, 1968). This may be undesirable in many cases, e.g., where the retardate is being taught to respond to some situation, and punishment is being used only to facilitate the development of differential responding rather than simply preventing responding. If punishment drives the retardate away from the training situation it has defeated the entire project. The first advantage is that by using a series of aversive stimuli of varying intensities the subject should continue to respond until he has received the aversive stimuli which have an intensity value that is optimally aversive for him; i.e., it stops his responding, but hopefully is not so intense that it will drive him away from the actual cite of punishment. Such a variable stimulus, if properly designed, should be suitable for a large number of retardates with fairly broad individual differences in their sensitivity to aversive consequences of any given value. The second advantage to this type of conditioned aversive stimulus is that, once conditioning (which is relatively rapid) is completed, the subject receives very few electric shocks. Because shocking people, even for their own benefit, is controversial, a conditioned aversive stimulus procedure should be more socially acceptable.

Other punishment procedures used with severely and profoundly retarded populations are response cost and time out from reinforcement. Lent eliminated food stealing in an institutional dining room using response cost and time out procedures. Hamilton, Stephens, and Allen (1967) also developed a time out procedure which successfully eliminated undesirable behavior among severely and profoundly retarded girls. One part of the ward was designated as a time out area. Four padded chairs, equipped with restraining belts, were placed in this area and bolted to the floor. Undesirable behavior, e.g., fighting, self-injurious behavior, window breaking, clothes tearing, and temper tantrums, was punished by restraining the delinquent person in a chair for 30 minutes to two hours. This procedure either totally eliminated the undesirable behavior or reduced the frequency of occurrence to a very low level. Henriksen and Doughty (1967) used such a procedure to eliminate undesirable mealtime behavior in the dining room with four severely and profoundly retarded young boys. The five behaviors of interest were eating too fast, eating with hands, stealing food from others' trays, hitting others at the table, and throwing trays on the floor. Whenever a child displayed any of this behavior he was immediately told by facial and verbal disapproval, "that's a bad boy!" If he continued, his movement was suddenly interrupted by restraining his arm. Conversely, when these children displayed proper eating behavior, they were told "that's a good boy!" along with facial approval and pats on the back. Training was conducted three meals a day, seven days a week, for 13 weeks. There was also an element of restraint in the time out procedure used by Hamilton, Stephens, and Allen.

This review of the MR literature suggests that electric shock, a conditioned aversive stimulus, response cost, and time out are all effective for eliminating undesirable behavior in the severely and profoundly retarded. Although these studies do not define the important parameters of punishment when used with this type of population, some tentative conclusions can be drawn from them. Highly intense punishment is probably more effective than moderate or mild intensities of punishment for suppression behavior. Time out from reinforcement is often effective, at least when an alternative response is available. Response cost should be effective with retardates (severely and moderately retarded, at least) in a token economy system (retardates receive tokens which they can exchange for candy, food and toys), and one factor determining the effectiveness of the procedure may be the fate of the monies obtained. Lent (1968a) found response cost to be effective for controlling aggressive behavior with one retarded girl when the tokens taken from her were given to the girl who was aggressed against, while simple response cost proved to be relatively ineffective with her. Much systematic research is needed to obtain a fuller understanding of the effectiveness of punishment and other aversive techniques with the severely and profoundly retarded.

There are three disadvantages to the use of punishment: the person may withdraw from the cite of punishment, aggression by the person being punished, and the controversy it creates. We have found in our own research at Columbus State School that response contingent electric shock may drive the subject away from the laboratory, i.e., the subject refuses to come back or refuses to work in the situation in which he was previously punished. This has happened with only one out of approximately 30 retardates in our laboratory with our conditioned aversive stimulus research and would be a problem only when the goal for the subject was to shape differential responding in the situation, e.g., operating a teaching machine or operating manipulanda that produce electric shock under some conditions but not under others. As Azrin and Holz and Colwell (1966) have pointed out, punishment may also interfere with social relationships—between the person administering punishment and the person being punished. Azrin and Holz state that punishment can produce aggression of two kinds: *operant* and *elicited*. In the case of operant aggression, the person being punished may attack or even destroy the person or thing inflicting the punishment. Elicited aggression may occur when another person is accompanying the person being punished, and the person being punished attacks the "innocent bystander." Another name for this is "displaced aggression." It would seem that one way to minimize the subject's operant aggression and withdrawal from the situation is for the person inflicting punishment also to administer positive reinforcement for socially acceptable behavior to create or maintain an emotional reaction that is incompatible with aggression and withdrawal. Thus if the subject is getting sufficient positive reinforcement from the administerer of punishment, he should still return for more positive reinforcement at the risk of being punished. There is insufficient evidence to predict the extent to which aggression and withdrawal from the person or situation providing punishment is a problem.

Finally there is the controversy. Many people feel that the use of punishment as a behavioral control technique is cruel and unethical—particularly in institutions for the psychotic and retarded. This reaction is due, in part, to the cruel treatment patients have received from time to time from sadistic institutional personnel as well as from past socially acceptable cruel disciplinary procedures. In an attempt to prevent such acts from recurring, rules have been made against punishing patients with physically painful stimuli. However, even a casual glance at modern social practices reveals that punishment, particularly of the time out type, is a common control procedure. People are fined, imprisoned, dismissed from their jobs, denied favors, and lose privileges. Physical punishment is also acceptable under certain conditions. Pupils receive corporal punishment in some elementary and secondary schools. Physicians require patients to undergo painful examinations and treatment to detect, palliate, and cure diseases of various kinds. There already exists in our society a rule that deems punishment to be acceptable under certain conditions, particularly those labelled as humanitarian. As Lovaas has argued so persuasively, punishment is justified if it will allow an emotionally disturbed child to be rehabilitated or cured or made normal—if he might not be otherwise. If a child engages in self-destructive behavior and is kept in restraints to prevent such behavior, he also is being maintained under relative stimulus deprivation. He is being prevented from interacting with his environment, and his normal development is being retarded. If, as a result of occasional, not constant or repeated punishment, a severely or profoundly retarded child can be taught self-help and social skills he might not learn otherwise, punishment would seem to be justified—particularly since there currently are no other alternative, effective, socially acceptable behavioral control procedures. By teaching this retardate such behaviors we are reducing his level of retardation, which in itself is humane. On the contrary, it would seem inhumane to leave him in his primitive state if his improvement depended, in part, on the use of punishment. By prohibiting the use of punishment for training where other procedures have failed habilitation of retardates may be markedly impaired.

STIMULUS CONTROL

Developing stimulus control over specific behavior is probably the greatest problem which must be considered with the severely and profoundly retarded in many institutions. Although they exhibit very little behavior, even the behavior they have is usually under inappropriate stimulus control. They defecate or urinate on the ward floor rather than in the toilet; they eat with their fingers, often from a neighbor's plate or tray; they engage in self-injurious behavior to obtain attention from ward staff, rather than call a person by name or tug at the person's hand or uniform; they eat string, wood, pieces of clothing, and feces in addition to food. None of these behaviors are inappropriate in and of themselves. Eating, eliminating and getting attention from others are all behaviors that are displayed by "normal" persons. Only the conditions under which these behaviors occur or the way they are manifested are inappropriate. The problem is one of stimulus control.

There are two basic ways to obtain stimulus control. The first and more traditional utilizes a differential reinforcement procedure. One waits until the desired behavior occurs in the presence of the appropriate stimulus and reinforces it. If it occurs at other times no reinforcement is given (assuming the trainer is controlling all reinforcement contingencies).

It has been our experience, at least in laboratory situations, that it is almost impossible to establish a successive discrimination using a simple reinforcement-extinction procedure. However, we have had some degree of success when a combination of reinforcement and differential reinforcement for low rates of response (drl) or time out were used, and we have been completely successful with the previously discussed conditioned aversive stimulus. The term *drl* refers to delaying the opportunity to obtain reinforcement for a specified interval. In contrast to time out, no external cue accompanies this event. Our laboratory findings suggest that if one uses the traditional discrimination procedure to develop stimulus control over behavior, he should use a combination of positive reinforcement to develop the desired stimulus control and a conditioned aversive stimulus to eliminate the undesired stimulus control.

"Errorless" discrimination training is the second kind of stimulus control procedure. Ideally, the subject can make the response of interest *only* in the presence of the discriminative stimulus and never in the presence of inappropriate stimuli. This procedure was developed by Terrace (1963a and b, 1966) and has been used effectively with normal children by Moore and Goldiamond (1964) and has been applied successfully to developing stimulus control in the severely and profoundly retarded by Sidman and Stoddard (1967) and by Touchette (1968). The general strategy is to prevent the behavior of interest from occurring in the presence of inappropriate stimuli while reinforcing it for occurring in the presence of the stimulus selected by the trainer. This can be done by physically preventing the behavior from occurring in the presence of other stimuli than the discriminative stimulus or by selecting as an initial discriminative stimulus one to which the retardate already has a high predisposition to respond and as the stimulus to which we do not want the retardate to respond, one to which he has a low predisposition to respond. After stimulus control has developed the initial discriminative stimulus is faded out and the particular stimulus that has been selected as the permanent controlling stimulus is faded in. An early phase of Terrace's (1963a) discrimination study with pigeons illustrates the first situation. Whenever a pigeon pecked at a disc it was of one color only—red—the stimulus selected to be the discriminative stimulus. He was reinforced for pecking at this stimulus. A second stimulus, the disc without illumination was presented only when the pigeon was some minimal distance from the key—too far away to reach it with his beak. Thus the pigeon could never peck at the unilluminated disc, and the red colored disc acquired stimulus control over key pecking.

The second way to establish errorless stimulus control is illustrated by Sidman and Stoddard's application to severely mentally retarded, autistic, and normal IQ children. They wanted to teach their subjects to discriminate between two kinds of visual form stimuli: a circle and ellipses of different shapes. They used as their training apparatus a console that contained nine two-inch square translucent keys arranged in a square with three keys along each side. Each panel was both a miniature screen upon which stimuli could be projected and a manipulandum which operated microswitches if it were pushed. The goal of training was to establish the circle as a discriminative stimulus and the ellipses as stimuli to which subjects were not supposed to respond. Sidman and Stoddard began in a manner similar to Terrace. Initially only one key was illuminated. The stimulus was a bright yellow background with a black circle on it. All other keys were dark. They began by teaching severely retarded subjects to retrieve M & M candies from a receptacle located at the bottom of the console so that delivery of the candy could serve as a reinforcement for panel pressing. Once the retardate learned to retrieve the candy when it was delivered, one experimenter pressed the lighted key as a demonstration and a chime sounded and an M & M was delivered to the food receptacle. Next he took the retardate's hand and pushed the lighted panel for three trials. Each time a lighted panel was depressed a chime sounded and an M & M candy was delivered. In addition, each time the lighted key was pushed there would be a brief blackout period and the lighted key would appear again in another one of the nine positions. Then the retardate independently selected a key—the lighted one. In this manner stimulus control was quickly established over panel pressing with little or no responding to stimuli other than the discriminative stimulus. At this point in training it was the intensity dimension rather than the form dimension (the dimension of interest) that was controlling key pressing. The subject pressed the *lighted* key. Now "fading" began to take place. Each time the subject pressed the lighted key the other keys became a little brighter. The brightness of these other eight keys increased gradually in a steplike fashion until brightness was equal across all nine keys. Now the subject was forced to select his key on the basis of form, but in this case the basis of the discrimination was the presence and the absence of form. Next the ellipses were gradually faded in on the other keys in a steplike manner. At first they were barely visible, but each time the subject pressed the key with the circle, the ellipses were a little clearer, until finally they were just as clear or distinct as the circle. Now all nine keys differed only on the basis of form. One contained a circle and the other eight contained ellipses. Thus, the brightness dimension was faded out and the form dimension was faded in. In this manner a form discrimination which is ordinarily very difficult to establish in a severely retarded individual was easily conditioned.

There are several critical factors to consider in this method. First, the response being conditioned should be brought under the desired stimulus control as early as possible. Sidman and Stoddard conditioned the key pressing response in the presence of the lighted circle stimulus (superimposed upon the key) resulting in the stimulus they selected acquiring stimulus control over key pressing from the very beginning of training. If the key pressing response had been conditioned in the absence of the lighted circle, other probably unknown stimuli would have developed control over key pressing and would have to be extinguished before the lighted circle could become the controlling stimulus (Terrace, 1963a). Second, the rate or size of the steps used to fade out the brightness dimension or fade in the form dimension are rather critical. If the rate of fading is too rapid or the steps are too large stimulus control may deteriorate (Sidman and Stoddard; and Watson and Sanders, 1966). A third important factor is the relationship between fading schedules for fading out the stimulus currently controlling behavior and fading in the one which will replace it. Sidman and Stoddard found that when the form dimension, i.e., the ellipses, were faded in while subjects still discriminated on an intensity basis, they evidently learned to ignore the ellipses, and when the light intensity dimension was faded and could no longer be used as a basis for discrimination, stimulus control had not transferred to the form dimension. To solve this problem, they faded out light first and then faded in form as the relevant dimension second in a sequential rather than a simultaneous fashion with only a brief overlap of the two stimuli. The moment at which transfer actually occurs appears to be critical to the procedure.

Another relevant problem to the establishment of stimulus control is *attention*. People do not attend to or look at all aspects of their environment. Similarly, when a person is presented with a stimulus intended to be a discriminative stimulus, he does not attend to all parts of the stimulus; rather he usually looks only at certain restricted components of the stimulus. For example, if a severely retarded child is presented with a black circle on a brightly lighted background, he may attend only to the brightness dimension. Actually there are other dimensions to such a stimulus: size, form, color and position, and so on. Some components or dimensions of a stimulus are more relevant to a severely or profoundly retarded child than other dimensions. Before a stimulus can acquire control over the behavior of the retardate, he must first attend to it.

Zeaman and House (1963) has used the attention concept to explain why retardates acquire discriminations more slowly than normal IQ humans, and why lower MA retardates acquire discrimination more slowly than higher MA retardates. It takes longer for low MA retardates to attend to relevant stimulus dimensions that are being manipulated by the experimenter than higher MA retardates, and it takes longer for higher MA retardates to attend to these cues than normal IQ persons. Once they have begun to attend to the relevant cues, the actual rate of discrimination acquisition is more or less equivalent across MA. Zeaman has analyzed the hierarchy of relevant cues from most relevant to least relevant. It seems that most retardates (moderately and mildly retarded) found multidimensional "junk" stimuli to be most relevant initially. These are common objects such as a toy truck, a plate, or a cup. Next in the hierarchy were stimuli that differed on the basis of both color and form. Next was form. The lowest or least relevant dimension in the hierarchy was color. Research by Watson (1966) with the severely retarded and by Suchman and Trabasso (1966) with normal IQ children suggests that the size dimension would be less relevant than either form or color for the severely and profoundly retarded. Zeaman's research suggests that attention should be a function of both the number of stimuli or stimulus dimensions used as the discriminative stimulus and the relevance of these dimensions for the retardate. Because attention is a major problem with retardates and especially with the severely and profoundly retarded, this problem should be considered first when attempting to develop stimulus control over their behavior.

There are two general approaches to solving the problem of attention. One can use a stimulus to which the retardate is highly likely to attend such as a multidimensional object or a bright light (probably a flashing bright light would be even more relevant) and let this serve as the permanent discriminative stimulus, or one could start with such a stimulus, and using the fading technique illustrated by Sidman and Stoddard, transfer stimulus control to a second stimulus dimension such as color-form.

In addition to developing stimulus control, another important problem with the severely and profoundly retarded is maintaining stimulus control under varying stimulus conditions. One aspect of this problem is more traditionally known as *transfer of training*. If specific behavior is brought under the control of one set of stimuli, behavioral control may begin to deteriorate when these stimuli are changed. Watson and Sanders (1966) found that when they began to fade stimuli, stimulus change beyond certain size steps resulted in a deterioration of stimulus control. Sidman and Stoddard also lost stimulus control during fading, when light intensity was faded out as the discriminative stimulus and the circle was faded in. Subjects were attending to or were under the control of light intensity differences between the discriminative stimulus and the stimulus which was never reinforced. They were not attending to the form dimension even though it was present. When they could no longer discriminate on the basis of light intensity (as this stimulus dimension was being faded out), stimulus control deteriorated. They found that their fading program itself led to the children ignoring the form dimension. A modification of the program eliminated this problem.

It appears that the context in which training occurs, as well as the discriminative stimulus itself, exert stimulus control properties. The room in which training takes place evidently exerts stimulus control over the behavior of severely retarded children (Baumeister and Klosowski, 1965). Behavior can be shaped in one room with a set of stimuli, test for stimulus control made in another room using the same set of stimuli, and one may find that the behavior will deteriorate. We observed such an effect upon stimulus control with moderately and mildly mentally retarded children when the context in which controlling stimuli were presented was changed (Watson, Clevenger, Hundziak and Sanders, 1964). Ferster (1961) reported a similar effect with autistic children when they were trained to operate vending machines. Because of the disruptive effects of stimulus change, either in the primary controlling stimulus or the context in which it is presented, all stimulus changes should be made very gradually, as demonstrated by Sidman and Stoddard.

Hamilton and Standahl's study illustrates the "failure to transfer" problem that appears to characterize the severely and profoundly retarded. As cited previously, they used response contingent electric shock to eliminate stereotyped screaming in a profoundly retarded female. Punishment was carried out during one half-hour daily sessions on the ward while the retardate was sitting on a bench. The effects of punishment were found to be specific only for the time and at the place where punishment was given. In addition only the vocal response being punished was affected. To extend or "generalize" the effects of punishment, it was necessary to extend the time and the number of places in which the contingency was effective. The time contingency was increased daily to one half-hour period in the morning and one in the afternoon. Place was extended to the entire ward. After 18 days of training screaming was reduced from a daily average of 44.7 to three responses for the two half-hour periods. However, screaming still occurred at its usual frequency at all times other than the two half-hour daily sessions. So punishment was extended to 24 hours on an intermittent punishment schedule. Under these conditions, screaming on the ward was eliminated almost entirely. The effects of punishment continued even after the contingency was eliminated. These results suggest that to gain broad stimulus control over specific behavior, contingencies of reinforcement must be maintained over a broad range of times and in many places rather than only for a brief period of time in a restricted place.

The study by Henriksen and Doughty provides an example of how stimulus control can be extended from one geographical location to another, i.e., between rooms or buildings. A combination of punishment and positive reinforcement was used to eliminate "misbehavior" during mealtime. Training took place in an area of the institution other than the regular dining area. When training was completed, the behavior was "transferred" to the regular dining area by maintaining the same contingencies of reinforcement in the regular dining room. Then the reinforcement contingency was faded out. For three days the trainers stood at the retardates' table, then they stood three steps away for two days, nine steps away for two days, and finally any place in the room for five days. The punishment contingency remained in effect throughout fading. If these retardates had simply been returned to the regular dining area without maintaining and then fading the punishment contingency, mealtime misbehavior probably would have returned.

It may be that one reason stimulus change disrupts stimulus control so markedly is because of the limited number of stimuli in the environment actually controlling the behavior of profoundly retarded persons (Ferster, 1961). If this is the case, then one is presented with two alternatives to the problem. Either keep the environment as homogeneous as possible or bring the behavior of interest under broader stimulus control. By making the institutional environment more homogeneous, e.g., having all ward rooms the same color, using the same curtains in all rooms, there should be less change in the stimulus context to disrupt the behavior. By bringing any given behavior under broader stimulus control, it may be possible to make the behavior more stable because behavioral control will not be so dependent upon any given stimulus. With respect to the first alternative, most of the behavior of retardates is either under the control of other persons or objects. By keeping the same attendants with a given retardate from day to day and having the attendants use a standard vocabulary, stimulus control from other persons should be more stable. The same rule should apply to items such as clothing and eating utensils such as plates, cups, and spoons.

The other alternative (and probably the preferred one) is to broaden stimulus control. Using fading procedures similar to those illustrated by Sidman and Stoddard, one can bring the behavior of interest under the control of a number of attendants, a number of articles of clothing and a number of plates, cups and spoons and a number of stimulus contexts.

One advantage the normal person and more adequate retardate has over the more severely retarded person is that he can generate his own stimulus control with language. He can use his own words to control his own behavior. If language can be taught to the severely and profoundly retarded, then they could be trained to use it to control their own behavior. As previously mentioned, Smaltz, at Parsons Training Center, is using such a technique with severely and moderately retarded girls—his bathing song. Such a procedure not only insures greater stimulus control in a given situation, but it also frees the retardate somewhat from external environmental controls, a factor which may create the transfer of training problems that plague those who attempt to train such individuals.

What should one do when stimulus control begins to deteriorate? Sidman and Stoddard have developed a useful "backup" procedure they use when they begin to fade out the existing controlling stimuli and fade in new stimuli. They simply reverse the fading procedure and move backward until they reach a point where the behavior again comes under the control of stimuli manipulated by the trainer. Then they resume fading. This is the same general procedure used with the successive approximation technique.

A very useful application of stimulus control to generate new behavior is to use an *imitation* technique, such as the one reported by Baer, Peterson and Sherman (1967). First, the retardate is trained to imitate the trainer when cued, e.g., the trainer says, "Do this!" and then executes some particular behavior. Once the retardate is conditioned to imitate the trainer following a vocal cue, "Do this!" he should respond to the discriminative stimulus by reproducing a response pattern similar to the one demonstrated by the trainer immediately following the vocal cue—although several trials may be required to improve the topography of each new response pattern.

To condition imitative behavior in the severely and profoundly retarded, successive approximation and fading procedures may be required. Baer, *et al.*, initially conditioned imitative behavior in severely and profoundly retarded children by means of an arm-raising response. The trainer would say, "Do this!" and then would raise his own arm. If the retardate did not respond he repeated the vocal cue followed by a demonstration and then lifted the child's arm into the proper position and immediately reinforced this response. Lifting of the arm by the trainer served as a prompt to facilitate communication. After several trials of this kind the trainer began to fade out the prompt gradually by raising the child's arm only part way and using successive approximation to complete the response. Gradually the prompt was faded until the child made an unassisted arm-raising response whenever the trainer presented the vocal cue "Do this!" followed by raising his own arm. Once the initial response pattern, imitation, is established to the vocal cue, it should be possible to generate new behavior fairly readily with this procedure, assuming the retardate already has the necessary fundamental behavioral components in his repertory.

Shaping and Maintaining Behavior: Institutional Personnel

Success or failure of a training program for the severely and profoundly retarded will depend to a great extent upon the effectiveness of the personnel involved in the program. This includes attendants, ward matrons, nursing supervisors, psychologists, teachers, recreational therapists, and other persons involved. For this reason, particular attention should be given to shaping and maintaining the behavior of these personnel. Their behavior should be carefully shaped using both successive approximation and chaining procedures. Effective reinforcement techniques should be employed during behavior shaping and should be continued beyond the training period of the future trainer to insure that the newly acquired behavior will be maintained. In order that the personnels' behavior will occur at the proper time, it should be brought under appropriate stimulus control. Careful attention to shaping and maintaining behavior in personnel is just as important as shaping and maintaining behavior in retarded residents. Many programs probably fail or are minimally effective because of problems of personnel.

SHAPING

Behavior shaping procedures should be used to teach attendants the various skills they will employ in shaping and maintaining the behavior of residents and other relevant institutional personnel. Just as with residents, the first step involved in setting up a program for institutional personnel is to identify all behaviors that they must carry out in their particular assignment, identify all terminal behavior that characterizes each behavioral pattern, and determine the attendants' present relevant behavioral repertory. Then the component behaviors involved in shaping the attendant's behavior from the existing to the terminal repertory should be determined. Once each behavioral unit has been identified, the terminal behaviors that characterize each unit have been isolated, the present relevant behavioral repertory determined, and the important behavioral components that will permit shaping the existing to the terminal repertory identified, one has the necessary basis for a training program.

The next step is to select a means of communication. There are two basic ways to train institutional personnel. One can either begin in the classroom, lecture and discuss training the mentally retarded with or without a variety of audiovisual aids, including retardates themselves. The main type of feedback the pupil provides to demonstrate his understanding is verbal, either vocal or written. Or one can take the personnel trainees directly to the ward, and using residents involved in the very behaviors to be shaped, let the attendants train the residents in a real-life situation. In this case there are two types of feedback available to determine how well the personnel trainee understands his task: verbal and behavioral. Because one is usually primarily interested in the actual behavior exhibited by the trainee when he attempts to control residents or other staff, this behavioral mode constitutes a more direct test of the trainee's skill in controlling such persons. The first means of communication is probably best suited for teaching principles of behavior modification, while the second one is most effective for teaching applications of the principles to actual behavior modification situations.

A ward management training program for institutional personnel should be oriented toward two goals: to teach the psychological principles that provide the basis for application of behavioral control techniques, and to teach the behavioral control techniques themselves. If trainees are not provided with a framework of principles, their knowledge of behavioral control may be limited to the specific context in which training occurred, i.e., they may not be able to generalize these procedures to novel situations that inevitably will occur. Similarly, if after the principles are learned, sufficient illustrations of applications of these principles are not given, then the precise manner in which they are applied may remain unclear.

An effective shaping procedure should adequately communicate information to the student, and provide both the student and the instructor with knowledge of results concerning how well the student is progressing. In addition, an ideal shaping program begins training at the educational level at which the trainee is presently operating—at his existing relevant behavioral repertory—and moves him toward the terminal repertory at a pace that is optimally suited for him. Further, the trainee does not progress in the educational program until fundamental steps or concepts are mastered, that is, progress in the program is made contingent upon sufficient understanding of all previous steps in the program. This last requirement prevents the person from leaving a step in the program until he has shown adequate comprehension. It also allows each successive step to serve as a reinforcement for each previous step in an application of the principles of chaining.

TEACHING PRINCIPLES

The following methods can be used to shape psychological principles: traditional lecture using a blackboard to provide visual examples and prompts; a lecture plus visual aids such as an overhead projector, a slide projector or movies; discussion with or without visual aids; conventional textbooks; programmed texts; written or oral examinations; and behavioral demonstrations. The conventional lecture with blackboard examples is probably the most ineffective and most inflexible communication procedure. Most student populations have rather diverse educational backgrounds. For this reason, the rate and extent to which they will comprehend lecture material will vary widely. While some students may find the lecture to move at a pace and be presented at a level of complexity that is both interesting and comprehensible, others will find the pace to be too slow and elementary, and still others will find it to be too fast and bewildering. The two latter groups will probably lose interest and will not learn the lecture material. In addition, many students find it difficult to be attentive for any length of time, probably because they play such a passive role. The instructor receives very limited feedback from the students and therefore usually does not know the extent to which they understand the material being presented.

If a lecture method is to be used, it would probably be more effective if accompanied by visual aids such as slides that present pictures and diagrams illustrating the subject matter of the lecture. Visual aids appear to maintain student attention better than a lecture alone, and if properly constructed and sequenced, can clarify the lecture greatly. An even more efficient procedure may be to prerecord the lecture on a tape recorder and present it with slides or a movie using a synchronizing device attached to the tape recorder. When the lecture is prerecorded it can be edited before final presentation.

If the lecture method is used, written or oral examination should be given to obtain feedback both for the instructor and the trainee. In addition, the lecture can be presented in "units," each of which is designed to teach certain concepts or terminal behaviors, with the most fundamental ones being presented first. Redundancy is one way to insure understanding of a particular concept when the lecture method is used. By presenting a concept or principle and then illustrating it in a variety of contexts, the likelihood of its being understood will be increased. Examinations should be given before the first lecture to determine the student's relevant verbal repertory and after each lecture unit to determine the extent of understanding of that unit. The students receive greater feedback if the examination is graded immediately and they can discuss the results. Results of the lecture indicate to the instructor which topics in the lecture need supplementation during the next lecture or revision if the lecture is to be repeated with other students. If students do not do well on the examination and poor performance appears to be related to certain topics or concepts the exam has indicated that the lecture needs revision and supplementation at these points. Poor test performance can also be a result of the test's not being an adequate sample of the student's understanding of the material (i.e., it is not valid), or the student may not be sufficiently reinforced for superior test performance. Cohen and Filipizak (1968) found they could increase test grades by charging students a penalty or punishing them for low grades. In addition they set up definite reinforcement contingencies for high grades—90 per cent correct. High grades were reinforced by permitting students to continue to progress through the program.

Cohen and Filipizak used a combination of textbook, lecture, discussion, and written examination in a manner that allowed them to employ shaping and reinforcement principles to teach a large class of college students. When a new class of students arrived at the beginning of the course, they first assessed students' relevant behavioral repertoires by giving them a written examination. Results of the pretest enabled the instructors to select more difficult subject matter which would need more emphasis and elaboration and to select other material with which students were familiar that would require less attention. The course was divided into a series of lecture units, each of which lasted for a week. Each unit was designed to produce certain terminal behaviors clearly defined to the student. During each week each student could attend as few as two or as many as five lectures, depending upon his examination scores. The lectures were either prerecorded presented via tape recorder in conjunction with slides or "live," presented by an instructor. Students were given a reading assignment before the first lecture of the week, and upon arriving for the lecture, were given a brief written examination to evaluate their comprehension of the reading assignment. The score on this test provided a given number of points that contributed to the final grade—the reinforcement for reading the text carefully. The prerecorded lecture accompanied by slides was then presented, followed by a written examination pertaining to the lecture. After the exam was completed it was graded in class, and the correct answers were discussed by an instructor with the students. If students passed the test at 90 per cent or higher they were eligible to attend the live lecture held later in the week. If they attained a lower score they had to repeat the prerecorded lecture, take a second examination, and receive a grade of at least 90 per cent to attend the live lecture. Thus admission to the live lecture was the reinforcement for attending the prerecorded lecture and achieving a satisfactory score on the exam. They could repeat the prerecorded lecture up to three times. In addition, a graduate student instructor was present during the third prerecorded lecture and would discuss the lecture material with students following the lecture and before the exam. If the exam was failed a third time the student would have received tutoring from a graduate assistant. No student ever required this private review. The live lecture was based on students' performance on the test following the prerecorded lecture. It was designed to supplement, integrate, and synthesize the week's study material in a manner most beneficial to student learning. After the live lecture, they took another written examination. Performance on this exam produced points which contributed to the final grade—another reinforcement. The entire subject matter of the course was programmed to allow the student to engage in behaviors that were successive approximations of the terminal behaviors selected as the final objectives of the course, all clear to the student. Thus lectures were set up in units, each unit was programmed so that each component of each unit was reinforced either by contributing to the final grade or allowing the student to move on to the next stage of the unit. Feedback for both instructor and student was obtained from written examinations which were graded immediately in class, and discussion of the examination results following each stage of a lecture unit. This program represents an elegant combination of the lecture method and principles of programming *a la* operant conditioning. Cohen and Filipizak also programmed "examsmanship." In order that they not frighten students unduly with the pretest, it was composed entirely of true–false items. As the course progressed, requirements for expression on the exams progressed to the point where on the posttest students were required to write essays about the interrelations of the subject matter. Exam trauma may be a particular problem with attendant level personnel and should be considered when preparing examinations for them.

There are few textbooks suitable for teaching principles of behavior modification to institutional personnel. Bensberg and his associates have written such materials (Bensberg, 1965). So, if one is planning to develop a program in which institutional staff are to be taught behavior modification principles, textual materials will probably have to be designed by the initiators of the program. The instructor can choose from two basic types of textbooks, the programmed text or the conventional text. The programmed text offers all of the advantages outlined earlier in this section: 1. ideally the text is designed for a specific population of individuals, with a specific classification of reading skills or vocabulary; 2. the subject matter is written in small, well-organized, optimum-sized steps; 3. the student is permitted to progress through the material at a pace which suits him; 4. the student is not allowed to progress to new material until he has demonstrated an understanding of early more fundamental material; 5. the student gets immediate knowledge of results; and 6. prompting or successive approximation principles can be used extensively to develop concepts or behavioral repertoires.

Conventional textbooks, written in the manner of *Behavior Principles* by Ferster and Perrott, also employ some principles of programming, although they are somewhat limited as compared with conventional programmed instructional materials. They can be written for a specific population or audience. Shaping principles can be employed by using prompts, fading procedures, and redundancy. The book can be developed for a specific population by having representative members read early drafts of the book, by testing them for understanding of the material, and by using these test results as a basis for revision. Sources of feedback for the reader would be a list of questions or "prompts" at the end of sections, which the student could use to drill himself, as in the case of Ferster and Perrott's text and written or oral examinations.

If one is developing textbook material for institutional personnel, certain data should first be collected to provide a framework for writing the text, whether it be conventional or of a programmed instructional type. First, students should be given a reading test to determine their level of reading sophistication. The material should be composed at a level of complexity indicated by such a test. Second, students should be given a vocabulary test that is relevant to the subject matter to be taught. Results of this pretest will provide a basis for choice of words to use in writing the material and words or terms to be taught as part of the problem. Third, a pretest should be given to determine the students' knowledge of the subject matter at the outset of training. Ideally, the subject matter will start at a level equivalent to their existing verbal repertory and shape their behavior toward the terminal behaviors identified as the goals of the program.

Discussion can be very useful for shaping verbal behavior when used with small groups. The instructor can determine various components of each student's verbal repertory by asking pertinent questions. He can reinforce them verbally for desirable verbal behavior and shape the student's behavior further through discussions of other aspects of the subject matter. By breaking his subject matter into small steps or units, the instructor can present a unit, sample each student's understanding of that unit, verbally reinforce correct verbal behavior, verbally supplement less than acceptable verbal behavior and move on to the next unit.

TEACHING BEHAVIOR MODIFICATION

Demonstrations, either by movie, or an instructor or trainee with a retardate are probably the most effective ways of shaping actual behavior modification skills. One of the most useful applications of these techniques may be to take a group of trainees who have learned principles of behavior modification and have them observe either an instructor or another trainee attempt to shape the behavior of a retardate, e.g., teaching him to dress or undress himself. There is an advantage to using a trainee to demonstrate shaping procedures, either instead of or in addition to an instructor demonstration. The trainee invariably makes mistakes during his initial attempts at shaping, and other students see these errors and criticize him. If criticism can be withheld until after the demonstration, other trainee's remarks can provide the basis for a lively discussion which allows the entire trainee group to become more involved and clarify its own thinking about shaping. By injecting role playing into the situation as soon as criticisms begin to appear, the exercise can be even more beneficial. We have tried this at Columbus State School. The first person to criticize the trainee participating in the initial demonstration is asked to show how he would teach the patient to dress or undress. As soon as someone criticizes the trainee playing the role of the behavior shaper, he is asked to demonstrate how he would do it. If no one criticizes the initial demonstration, a behavior shaping problem can be posed and two trainees can be selected to demonstrate the correct procedure through role playing with one acting as a patient and the other as an instructor.

Demonstrations and role playing provide trainees with an introduction to behavior modification itself. Following this kind of instruction, they should be ready to practice directly with a patient. To facilitate shaping and insure that application of behavior modification principles are thoroughly understood, it may be desirable to catalog all terminal behaviors one wants to develop in trainees, i.e., behaviors relevant to shaping and maintaining behaviors in both institutional personnel and residents, develop well-defined steps for shaping each behavior, and have trainees shape some of these behaviors in a patient. By standardizing the shaping procedure for reaching each terminal behavior, it may be simpler both to show and criticize trainees during behavior shaping exercises, because each will know which steps have been identified as being essential. If one is to evaluate their actual behavior-shaping procedure, trainees should be given real-life behavior modification tests before and after training, either with a trainee or a staff member playing the role of a patient. One simple test to give is to have trainees attempt to shape the terminal behaviors that constitute the goal of the training program.

REINFORCEMENT

Salary increases and promotions seem to be paramount reinforcement for personnel in institutions. Money is a powerful reinforcer and like all generalized reinforcers, is relatively independent of specific deprivation states, and therefore, nearly always effective. Unfortunately, it is probably the least accessible and least manipulable reinforcement (from the trainer's viewpoint) in the institutional environment. Most state institutional beaucracies maintain a rigid control over this particular reinforcement and are very reluctant to relinquish control to others, such as holders of training grants and training supervisors. The same situation may often exist for promotion. Fortunately, there are other reinforcements which can be used. As Herzberg (1966) has pointed out, money or the lack of it makes an important contribution to job dissatisfaction but contributes very little to job satisfaction. Factors such as individual attention or recognition, increased responsibility in making decisions concerned with one's own job and taking part in policy making should make a significant contribution to job satisfaction. These are, of course, social reinforcements and can be used by supervisors in conjunction with various contingencies to shape and maintain behavior in ward personnel.

The first step in establishing a reinforcement procedure for ward personnel is to identify the specific contingencies that will serve as a basis of reinforcement. Contingencies can be considered from two points of view. First, as already pointed out, the terminal behaviors that constitute the duties of each job classification should be determined. Either these behaviors themselves are made reinforcement contingent or components that approximate them become the basis for receiving reinforcement. Once the reinforcement contingencies are identified they should be clearly specified to each attendant and supervisor. "These are your 'duties'." When he has fulfilled a contingency he should be reinforced with attention or recognition or whatever reinforcement is being employed. As the reinforcement contingencies are specified for all personnel, it will become clear who is responsible for providing reinforcement and for shaping and maintaining behavior in whom. It is usually the attendant's responsibility to shape and maintain behavior in residents. They are responsible for reinforcing residents when they have satisfied different reinforcement contingencies. Similarly, it is usually the responsibility of the attendant's immediate supervisor to shape and maintain behavior in the attendant. Thus, this supervisor is responsible for reinforcing attendants when they have satisfied different reinforcement contingencies. And on and on it goes. The attendant's supervisor should be reinforced by her supervisor (who may be the cottage supervisor) when she satisfies different contingencies, and this supervisor should be reinforced by the division supervisor (who may be the chief of nursing or cottage life), who should be reinforced by the clinical director, who should be reinforced by the superintendent, who in turn should get his reinforcement either from the state central office or from his own section heads. Such a reinforcement contingency hierarchy needs to be established if a reinforcement system is to be used with personnel. This involves not only clearly determining reinforcement contingencies for each job classification but also establishing lines of authority for each person. (Which is simply part of the reinforcement contingency.) If an attendant is responsible for certain residents and has certain specific duties which no other person has, then if the contingencies are met it is quite clear who did it, and if they are not met it is also quite clear who was negligent. Then it is simple enough to determine who is responsible and who is to be either positively or negatively reinforced. The same should also be true for supervisory personnel.

A second way to view reinforcement contingencies is as a reinforcement —as done in applying the Premack Principle. To engage in certain higher probability behaviors the attendant must first engage in other lower probability behaviors. If the daily schedule could be divided into high probability (duties attendants like to engage in) and low probability behaviors (duties attendants do not particularly like) and alternate them with low probability behaviors preceding the high probability ones and then engaging them in the high probability behaviors contingent upon first completing the low probability ones, the day's work might go faster and more efficiently and be less monotonous as well. If the existing behaviors that constitute the daily duties of the attendant are all low probability behaviors, the attendants' duties could be reorganized and some high probability behaviors or desirable duties created to provide this form of reinforcement. When arranged in this fashion the entire daily schedule could be viewed as one long chain from the time the attendant arrived until she went home. The same contingency arrangements should also apply to other personnel.

The main form of reinforcement available in an institutional setting, attention or recognition, can be used by both supervisors and subordinates to shape and maintain behavior in one another. When teaching shaping principles to an attendant, for example, correct performance can be reinforced with a nod indicating correctness, a smile, or a vocal "That's right!" or "That's correct!" or "Well done!" Physical contact, such as a pat on the back, can serve a similar function. Such reinforcements should be presented in a natural manner which may suggest to the recipient that the reinforcer is sincere. It goes without saying that they should be given with the appropriate emotional affect that normally accompanies such verbal reinforcement. Other forms of recognition may be based on competition, where the outstanding attendant of the week or the month receives some type of commendation or simply has her name and picture with an appropriate caption posted in a conspicuious place. The disadvantage of this type of reinforcement is that only one individual can receive it at a time, and the award or recognition may even be aversive to some of the persons who do not receive it, particularly if it a highly reinforcing event for them.

For attention from a supervisor to acquire greater reinforcement value and thus be more effective, the supervisor should attempt to increase her own reinforcement value through conditioning. Attention is a generalized reinforcement, and as such, its reinforcement value should be positively related to the value of other reinforcements with which it is associated—in this case, the person giving the attention. Attention from a supervisor who is well-liked and respected should be greater than from one who is less well-liked and less respected. Respect is probably based on such vague concepts as "being fair," "consistent," and "effective in" or "good at" one's job. Being liked is probably determined, to a great extent by the interest the supervisor takes in the subordinate and the extent to which he permits the subordinate to know he likes him, is concerned about him, and feels he is a worthwhile person. A supervisor who takes the time to stop by each day to chat with and show a personal interest in his subordinates should be more effective as a generalized reinforcer than one who does not, particularly if he is also already liked and respected. It also helps if the subordinate feels the supervisor "understands" his problems relevant to his work.

One factor which may be related to being liked is the degree of communication that exists both within and between supervisors and subordinates. Once subordinates begin to feel supervisors do not understand their problems, they may stop communicating with them, and this may lead to the development of factions—the subordinates versus the supervisors. This often occurs when a conflict or disagreement develops between supervisors and subordinates or when some individual or group of subordinates are penalized for violating an institutional rule.

One way to decrease the possibility that communications will break down is to have weekly meetings in which supervisors and subordinates can get together and let the subordinates (and their supervisors) air their views and their grievances openly and frankly without fear of reprisal. This is an excellent opportunity for supervisors to show subordinates that they both understand and are sympathetic to their problems even if they do not agree with them completely. It also is an opportunity to let subordinates express their grievances toward one another, grievances that invariably develop and recur, and work them out in the meeting. Such discussions may and should lead to some changes in institutional policy concerning ward operation— if it becomes obvious that either some rule is obsolete or that no rule or convention has been created to deal with certain problems. If subordinates are allowed to contribute to the development of institutional policy they may be more willing to abide by it as well as being reinforced for participation in policy development. It may be that in many cases they are better qualified to develop institutional policy than anyone else if the problems are related to ward function.

The more attendants and other ward personnel can be given responsibility to make decisions related to carrying out their own job assignments, the better they may like their work. In addition, if they can be shown the value of their own presence for the ward operation as a whole, i.e., see clearly the role they play and the specific contributions they make, they should feel more worthwhile and enjoy their jobs even more.

By letting attendants know as well as showing them he is trying to keep working conditions as good as possible, the supervisor should improve his image with them and be better liked and more respected, thus contributing to his generalized reinforcement value, or making attention from him a more effective conditioned reinforcement.

As with residents, either extinction or punishment may be necessary to eliminate undesirable behavior in institutional personnel. Punishment can be in the form of disapproval from a supervisor, or "chewing him out," or something as extreme as docking the employee's pay. Firing an employee has no value as far as changing his behavior on the job at the institution. Side effects of punishment should be carefully considered before using it. The clever supervisor will attempt to change undesirable behavior in subordinates by conditioning incompatible responses.

STIMULUS CONTROL

Developing appropriate stimulus control in institutional personnel is probably the greatest training problem. They already have most of the behavior in their repertoires that is relevant to their duties as attendants or ward supervisors. The greatest problem, therefore, is teaching them just what they should do under different circumstances. If they are new inexperienced employees the problem is one of evaluating their relevant behavioral repertoires, developing whatever necessary behavior appears to be missing, and bringing all relevant behavior under appropriate stimulus control. If they are seasoned experienced institutional personnel the problem is greater. Most of their relevant behavior is already under institutional stimulus control and much of it may be inappropriate from a behavior modification point of view. Now, the problem is one of eliminating old stimulus control and substituting new stimulus control. Unfortunately the old stimulus control may be rather difficult to eliminate. "Old timers" first have to be convinced that the new method is more effective than the techniques they are accustomed to using. Some are very skeptical about innovations. In addition, even if they are convinced the new method is better, old patterns of responding to specific ward stimuli still have to be replaced by new ones and this may be a rather difficult time consuming task. It seems far simpler simply to develop only new institutional stimulus control over the behavior of ward personnel rather than first eliminating the former institutional stimulus control and replacing it with the control selected by those training personnel. If one is training experienced personnel the problem is actually one of conditioning incompatible responses to stimuli controlling inappropriate behavior. The stimulus condition remains the same, i.e., children have to be cleaned, dressed, fed, their elimination activities have to be dealt with, and some kinds of daily activities have to be generated. Formerly, the seasoned attendant washed and dressed the retardate when he got up in the morning, led him to breakfast and either fed him or let him finger feed himself, then returned him to the ward where he was required to spend most of the day sitting relatively quietly on a bench or in a chair, and changed him when he soiled or wet himself. Under the innovative conditions she would wake the retardate in the morning, let him wash and dress himself with little or no assistance, let him eat his breakfast with a spoon, perhaps generate some social activities such as different kinds of games which he could play with peers, perhaps let him do some simple ward chores, and let him go to the toilet when elimination was impending. All of these innovative retardate responses are incompatible with the old responses. Whether they will occur after the retardate is trained depends primarily on the attendant and her supervisor. They must allow the retardate to carry out these new behaviors and may even need to reinforce them when they occur. If the attendant locks the bathroom door the retardate cannot eliminate in the toilet. Some response incompatible with bathroom door locking needs to be conditioned in attendants. If the attendant who has just learned the new behavioral control techniques finds, following her reassignment to a ward, that her supervisor does not want the new procedure to be used on the ward, she will probably revert to the old established patterns of resident control. Responses incompatible with coercing newly trained attendants to use only old traditional behavioral control procedures need to be established in ward supervisors if new behavioral control techniques are to be used effectively.

Verbal and behavioral procedures are the primary ways stimulus control is established in personnel. Some stimulus control can be brought about through textual materials—reading, and through lectures, discussions, audio-visual demonstrations, and live demonstrations. The other, and probably more effective way to bring about stimulus control is by having the attendant actually attempt to control a retardate's behavior and be both shaped and reinforced by a trainer. Because stimulus control develops as a result of behavior being reinforced in the presence of a stimulus, it is important that the trainer provide reinforcement to the trainee for appropriate behavior under a given set of stimulus conditions. The attendant will, of course, provide some of her own reinforcement if she knows her own behavior is appropriate to the situation, but she initially needs knowledge of results from the trainer to inform her she is correct, and she still needs reinforcement from her trainer to further facilitate her behavior shaping and later from her supervisor to insure the appropriate behavior will be maintained.

It would be highly useful to catalog as many institutional situations in which attendants interact with retardates as possible, work out appropriate solutions to these situations, have attendant trainees first role-play these situations with other attendant trainees playing the role of patients, and then repeat the process in the ward situation with residents with a trainer available to provide knowledge of results or reinforcement for appropriate trainee behavior.

Summary

This chapter has reviewed behavior modification techniques based on principles of operant conditioning. From this point of view, the mentally retarded person is depicted as one with a relatively impoverished behavioral repertory as compared with a "normal" person. In addition, much of the behavior within his repertory is under inappropriate stimulus control. The task for the behavior modifier is to build up the retardate's behavioral repertory and bring all behavior under appropriate stimulus control. New behavior is generated employing shaping and reinforcement principles, while reinforcement and stimulus control principles are used to bring behavior under appropriate stimulus control. To accelerate desirable behavior positive reinforcement is recommended while punishment is suggested for decelerating undesirable behavior.

The evidence to date indicates that operant conditioning procedures constitute an effective behavioral control technique. However, the extent to which the behavior modifier will be effective with these procedures will depend upon how carefully he identifies the terminal behavior he wants to shape, how well he determines the retardate's existing relevant behavioral repertory and the effectiveness with which he programs the existing behavior so it will approximate and finally become the desired terminal behavior. If the behavior modifier finds he is not successful, he should reassess his analysis of the behavior problem and carefully reevaluate his programming procedures. Most behavior modification fails because of improper programming.

References

Ayllon, T. Intensive treatment of psychotic behavior by stimulus satiation and food reinforcement. *Behavior Research Therapy,* 1963, 1, 53–61.

Azrin, N. H. and W. C. Holz. Punishment. In Honig, W. K. (Ed.), *Operant Behavior: Areas of Research and Application.* New York, Appleton-Century-Crofts, 1966.

Baer, D. M.; R. F. Peterson, and J. A. Sherman. The development of imitation by reinforcing behavioral similarity to a model. *Journal of Experimental Analysis of Behavior,* 1967, 10, 405–416.

Baer, D. M. and M. M. Wolf. The entry into natural communities of reinforcement. Paper read at meeting of American Psychological Association, Washington, D. C., 1967.

Baumeister, A. and R. Klosowski. An attempt to group toilet train severely retarded patients. *Mental Retardation,* 1965, 3, 24–26.

Bensberg, G. J. (Ed.) *Teaching the Mentally Retarded,* Atlanta, Southern Regional Education Board, 1965.

Bensberg, G. J.; C. N. Colwell, and R. H. Cassell. Teaching the profoundly retarded self-help activities by behavior shaping techniques. *American Journal of Mental Deficiency,* 1965, 69, 674–679.

Birnbrauer, J. S. Personal communication, 1967.

Cofer, C. N. and M. H. Appley. *Motivation: Theory and Research.* New York, John Wiley and Sons, Inc., 1964.

Cohen, H. L. and J. Filipizak. An application of contingency programming to mass education in a college classroom. In Cohen, H. L.; I. Goldiamond, J. Filipizak, and R. Pooley. (Eds.) *Training Professionals in Procedures for the Establishment of Educational Environments.* Silver Springs, Md., Educational Faculty Press, 1968.

Colwell, C. N. The role of operant techniques in cottage and ward life programs. Paper read at meeting or the American Association on Mental Deficiency, Chicago, 1966.

Dayan, M. Toilet training retarded children in a state residential institution. *Mental Retardation,* 1964, 2, 116–117.

Ellis, N. R. Toilet training the severely defective patient, an S-R reinforcement analysis. *American Journal of Mental Deficiency,* 1963, 68, 98–103.

Ferster, C. B. Positive reinforcement and behavioral deficits of autistic children. *Child Development,* 1961, 32, 437–456.

————. Arbitrary and natural reinforcement. Paper read at meeting of the American Association for the Advancement of Science, Washington, D. C., 1966.

Ferster, C. B. and M. K. DeMyer. A method for the experimental analysis of the behavior of autistic children. *American Journal of Orthopsychiatrics,* 1962, 32, 89–98.

Ferster, C. B. and M. C. Perrott. *Behavior Principles.* New York, Appleton-Century-Crofts, 1968.

Ferster, C. B. and B. F. Skinner. *Schedules of Reinforcement.* New York, Appleton-Century-Crofts, 1957.

Fuller, P. R. Operant conditioning of a vegetative human organism. *American Journal of Psychology.* 1949, 62, 587–599.

Giles, D. K. and M. M. Wolf. Toilet training institutionalized severe retardates: An application of operant behavior modification techniques. *American Journal of Mental Deficiency,* 1966, 70, 766–780.

Girardeau, F. L. and J. E. Spradlin. Token rewards in a cottage program. *Mental Retardation,* 1964, 2, 345–351.

Goldiamond, I. Behavior analysis and programming. Paper read at symposium held at the Veterans Administration Hospital, Breckville, Ohio, 1968.

Gorton, C. E. and H. H. Hollis. Redesigning a cottage unit for better programming and research for the severely retarded. *Mental Retardation,* 1965, 3, 16–21.

Hamilton, J. and M. A. Standahl. Suppression of stereotyped screaming behavior in a profoundly retarded institutionalized female. *Journal of Experimental Child Psychology,* 1967.

Hamilton, J.; L. Stephens, and P. Allen. Controlling aggressive and destructive behavior in severely retarded institutionalized residents. *American Journal of Mental Deficiency,* 1967, 71, 852–856.

Henriksen, K. and R. Doughty. Decelerating undesired meal-time behavior in a group of profoundly retarded boys. *American Journal of Mental Deficiency,* 1967, 72, 40–44.

Herzberg, F. *Work and the Nature of Man.* New York, World Publishing Co., 1966.

Hollis, J. H. Development of perceptual motor skills in a profoundly retarded child. Paper read at the 90th annual meeting of the American Association on Mental Deficiency, Chicago, Ill., May, 1966.

Kish, G. B. Studies of sensory reinforcement. In Honig, W. K. (Ed.), *Operant Behavior: Areas of Research and Application.* New York, Appleton-Century-Crofts, 1966.

Lawson, R. and L. S. Watson. Learning in the rat (*rattus novegicus*) under positive versus negative reinforcement with incentive conditions controlled. *Ohio Journal of Science,* 1963, 63, 89–91.

Lent, J. R. Modification of food stealing behavior of an institutionalized retarded subject. Parsons Working Paper No. 175, 1967.

————. Mimosa cottage: experiment in hope. *Psychology Today,* 1968a, 2, 51–58.

————. Personal communication, 1968b.

Lindsley, O. R. Direct measurement and prosthesis of retarded behavior. *Journal of Education,* 1964, 147, 62–81.

Lovaas, I.; G. Freitag, M. Kinder, B. Rubenstein, B. Schaeffer, and J. Simmons. Developing social behaviors in autistic children using electric shock. Paper read at meeting of American Psychological Association, Los Angeles, 1964.

Moore, R. and I. Goldiamond. Errorless establishment of visual discrimination using fading procedures. *Journal of Experimental Analysis of Behavior,* 1964, 7, 269–272.

Morse, W. H. Intermittent reinforcement. In Honig, W. K. (Ed.). *Operant Behavior: Areas of Research and Application.* New York, Appleton-Century-Crofts, 1966.

Nicosia, D. Teaching the profoundly and severely retarded. Symposium held at Pinecrest State School, Pineville, La., 1968.

Powell, J. and N. Azrin. The effects of shock as a punisher for cigarette smoking. *Journal of Applied Behavioral Analysis,* 1968, 1, 63–71.

Premack, D. Toward empirical behavioral laws: I. Positive reinforcement. *Psychological Review,* 1959, 66, 219–233.

Reese, E. P. *The Anlysis of Human Operant Behavior.* Dubuque, Iowa, Wm. C. Brown Company, 1966.

Sidman, M. Personal communication, 1967.

Sidman, M. and L. Stoddard. Programming perception and learning for retarded children. In Ellis, N. R. (Ed.), *International Review of Mental Retardation.* New York, Academic Press, 1967.

Skinner, B. F. *Science and Human Behavior.* New York, MacMillan, 1953.

Smaltz, J. Personal Communication, 1968.

Spradlin, J. E., F. L. Girardeau, and E. Corte. Fixed ratio and fixed internal behavior of severely and profoundly retarded subjects. *Journal of Experimental Child Psychology,* 1965, 4, 340–353.

Suchman, R. G. and T. Trabasso. Color and form preference in young children. *Journal of Experimental Child Psychology,* 1966, 3, 177–187.

Tate, B. G. and G. S. Baroff. Aversive control of self-injuring behavior in a psychotic boy. *Behavioral Research Therapy,* 1966, 4, 281–287.

Terrace, H. S. Discrimination learning with and without "errors." *Journal of Experimental Ananlysis of Behavior,* 1963a, 6, 1–28.

————. Errorless transfer of a discrimination across two continua. *Journal of Experimental Analysis of Behavior,* 1963b, 6, 223–246.

————. Stimulus control. In Honig, W. K. (Ed.). *Operant Behavior: Areas of Research and Application.* New York, Appleton-Century-Crofts, 1966.

Touchette, P. E. The effects of a graduated stimulus change on the acquisition of a simple discrimination in severely retarded boys. *Journal of Experimental Analysis of Behavior,* 1968, 11, 39–48.

Watson, L. S. The relationship between discrimination and stimulus generalization in severely retarded children. Unpublished doctoral dissertation, Ohio State University, 1966.

————. Application of operant conditioning techniques to institutionalized severely and profoundly retarded children. *Mental Retardation Abstracts,* 1967, 4, 1–18.

————. Applications of behavior-shaping devices to training severely and profoundly mentally retarded children in an institutional setting. *Mental Retardation*, In Press, 1968a.

————. Unpublished research conducted at Columbus State School, 1968b.

Watson, L. S.; L. Clevenger, M. Hundziak, and C. Sanders. Transfer of training of ward-recognition performance by brain-injured mentally retarded children. Paper read at Great Lakes Regional Meeting of American Association on Mental Deficiency, Columbus, Ohio, 1964.

Watson, L. S.; R. Orser, and C. Sanders. Reinforcement preferences of severely mentally retarded children in a generalized reinforcement context. *American Journal of Mental Deficiency*, 1968, 72, 748–756.

Watson, L. S. and C. Sanders. Stimulus control with severely and profoundly retarded children under varying stimulus conditions. Paper read at meeting of the American Association on Mental Deficiency, Chicago, 1966.

————. Reinforcement preferences of severely and profoundly mentally retarded children. Paper read at Gatlingburg Conference, Gatlingburg, Tenn., 1968.

Whaley, D. Eliminating self-injuring behavior in children. Paper read at symposium at Veterans Administration Hospital, Breckville, Ohio, 1967.

White, J. C. and D. J. Taylor. Noxious conditioning as a treatment for rumination. *Mental Retardation*, 1967, 5, 30–33.

Whitney, L. R. and K. E. Barnard. Implications of operant learning theory for nursing care of the retarded child. *Mental Retardation*, 1966, 4, 26–29.

Zeaman, D. and B. J. House. The role of attention in retardate discrimination. In Ellis, N. R. (Ed.). *Handbook of Mental Deficiency*. New York, McGraw-Hill, 1963.

Functions and Problems of
Social Workers in Institutions
for the Mentally Retarded

Social workers, like others in the helping professions, have recently shown much more interest in the problem of mental retardation. Where once the prevailing attitude was a pessimistic feeling that mental retardation was a hopeless condition, now there is an optimistic conviction that many of the retarded and most of their families can be helped. The current emphasis on comprehensive, community-based services is particularly appealing to social workers, and increasing numbers of them are participating in the development of new programs and services designed for retarded persons and their families.

The enthusiastic emphasis given to the development of these new community services may overshadow the importance of the older institutional programs. But institutions are changing too, and it is certainly possible to make a case for the "new" institution as a most exciting setting for the practice of social work in the area of mental retardation.

Supporting evidence is found, in part, in the great diversity of services that are performed by social workers in institutions for the mentally retarded, necessitated by the great variety of problems that need social work help.

This diversity of services contributes to making the institution an interesting place to practice social work. But the real excitement of working in the institution is found in the challenges that are related to the nature of the client and to the problems of the interdisciplinary setting.

Social Work Services to Applicants, Residents and Their Families

Services in this category can be most efficiently considered in a chronological sequence, that is, services offered to the retarded person and his family from the time of the initial contact through final separation from the institution.

PREADMISSION SERVICES

Institutional placement *per se* should not even be considered until the necessary preparation has been accomplished. To ignore or avoid this issue is simply to invite problems such as abortive placements, complaints, and generally disillusioned parents and unhappy residents.

The purposes of preadmission services include: helping parents to understand the facts of their child's condition and to deal with the emotional and social problems related to having a defective child; assisting them in realistic planning, and in considering institutional placement in relation to their plans; interpreting fully the positive and negative aspects of placement; and helping the family to implement their decision. Many activities are subsumed in this brief listing, and the specific nature of the preadmission service offered is determined by the individual family's needs.

Most of these services are needed by virtually every family with a retarded child, but it may be questioned whether the institution's social work staff should be responsible for providing them. Where community facilities for comprehensive diagnosis and family counseling are available, it may be more appropriate to refer families to them for needed service. Certainly, the institution's social workers should encourage contacts between community agencies and families with retarded children, both in regard to preadmission counseling and for possible exploration of alternative resources for care and treatment of the retarded child. But the unfortunate fact is that some community agencies are not very objective when it comes to helping parents consider institutional placement; perhaps because they feel the pressure of other clients clamoring for their service, or because they share with much of the general public the lingering notion that retarded children *should* be institutionalized, community agencies occasionally recommend placement before a family is ready for it. Talking with a bewildered parent, who appears at the institution's doorstep to see about placing his child because "they" at some hospital or clinic or at some school or community agency told him he should do so, is a common experience for most institutional social workers. Even if he fervently believes that comprehensive preadmission counseling should be offered by community agencies, the institution's social worker must be ready to accept the reality of an "unprepared" parent.

Additionally, there are a few instances in which there is no appropriate resource to help a family consider institutional placement. Fortunately, community resources are proliferating rapidly, but in some states, particularly in rural areas, no resource is available to provide comprehensive diagnosis and knowledgeable counsel about the problem of mental retardation. In these cases, the institution often has to fill the gap.

Thus, the first task of the social worker, at the time of the initial contact with a family, is to find out "where the client is" in the process of understanding and dealing with the problem of having a defective child. In many cases, the parents will have made the rounds of diagnostic centers, will have received some help in dealing with their emotional reactions, will have thought a great deal about the long-range needs of their child, and will have been constructively using various resources in the community to meet these needs. For various reasons, they feel that the time for institutional placement has arrived, and they come seeking confirmation for and implementation of a decision they have already been helped to make.

In cases such as these, the social worker may be able to proceed directly to planning the details of placement by recognizing and accepting the preparation these parents have already received. In other cases, the "they-told-me-to-come-here" type and those in which no resource for counseling is available, the institution's social workers must assume the responsibility for interpreting the facts of the child's condition to the family and helping them to deal with their emotional reactions.

A veritable glut of material has been written about the emotional reactions of parents of retarded children. Most of it consists of descriptive reports based on the clinical observations of the various authors, and these are largely focused on such topics as guilt and rejection (either overt or disguised, as in over-protection). While many parents undoubtedly do manifest these emotional reactions, the literature's repeated emphasis on such behavior has led many social workers to the pseudo-panacea of "acceptance" as the key to absolving guilt and mitigating or eliminating rejection. Olshansky (1962) has discussed the consequences of social workers' uncritical use of "acceptance" as a treatment technique. In general, it may be said that the inevitable conflict between two basic social values—that all expectant parents should want a normal, healthy baby (and should *not* want a defective one), but that all parents are supposed to accept and love the child they have, regardless of his normality—is so complex, that, as Heilman (1950) notes, "parents have a right to be disturbed."

Once these emotional responses have been recognized, if not "resolved," the social worker can begin to help these families to consider institutional placement. There is also much that has been written about those factors which make institutional placement appropriate or helpful, or which affect the parents' decision to seek placement. Once again, much of this work is opinion based on the author's clinical observation. There are also, however, the extensive sociological analyses of Bernard Farber and his associates (Farber, 1959; Farber, *et al.,* 1960).

Farber's staff studied 268 families in which there was a severely retarded child. They identified several variables which were associated with the family's reaction to the "crisis" of having a retarded child and with their willingness to place the child in an institution. The most important of these variables were: age and sex of the retarded child; social status of the family; relationships between the defective child and his siblings; and the degree of marital integration of the parents, defined as their agreement on family values and their coordination of family goals. A few of the more significant findings were that in infancy and early childhood the presence of a retarded son had the greater emotional impact on fathers, with sons and daughters being equal in emotional impact on mothers; in later childhood and beginning adolescence, however, the emotional impact was greater on mothers and was greater for sons than for daughters. In families of high social status, fathers were more willing to institutionalize the child than were mothers; in low social status families, mothers of retarded sons were more willing to institutionalize their child than were mothers of retarded daughters.

These and the rest of Farber's findings clearly indicate that a parent's decision to consider placing his child in an institution is the result of a dynamic interaction of several factors, and that the importance of any one factor can vary from situation to situation and from time to time. The major implication of these findings for the institution's social worker is that he must be careful not to overgeneralize in helping parents consider their need for placement; rather, he must help each family to look at those factors in their particular situation which are relevant to this decision. To the decision-making process the social worker contributes a factual explanation of what the institution can and cannot do for a family and how this relates to the family's goals and needs. Reaching a decision in this way challenges and can eliminate unrealistic expectations and help to avoid undermining the parents' sense of responsibility for their child. It is important for the social worker to be aware that institutional placement of a child was once described as "putting him away," with the connotation of abdication or termination of parental responsibility. It is vitally important that this notion be dispelled; the social worker must assure the parent that his rightful responsibility does not cease with placement. The stress during this preadmission phase is on helping the parents make *their* decision regarding placement.

There is another group of parents for whom many of these aspects may be irrelevant. The existence of the disadvantaged, or lower-class group of parents, especially those for whom institutional placement of their child is not a voluntary act, is virtually unrecognized in the literature, but they should be a primary concern to the institution's social work staff. For example, a child may have been neglected or physically abused, so that a welfare department has intervened and removed him from his parents' custody; an older child may have been involved in some delinquent behavior and placed under the jurisdiction of a probation department. Even when parental rights have not been removed by a court, community agencies, especially those concerned with law enforcement, may be able to exert considerable pressure on a poor family to place their child in the institution.

In cases such as these, there may be no preadmission service to the family involved. Where there has been court action, the institution obviously has little choice other than to work with the agency to which custody has been awarded. Unfortunately, some of these agencies may have a very antagonistic attitude toward the child's parents and may discourage or even try to prevent the family from establishing any contact with the institution. In those few cases in which the disadvantaged family does visit the institution before placement, the nature of the social worker's service may be considerably different.

Many of these children will be only mildly retarded, and the family may not perceive that there is anything "wrong" with their child. Should the social worker attempt to explain the child's condition to them? Perhaps so, but he should also realize that often the mild degree of retardation of the child is not really the reason he is being placed; it simply serves to help the community agency decide which resource could be used for the care and supervision of the child. The fact of retardation is somewhat irrelevant, and it could be legitimately argued that no good purpose will be served by a lengthy explanation of this condition to the parents; this is not the primary reason their child is being placed in the institution, and they know it. Further, how realistic is it to think in terms of helping these parents "reach a decision" about placement when the fact is that they really have little or no choice in the matter?

There are two major reasons why these families should be a primary concern for the institution's social work staff. First, except for the very few cases of extreme pathology, a continued relationship is probably meaningful to both the parent and the child, and such a relationship is legitimate regardless of what caused the placement. That is, the right of a parent and his child to maintain some relationship should not be abrogated by institutional placement of the child, even though it may have been entirely appropriate and very necessary for the child to be removed from the home. A second reason for concern is that it is precisely this group of youngsters who have the most potential for return to the community through vocational training programs. Having maintained contact with the family throughout the placement is indispensable when the time comes to consider placing the child outside the institution; for example, factors may have changed so that the home is now a suitable place to which he may return.

Once the decision for placement has been made, voluntarily or otherwise, the social worker participates with other staff members, most frequently psychologists and physicians, in evaluating the application for admission. In most cases, the applicant's mental retardation will already be well documented, and this aspect of the determination of eligibility will be rather automatic. Depending upon what the institution's admission policy is, there will be a few cases in which eligibility is doubtful, either because the applicant's measured intelligence is near the upper limit accepted by the institution or for various other reasons. In these cases, consideration of other variables may determine whether he is to be declared eligible for admission. School or community problems, poor academic achievement, and the nature of the family situation are some of the factors that may be important in influencing this decision. The social worker has an obviously important role to play in these cases, both in gathering important information about the client from schools, clinics, and all other resources, and in contributing his understanding of the total social situation.

Some institutions routinely provide a diagnostic evaluation of all applicants; others do this only when there is no diagnostic information available from other sources and there is no other way for the applicant to get an evaluation. The social worker naturally plays a part in this process, contributing information to the diagnostic team and interpreting findings and conclusions to the family. In those cases in which it is decided that the applicant is not eligible, the social worker has a special responsibility to refer the family to an appropriate resource for further service.

Once eligibility has been determined, and all application procedures are completed, there is usually a waiting period, sometimes lengthy, before space becomes available to admit the applicant. This waiting is often a very difficult time for the family; they have agonizingly made the decision to institutionalize their child, and they may feel a need to get it over with as quickly as possible. Too, the family may have waited until a real crisis developed before they decided to apply for placement. The social worker will need to help the family throughout the waiting period, perhaps referring them to other agencies for short-term help or emergency service if needed. The social worker may face the troublesome problem of determining the order for admission of applicants. The pressure is often great, from agencies and parents alike, to provide admission as soon as possible. Many institutions maintain a separate top-priority waiting list in an attempt to provide admission first to those who need it most. Social workers should be responsible for adopting criteria for priority status.

THE ADMISSION PROCESS

The admission process actually begins before the applicant comes to stay at the institution. When the social work staff determines that space will soon become available to accommodate an applicant, the family should be notified, beginning the process of preparing for admission. Some sort of final orientation and information exchange session should be scheduled a few weeks before the actual date of admission. Many institutions schedule groups of parents for such sessions, and a group situation can be very helpful to many parents if handled properly. At these meetings, parents can ask questions and can be informed on institutional policies and procedures. Tours to various places on the campus can be provided, and parents should especially have the opportunity to visit the living unit to which their child will be assigned and to meet the child care workers who will be caring for him. This may help to relieve some of the parents' natural anxiety by reducing some of the "unknown" factors of placement, and it may provide an opportunity for some informal sharing of information about the child which will later help the child care workers to establish a relationship with him.

In addition to the group question-and-answer session and the tour, each family should be seen privately to permit them to bring up any questions or problems they want to discuss and to give the social worker the opportunity to update and complete his case record. Unfortunately, it is the practice in many institutions to wait until the day of actual admission of the child to try to exchange information with parents. Such a last minute information exchange is limited by the tension, anxiety, and emotional impact of the separation. Parents may not be able to concentrate on asking their questions or on giving important information. There is little reason for this torturous ordeal; if parents can be interviewed before the actual date of admission, why cannot this exchange of information take place then? In addition to seeing the social worker, the parents might also be scheduled for interviews with a staff physician, with the business office, and with anyone else whom they need to meet; the ubiquitous multitude of forms could be completed, so that all of the "work" of admission involving the parents would be completed.

It is important also to involve the child to the maximum extent possible in preparation for admission. Even the rather severely retarded child, who could not understand a verbal explanation of placement, could possibly be helped to prepare for it by a preadmission visit to the unit on which he will be living, by helping or watching the parent pack his clothing, and by other such nonverbal activities. (See Adamson, *et al.,* 1964, for an elaboration of some methods of preparation). The moderately or mildly retarded child should be able to profit from these methods and from a simple explanation of what his life will be like in the institution. This may be difficult for some parents, and the social worker should be prepared to give them some suggestions, but it is probably very important to the child's initial adjustment that he have some degree of understanding, however limited, about what is happening to him.

If these procedures are followed, then there is little work to be done with the parents on the day of admission. The social worker can simply be supportive to the parents throughout the separation process and can observe their reaction to the separation for any possibly significant implications. Many parents experience a post-placement syndrome of relief that leads to guilt, and the social worker can help them to anticipate this reaction by discussing it with them. The child too may be able to understand the social worker's explanation of how he will probably feel during the first few days of placement.

The first few days or even weeks after the child is admitted can logically be considered a part of the admission process. There should be some contact between the institution and the parents and soon after admission, possibly initiated by the social worker. There may not be much that he can say, but the reassurance of the first letter from the institution can be very meaningful to the parent. Likewise, the social worker's visit with the child, perhaps on the day after admission, can be very important. The child's association of the social worker with his parents might be comforting during this difficult period.

POST-ADMISSION SERVICES

Social workers in institutional settings have a long tradition of services to the families of the institution's residents. Much of this service is implied in the frequently used description of the social worker as the "liaison" between the institution and the family. Parents' letters regarding their children's adjustment and progress are important; because they often come in torrents, they may be handled too routinely by the social work staff. Brief reflection on the importance of such communication will usually justify the considerable amount of time spent in answering this correspondence. Social workers also continue to offer casework help to parents, as appropriate and needed, and are responsible for communicating to them the staff decisions and plans that concern their child. This should be a two-way street; the parents should be kept involved in the planning for *their* child. Their ideas should be important to the staff and realistically may have some effect on the decisions reached.

Perhaps the most important activity of the social worker in his service to parents is in the area of visiting. Parent visiting is now widely accepted as the most important element in maintaining the family relationship essential for good adjustment of parents and child (Porter, 1961; Tarjan, 1966). In most institutions the social work staff is assigned the responsibility for administering visiting policy, and their recognition of the importance of visits should lead to careful consideration and planning of them. The timing of the first visit deserves special consideration. Social workers have generally assumed that the first parent visit should be very soon after admission, basing their feeling on a psychoanalytic interpretation of separation and its meaning to the child and to the parents. Some institutions, however, prohibit parent visits for an arbitrary number of days or weeks immediately after admission, on the assumption that both the child and the parents need some time to adjust to the new situation. There does not seem to be any research evidence to categorically substantiate either position, and it is probable that numerous factors affect the timing of the first parent visit in such a way that decisions can be made only on an individual basis. In any event, the first few visits after admission are particularly important, and the social worker must help prepare the family and the child for the visit and later determine the effect of the visit on both.

In addition to helping families, the institution's social workers give direct service to many of the residents. Obviously there is little that the social worker can do in terms of direct service to profoundly and severely retarded residents of the institution. He may visit their living units to keep informed of their adjustment; he may help to obtain the assistance of a volunteer "friendly visitor" for some child who seems to need a little extra attention; but social workers generally have no useful service to offer most of these children. For the moderately retarded child, the social worker may expand the services offered to the more severely handicapped to include help in preparing the child for visits, and he may serve by passing along messages from the child's family. In a few cases, casework or group work service may be of help in dealing with adjustment problems, but in most institutions there is probably little direct social work service extended to this group.

One small and very special group of residents deserves special attention and service from the social workers as well as other professionals in the institution. These are children with multiple handicaps, whose physical functioning is perhaps even more limited than their mental abilities, and who, for this reason, may not be able to participate in all the activities and programs that would be available to them on the basis of their mental level alone. For example, the requirements of their physical care may cause some of these children to be placed on living units with children of significantly lower mental ability. The unique problems these children face in adjusting to the institution may demand extra service from the social work staff.

The greatest proportion of direct social work services will be offered to the mildly retarded and borderline group of institutional residents, simply because these residents are more likely to have the kinds of problems that are appropriate for social work service. They are the future vocational training candidates, and social workers can help in assessing their readiness to return to the community and in preparing them for it. Because they are more nearly normal, these residents can be expected to have more problems in adjusting to the impositions of the institutional environment, and the services of the social work staff can be helpful in ameliorating these adjustment problems. By the default of tradition, most of the social worker's service to these residents has been through a casework counseling approach. There is much undeveloped potential in the use of group work methods with the mildly retarded, especially since the failure of retardates in vocational training is widely attributed to problems in interpersonal relationships rather than to inability. Recent interest in group work methods (Begab, 1962; Scheer and Sharpe, 1963; Scheer and Sharpe, 1965) will hopefully be manifested in more group work specialists being added to the social work staffs of institutions for the retarded.

Along with services to parents and direct social work with residents, the third major area of the social worker's responsibility is as a staff member, as a participant on the "team." It is in this team member role that the social worker can best fulfill his obligation to the profoundly and severely retarded and those with multiple handicaps. He can keep the institution's administrators and other staff members aware of the special needs of some of these children, and he can work together with representatives of the institution's various disciplines to develop new programs to meet these needs. The social worker also participates in planning programs for the residents and in making decisions about them. For example, diagnosis of individual cases, including determination of the etiology of the retardation, will usually be the concern of the psychologists and physicians, although the social worker's reports of the child's medical and developmental history and his knowledge of social factors in the child's early life will be necessary and valuable for reaching some conclusions. But when the cause of the child's retardation is presumed to be his cultural-family background or severe environmental deprivation (see Heber, 1961, pp. 39–40), the information provided by the social worker and his evaluation of cultural, familial, and environmental factors is of critical importance. Likewise, in staff planning for residents, especially the mildly retarded who are or may become involved in vocational training programs, the social worker's prognosis for return to the home or success in community adjustment can be very important. The social worker can contribute to the understanding and amelioration of behavior problems through his knowledge of significant cultural and social factors that may be related to the problems; this interpretation of the effects of socio-cultural variables can be especially helpful and important to the nonprofessional child care staff.

The most important contribution of the social worker as an institutional staff member is realized when he leaves his office and goes into the children's living units. The major impact of institutionalization on residents is undoubtedly found in the day-to-day management of them in their living units. Substantiating this conclusion are the observation by Butterfield and Zigler (1965) that institutions vary in social "climate" and their finding that the social climate of an institution can have a significant effect on the residents' performance of certain tasks. Any professional who feels that he can significantly affect an institutionalized child's behavior without confronting directly the nature of the environment in which the child lives daily is engaging in a most futile exercise of unrealistic behavior. Putting a staff-determined program into operation may be less important in effecting a youngster's rehabilitation than how the child care workers on his unit relate to him, whether he is treated as a worthy human being with present assets and even greater future potential, or whether realistic expectations are made of him. In short, the little details of daily living communicate much to the retarded youngster that affects his self-perception, his motivation, and his present adjustment. Thus, the great task of the professional staff of the institution, social workers and others, is to work to influence the institutional milieu. This is achieved not by control or coercion of the child care staff but by the slow process of establishing and maintaining real communication; the professionals must spend time in the living units, not to "check" on the child care staff nor to usurp their responsibilities, but to establish relationships that will permit the communication of knowledge and values in such a way that they can be used by nonprofessional workers.

SERVICES OUTSIDE THE INSTITUTION

A most striking change of the past few years has been the emergence of the social work staff from their formerly rather cloistered existence within the institution. Actually, the social worker's emergence is only one part of a general trend that is now integrating the once-isolated institution into the total pattern of community services for the mentally retarded. This has expanded considerably the scope of the activities of the social work staff, the nature of the clients whom they serve, and the range of problems which they may be called upon to handle.

EXTRAMURAL PLACEMENT SERVICES

One important area of social work activity outside the institution is not really very different from traditional service because the client is the same and the service has existed for quite some time. This is the placement of residents outside the institution. Foster family care of former institutional residents has been provided by a few institutions for some time, but recent data (Morrissey, 1966) indicate that it is still not a part of the institutional program in many states, and in those where it is offered (with the exception of California), it has been extended to only a few children. It is possible that increasingly better funding of enlightened child welfare agencies has led to provision of foster family care to significant numbers of retarded children who never come to the attention of the institution. But, as noted above, some mildly retarded children are still being institutionalized solely because they have inadequate parents; it can hardly be questioned that foster family care of these children would be better from almost any standpoint—psychological, social, and economic. What can be questioned is whether the institutions should develop or expand their own foster family care programs or whether this should be the responsibility of welfare departments. A continuing dialogue over relative responsibility in this matter may be necessary or helpful in some states; however, the children should not have to wait until the final resolution of these problems, and thus some kind of foster family care program is needed in virtually every institution for the retarded. Social workers play an important role in the operation of family care programs where they already exist, and they assume much of the responsibility for developing programs in institutions not now having them. The typical social work functions in such programs are to participate with other members of the institution's staff in selecting children who would be good candidates for foster family care, to find and prepare foster families, and to supervise placements. In states where cooperative agreements between institutions for the retarded and public welfare agencies exist, some of these functions may be shared with a welfare agency's social worker. Small group foster care, with the foster parents being full-time employees of the institution, has been virtually untried (again with the exception of California). Especially with the increased availability of Social Security benefits that may be used to finance placements (Popick, 1966), it must be recognized that development of imaginative foster care programs should be one of the greatest challenges to the institution's social workers in their extramural activities.

At the other end of the age continuum are nursing home placements of the aged institutionalized retarded. Recent amendments to the Social Security Act have increased the availability of funds to support nursing home placements, and there are probably many aged residents in most institutions who could be cared for just as well, if not better, and at possibly lower cost, in such settings. Again, the social work staff of the institution, possibly in cooperation with local Social Security Agency staff and adult service public welfare workers, should participate in screening residents for nursing home placement, in finding nursing homes and interpreting to their staffs the special needs of retarded patients, and in supervising placements.

The third group of former residents of the institution whom the social workers help in extramural settings are those in work placements. Problems of reintegrating mildly retarded youngsters into the community have been discussed by several writers (e.g., Parnicky & Brown, 1964); while these are often the concern of the institution's vocational rehabilitation counselor, social workers may be able to give considerable assistance, both in preparing the residents to move out of the institution and in the supervision of outside living arrangements. Placement may be in the client's own home or in some group setting such as a halfway house. Depending on the division of responsibility between himself and the vocational rehabilitation counselor, the social worker may provide individual or group counseling to help resolve readjustment problems and to promote increased independence.

DISCHARGE

Retardates leave the institution in one of two ways: they return to the home of their parents who, for a variety of reasons (see Mercer, 1966), feel that they no longer need the assistance of the institution in providing care for their child; or they "graduate" into being on their own, through success in vocational training programs. The former group is by far the larger. Some in this group will have been in institutional job-training programs and will be considered employable; others will have varying degrees of dependency on their families for care and support. For all of them, the social worker should provide some sort of follow-up service for a period of a few months, to assist the family in working out problems caused by the return of the retarded child. It may be necessary, and in any case it is extremely important to involve local community agencies in helping the family in its readjustment; thus the basis for future service, if needed, is established. This provides an alternative resource for the family when problems arise that they do not know how to handle; otherwise, they may automatically think of returning the child to the institution. Discharge of the child from the institution should be recommended only after several months of readjustment experience, and optimally should follow full discussion and mutual accord of the family, the institution's social worker, and the social worker from the community agency.

The "graduating" group can be further divided into two categories—the few who actually or for all practical purposes have *no* family and who will be living by themselves or with friends, and the majority who will function rather independently even though they may reside with some family member. Many, perhaps most of these youngsters, will have come from very disadvantaged environments, and whether they live alone or return to the deprived home of some relative will make no practical difference in their need to be able to function independently in the community. In these cases it is even more important that the social worker enlist the aid of some community agency in helping his client during the first few months of independent living; thus is established the channel for future help with those problems that the mentally retarded person will inevitably encounter. Also, these clients should be allowed quite some time to develop security in their ability to function independently before they are discharged from the institution; many months, or even a few years, is not too long for the institution's social worker to observe their ability to handle daily problems. When the former resident has demonstrated the ability to be basically independent and to use constructively and appropriately the services of community agencies for those problems he cannot handle alone, he may be considered for discharge from the institution, again with the knowledge, and hopefully with the full approval of the community agency.

SERVICES TO THE COMMUNITY

Extramural services of the institution's social workers are not limited to former residents. The trend that has developed over the last few years of integrating the institution into the total pattern of services to families with retarded persons has had considerable impact on the activities of the institution's social work staff. Emphasis on the development of comprehensive services for the mentally retarded and elaboration of the concept of a continuum of care and service has led to fresh consideration of what the role of the residential institution should be in the total pattern of services. The institutions have been asked to develop new services and to coordinate their programs with those of community agencies which also serve the mentally retarded. Because of their professional kinship to the social workers who staff these various community agencies and their traditional interest and *expertise* in utilizing community resources, the institution's social workers have been given much of the responsibility of implementing these recent developments. Social workers have served on committees studying gaps in the pattern of services for the mentally retarded and discussing by whom and how these gaps should be filled. They have also tried to define clearly, both for local social agencies and for the general public, the proper role of the institution, explaining its assets and its liabilities, and suggesting when it should and should not be used.

One aspect of the institution's moving into the community is the increased opportunity afforded for the use of community services by the institution's residents. An unfortunate consequence of the institution's long isolation has been a lack of knowledge about and a reluctance to use services which already exist in the community. Indeed, institutions attempted to be self-sufficient by developing their own programs and resources. This may have been necessary at an earlier time, but today the integration of the institution into the total pattern of social services, coupled with the recognition that maintaining contact with the "outside world" is important for most of the institution's residents, seems to have led to some abandonment of striving to achieve self-contained sufficiency, with a concomitant increase in creative use of community resources. For example, increased use of community public and private recreation facilities and programs not only provides pleasureable activity for the children but also serves to facilitate their having some experience outside the institution, laying the basis, for those moderately and mildly retarded residents who may leave the institution in the future, for the ability to use leisure time constructively. Indeed, the latter is one of the most important reasons for use of community resources by the institutions residents: reintegration of the retarded into the community must begin while they are still in the institution. By providing supervised experience in the use of community services and resources, the institution helps to assure that its residents who will be returning to the community will be better prepared to function there. Any number of community resources are important for this purpose. In addition to using recreation facilities and programs, attending services in local churches, depending on public transportation rather than that offered by the institution, and learning how to utilize public sources of information are examples of ways in which the use of community facilities can enrich the experience of the institution's residents. The establishment and expansion of programs designed to provide these experiences may be primarily the responsibility of the institution's social work staff, but the social worker's interest in community resources and his knowledge about the importance of these experiences for the institution's residents should make him a stimulating advocate or advisor of these programs, regardless of who is directly responsible for them.

Another aspect of the institution's moving into the community is the increased use of the institution's resources by appropriate segments of the community. Another aspect of the reintegration of the institution into the community is the development of the idea that the institution, as one part of the total pattern of services to families with retarded persons, should offer certain services to all such families. There is increasing use of the institution's services by families who have no present desire or intention to institutionalize their child, but who simply need some assistance that the institution can offer in dealing with the problem of retardation. Several kinds of services are prominent among those now being extended by the institution to any person in the community. Comprehensive diagnostic evaluation is often included, especially in areas where it is not otherwise available, with the institution offering the medical and psychological diagnostic *expertise* of its staff to any who need it. Complementing the use of community recreational facilities by the institution's residents, there is the opening of the institution's recreational program to those retarded in the community, particularly the teenage and adult retarded who have difficulty or feel discomfort in using the community's facilities. There are even more divergent developments: sheltered workshops and day care centers for the retarded are being established on some institutional campuses; cooperative agreements for exchange of students between the institution's school and the local public school's special education department are being studied. More institutions are developing programs of short-term residential care for families who need it during some crisis or for periodic relief, but who do not need or want full-time institutional placement of their child (Savage, *et al.*, 1967). Social workers on the institution's staff are usually involved in all these developing programs, especially in interpreting to families who do not desire full-time placement what other services the institution can make available to them, in helping the families deal with the problems of retardation that are relevant to the institution's services, and in generally working with some of the retarded persons making use of these services. In this situation too, the social workers may not be primarily responsible for all of these new programs, but the breadth of their activities and the difference in the nature of the problems they are presented with by noninstitutionalized clients significantly affects their work and challenges their creativity.

Problems, Issues, and Conflicts

Descriptions of activities cannot convey all of the excitement and vitality of a work setting; for this, to communicate "what really goes on" in the social work department of the institution, one must examine the problems of practicing social work and of being a social worker in such a setting, the issues of policy that social workers must resolve, and some of the conflicts generated by the dynamism of modern institutions.

IMPLICATIONS OF THE SETTING FOR CASEWORK PRACTICE

Social work students are nurtured on client self-determination; their job, in whatever setting, is to help the client deal with his problem, not to solve it for him. This is certainly appropriate in dealing with the family considering institutionalization of their child: the social worker's task is to help them reach a decision that is their own. But when the client is the mentally retarded resident of the institution, the social worker needs to reassess his technique. As Begab (1959) has noted, the retarded client's limitations in verbal comprehension, capacity for insight, and communicative skills limit the efficacy of the traditional casework counseling approach. The social worker must rely on careful selection of language and frequent repetition in communicating with his retarded client, and he frequently must be rather explicit and directive in giving advice. This limitation of traditional counseling methods is faced not only by social workers, but by psychologists as well. Although a survey of clinical psychologists who were members of AAMD indicated that many did try to provide traditional psychotherapy (Woody and Billy, 1966), others have felt that this was inappropriate (Gardner, 1967), and the merits of a behavior-shaping therapy as a more realistic alternative to insight therapy have been propounded (Doubros, 1966). The client's limitations also affect the making of decisions; the retardate cannot make many of the decisions about his program that must be made; others must make them for him.

The danger in all of this is that the limitations of the client will be overemphasized, and he will not be communicated with at the highest possible level nor allowed to make those decisions that he could. This is partly the result of the social worker's failure to individualize and constantly reevaluate his client, a mistake that is important but one which can be corrected by thoughtful consideration and good supervision. Far more dangerous is the insidious effect of the authoritarian nature of the institutional setting. Even in the best of the "good" institutions, where administrative flexibility and resident self-determination are maximized, there is an atmosphere of authoritarian control and regulation. There are "rules" which must be explicit to be effective for the retarded residents, but which, by their very explicitness, emphasize the distinction between the regulated institution and the "free" outside. Obviously, some degree of authoritarian control is essential to the functioning and purpose of the institution, but it is all too easy for social workers and other staff to internalize this authoritarianism, to unconsciously relate to their clients on the basis of it, to automatically support it when it may not be necessary to do so. Social workers must strive continuously to remain aware of this problem, to strike an appropriate balance between the realistic need of their retarded client for more-than-usual control and direction and the inherently regulating and controlling atmosphere of the institutional setting.

The nature of the setting also causes some problems in working with parents. Many of the families live far from the institution; so there is little possibility of continuing frequent contacts with them. In some instances, this problem can be alleviated by enlisting the aid of social agencies in the parents' home community; it might also help for the social workers to be on duty on weekends and holidays, when parents are most able to come for a visit and a conference. Another technique, probably not widely used, would be to provide the social work staff with sufficient travel funds so that occasional "home visits" could be made, either to individual parents, or to several parents meeting as a small group. But even with the use of these and other methods designed to reduce it, the problem of maintaining a helpful and constructive relationship with distant families is another challenge to the creativity of the institution's social work staff.

A second problem in working with families is found with those socially disadvantaged parents who did not voluntarily place their child in the institution. When placement of a mildly retarded teenager is precipitated by some delinquent act, it is not uncommon, nor is it entirely inappropriate for parents to view the institution as a reformatory. After a certain period of time the parents may feel that their child has paid his debt to society and should be released. In most states institutions have the legal authority to refuse parents' requests for release of their child, even though the institution's authorities may not exercise this prerogative in most cases. When they do, as they might in the case of a disadvantaged family, the social worker has an especially difficult task in maintaining any kind of constructive relationship with the parents. They may not understand the mental retardation aspect of their child's condition or if they do, they still may feel that institutionalization is not required. They may feel that they are being discriminated against because of their impoverished or minority group status and be totally unable to recognize or accept the possibility of any positive gains resulting from the institutional placement. In such cases the social worker may hide behind the legal authority of the institution or he may try to interpret the institution's position to the parents and try to reason with them about it. Whatever the outcome of his efforts, the social worker will again have to face the fact that the authoritarian nature of the institutional setting inescapably affects the practice of his profession, and he must creatively deal with the consequences.

PROBLEMS IN FORMULATING INSTITUTIONAL POLICIES

The social workers on the institution's staff, and particularly the director of the social work department, naturally participate in the formulation of most of the policies that govern the operation of the institution. But there are certain areas of policy making in which they are or should be especially involved, particularly in the area of admission policy. There is, of course, variation among the states in the extent to which admission criteria are defined by statute. There is probably no instance, however, in which these criteria are so specific and complete that there is no discretion left to the institutional administration; thus there is the need for some policies as to who shall be eligible for admission. It has been suggested here and elsewhere (Olshansky, 1966) that parents' expression of need for placement should have considerable influence in this determination of eligibility; that is, if the child meets the standard criteria for a diagnosis of mental retardation, and if the parents, after careful consideration in preadmission conference, feel that placement is the best solution, then the child should be accepted for admission. This view is not unanimously accepted. Others (Jaslow, *et al.,* 1966) have suggested that the institution should define its admission criteria on the basis of some determination of relative need and in relation to the existence of alternatives; thus, the more severely retarded child, especially if he has additional physical handicaps, is seen as more in need of placement than the nonhandicapped mildly retarded child, and children who can be served by community resources are seen as less in need of institutionalization than those who cannot. Those applicants not having a sufficient degree of need, as determined by these objective criteria, would not be considered eligible for admission to the institution. Kott (1967) has questioned this latter position, pointing out that parents' reaction to the problem of mental retardation and their resulting ability to care for their retarded child may not be correlated with any objective measure of the severity of the handicap, and also noting that many mildly retarded youngsters who might be excluded by such criteria have been and can be helped by institutional placement.

But Jaslow and his co-authors probably reflect majority opinion when they note that "institutionalization is not the ideal solution for strictly environmental problems—for instance, problems of parental neglect" (1966, p. 34). Social and law enforcement agencies in the community frequently seek institutional placement for retarded children who are socially disadvantaged, come from inadequate homes, or have been involved in some illegal behavior. Consistency would demand that if these youngsters can be diagnosed as mentally retarded, and if the community agency is legally responsible for them and feels that institutional placement is the best solution to the problem, these children should be accepted for admission to the institution, just as they would be if the parents made the decision. Social workers who feel that such admissions are not appropriate should try to "educate" the responsible community agencies. Or the youngster may be accepted for admission, with the plan to make the placement as short and as intensively therapeutic as possible. The frequency of cases of this type supports the need for comprehensive institutional programs of extramural placement; thus the institution can more appropriately care for those children whom they are forced to accept, but whom they feel are not in need of residential care.

Admission policy is only one of several policy-making areas that the institution's social workers are concerned about and affected by. But it serves as a good illustration of how important policies have many implications—in this case, for application of state statutes, for institution-community agency relations, and for development of institutional programs—for other areas which also affect the interests of the social work staff.

ROLE PROBLEMS

Some of the conflicts for the institution's social workers are caused by problems in defining their "role." This is easy to illustrate by example. For instance, should the institution's social worker be the representative of the parent to the institution or of the institution to the parent? The question implies that there is some inevitable conflict between the interests of the parent and the interests of the institution. A natural response is to deny the existence of such a conflict, to accept at face value the statements of all the institutional brochures that parents are wonderful, necessary, and welcome. In actual fact, the feeling that parents are intruders is frequently found in institutions. They may never express it, but child care workers may feel that parents somehow surrendered their rights when they placed their child in the institution; when this is added to the natural parental feelings that many of the child care workers have for "their" children, then the parent may be viewed as an unentitled interloper. Child care workers may resent parents' suggestions, wondering why this parent, who admitted by placement that he could not care for his own child, should have any right to suggest what might be done for his child or how to do it.

Indeed, the parent must walk a very thin line to avoid condemnation. If he says little in an effort not to interfere, the impression that he has abandoned his parental responsibilities may be reinforced; if, however, to reassure himself or the staff that he is concerned and responsible, he tries to get involved through offering suggestions or by asking questions, he will probably be seen as another "troublemaker parent" who is interfering in the operation of the institution. And, of course, it is true that when too few child care workers have a large group of children to manage, the disruption of a parent's visit can be disconcerting. Many children are upset after their parents visit or after they return to the institution from a few days leave; the extra attention demanded by an upset child may lead some of the child care staff to feel that the child would be better off if the parents never came again, thus reinforcing the perception of the parents as intruders.

For these and other reasons parents' contacts with their children in the institution may be viewed with considerably less than complete enthusiasm by many of the institution's personnel. This may lead to conflicts between these staff members and the social workers, who, because they are responsible for providing services to parents, may be identified with them, and who probably feel some obligation to support the parents and present their side of the problem. These conflicts may not always be intense. If the social workers and the institution's administrators are really committed to the belief that parent-child contacts must and should be maintained, and if they energetically and continually try to communicate this commitment and their rationale for it to all the institution's personnel; then slowly but surely the attitude toward parents can become increasingly positive. In especially difficult cases the social worker may arrange to be present during the visit or the visit can be scheduled for some place other than on the living unit; thus, an angry confrontation may be avoided. But no millenium can be realistically expected, and social workers should anticipate that their support of parents will lead to an occasional conflict with some other staff persons. Indeed, such minor conflicts are so inevitable that an absence of them raises the question of whether the social workers are adequately fulfilling their responsibilities to the parents.

In like manner, the social worker may find himself in conflict over supporting the institution or supporting the retarded resident who is his client. There are among the institution's staff the "bad guys" and the "good guys" (the social workers, naturally, being the forefront of the "good"). This obvious oversimplification may be the way in which the retarded resident views the very real division, in the institution as in society, between those who are chiefly concerned with order, security, and the good of the group as a whole and those whose concern is more for a minimum of restraints, a maximum enhancement of individual development, with an appreciation of individuality and divergence. The task of the administrator is to bring these groups together in some kind of consensus, but the fact that the different points of view do exist suggests that conflicts will develop over who shall "give" how much in the process of arriving at a compromise. The social worker may be able to accept his client's acting-out behavior and may feel that, for casework purposes, he must support him in spite of it; problems will develop if other staff members cannot accept this behavior and either do not understand or will not accept the social worker's position of support for his client.

It is simultaneously very correct and somewhat useless to say that there are merits on both sides of such conflicts and that all the participants should cooperate harmoniously to arrive at mutually acceptable solutions. This is essentially what usually happens, but there are several significant factors that affect this process. Institutions are staffed by very real people, and very real people do not always behave in the way textbooks on institutional administration indicate they should. Differences in ability, desire for personal or departmental power or influence, and characteristics of individual personalities are only a few examples of variables which can have powerful effects on the processes of conflict resolution. The social workers in the institution are affected by these variables just as other personnel are. The conflicts may be resolved and constructive interpersonal and interdepartmental cooperation may be maintained, but the fact that these problems do occasionally arise is yet another contribution to the vitality that flavors social work in the institution.

A third problem of role that the social worker faces is even more basic, namely, showing the institution what social work really is. The institution's administrators will have a general idea of what social workers can and should do, but when it gets to detailed implementation of the social work program, there may be all sorts of clues that they either do not really understand what social work is or they do not accept the social workers' protestations of what their role should be. In a study of role expectations for social workers in a medical setting (Olsen & Olsen, 1967), physicians and social workers, some of whom had worked together for years, were found to have very different perceptions of what the role of the social worker should be. In general and as might be expected, the physicians were willing to grant considerably fewer responsibilities to social workers than the social workers thought they should have. In like manner, the institution's administrators may demonstrate, through work assignments, expectations, and budgetary priorities, that they perceive the function of the social work department differently from what the social workers themselves do. Time and patient reinterpretation are probably the main ingredients in the solution of this problem. Here again, some compromise is probably essential. The professional social worker needs to achieve much of what his training enables and encourages him to do; he also will probably have to forego some of the activities he would like to pursue and to accept some of the chores which are necessary to the operation of the institution. But he will be constantly striving to upgrade his service, to obtain new professional challenges and responsibilities, and in his striving will be the excitement of defining his role in an interdisciplinary setting.

MANPOWER PROBLEMS

Whenever any of the institution's social workers desire some frustrating amusement, they can turn to the recommendations for staffing of social work departments in institutions for the retarded published by the American Association of Mental Deficiency (1964, pp. 81–82). There may be a few institutions which employ the recommended number of social workers; it is undoubtedly true, however, that most do not, and many fall far far short of meeting this standard. This is not to say that the standards themselves are unrealistic; if all of the social work services described above were adequately extended to all of the clients who need and could use them, the size of the staff recommended by the AAMD would probably be found to be minimal. The brutal fact is that because there are too few social workers in most institutions, their service must be curtailed, in its scope or in the number of clients reached.

There are several ways in which social workers can try to compensate for the limitations caused by this shortage of staff; none of them alone can overcome the effects of too few personnel, but taken together they can be significantly helpful. One of these is the use of volunteers. Teenage volunteers have been found to be very useful as social work aides in working with retarded groups (Schreiber & Bromfield, 1966). Some Foster Grandparents programs, funded through the federal government's OEO, have been based on the principle that older adult nonrelative visitors can be constructively used in the care and treatment of the institutionalized retarded. Standifer (1964) has described the creative use of parent volunteers in helping other parents who were considering placement or were making application to the institution for the admission of their child. These are only a few of the ways in which different types of volunteers have been enlisted to complement the services of the social work staff. The pool of potential volunteer manpower has probably not yet been fully tapped, and it behooves the institution's social workers to develop creatively ways in which this resource may be used to alleviate the shortage of personnel.

Of even greater importance is the need to study the services offered by the social work department to determine those which need the attention of professionally trained social workers and those which can be adequately performed by social work aides. This question is not restricted to the institution, rather it is endemic throughout the profession of social work. The institution has much to offer as a resource for experimentation and research on this issue, however, because institutions have always, and to a large extent still do rely on nonprofessional personnel to do social work-type jobs. Indeed, an honest critical assessment would undoubtedly indicate that many, perhaps even most of the activities performed by the social work department's staff can adequately be done by non-professional social work aides. The key to the success of their efforts is found, of course, in the selection, in-service training, and supervision of the aides by qualified and experienced social workers. And there can be more than one type of social work aide: most will probably be bachelor's degree level college graduates, but examination of the social work department's tasks might indicate that some of the work could be performed by persons with junior college, or even only high school education.

The problem is of more than academic interest. Professionally trained social workers are scarce, and scarcity leads to higher salaries. For the amount of money needed to pay five social workers with a master's degree a department could hire six, seven, or possibly even eight social work aides. For large social work departments, this means that, with no additional salary cost, 15 positions designated for professionally trained workers could be expanded to 20 or more by the use of aides. Professionally trained workers could be used in supervisory positions and for direct service in sensitive areas or for cases of special difficulty.

But no major problem is so simply solved, and there are difficulties that must be faced in the use of nonprofessional aides. Differentiation of social work duties into some hierarchy of professionalism suggests that any one client may simultaneously or over a short period of time be receiving services from more than one member of the social work department's staff. Followed to its logical conclusion, a functional division of workers' activities incorporating the degree of professionalism required might lead to one family's having one worker for preadmission counseling, another on admission day, a third for routine post-admission contacts concerning visits and general adjustment of their child, a fourth for any intensive post-admission counseling they might need, and so forth to the ridiculous. Likewise, the child could be served by one worker who specialized in group work, another who regularly visited on the living unit to consult with the child care workers and to handle minor adjustment problems, and a third for intensive counseling or for preparation for an extramural rehabilitation placement. This obvious exaggeration suggests some of the problems in communication and coordination, and in delegation of responsibility for case management that accompany and counterbalance the significant advantages of differential use of the social work department's personnel.

Solving this problem is only one of the challenges that confront the institution's social worker. There are many other challenges, only a few of which have been noted above. The stimulation of groping with these problems is yet another bit of support for our original assertion, that the diversity of the services performed by social workers in institions for the mentally retarded, and the challenge of the problems they encounter in their work make the institution an especially interesting place for them to work and serve.

References

Adamson, W. C., Dorothy F. Ohrenstein, Dolores Lake, and A. Hersh. Separation used to help parents promote growth of their retarded child. *Social Work*, 1964, 9 (4), 60–67.

American Association on Mental Deficiency. Standards for state residential institutions for the mentally retarded. *American Journal of Mental Deficiency*, Monograph Supplement, 1964, 68, No. 4.

Begab, M. J. Some basic principles as a guide to more effective social services. *Mental retardation content in the social work curriculum.* Salt Lake City:

Graduate School of Social Work, University of Utah, 1959, Pp. 33–38. Reprinted in M. Schreiber (Ed.), *Source Book on Mental Retardation for Schools of Social Work*. New York: Selected Academic Readings, 1967.

————. Recent developments in mental retardation and their implication for social group work. *Training School Bulletin*, 1962, 59, 42–52.

Butterfield, E. C. and E. Zigler. The influence of differing institutional social climates on the effectiveness of social reinforcement in the mentally retarded. *American Journal of Mental Deficiency*, 1965, 70, 48–56.

Doubros, S. G. Behavior therapy with high level, institutionalized, retarded adolescents. *Exceptional Children*, 1966, 33, 229–232.

Farber, B. Effects of a severely mentally retarded child on family integration. *Monographs of the Society for Research in Child Development*, 1959, No. 71.

Farber, B., W. G. Jenne, and R. Toigo. Family crisis and the decision to institutionalize the retarded child. *C.E.C. Research Monographs*, 1960, No. 1.

Gardner, W. I. What should be the psychologist's role? *Mental Retardation*, 1967, 5 (5), 29–31.

Heber, R. A manual of terminology and classification in mental retardation. *American Journal of Mental Deficiency*, Monograph Supplement, 1961, (2nd ed.).

Heilman, A. E. Parental adjustment to the dull handicapped child. *American Journal of Mental Deficiency*, 1950, 54, 556–562.

Jaslow, R. I., W. L. Kime, and Martha J. Green. Criteria for admission to institutions for the mentally retarded. *Mental Retardation*, 1966, 4 (4), 2–5.

Kott, M. G. Who sets admission policies? *Mental Retardation*, 1967, 5 (3), 35–36.

Mercer, Jane R. Patterns of family crisis related to reacceptance of the retardate. *American Journal of Mental Deficiency*, 1966, 71, 19–32.

Morrissey, J. R. Status of family-care programs. *Mental Retardation*, 1966, 4 (5), 8–11.

Olsen, K. M. and M. E. Olsen. Role expectations and perceptions for social workers in medical settings, *Social Work*, 1967, 12 (3), 70–78.

Olshansky, S. Chronic sorrow: A response to having a retarded child. *Social Casework*, 1962, 43, 190–193.

————. Parent responses to a mentally defective child. *Mental Retardation*, 1966, 4 (4), 21–23.

Parnicky, J. J. and L. N. Brown. Introducing institutionalized retardates to the community. *Social Work*, 1964, 9 (1), 79–85.

Popick, B. Social Security benefits for retarded children. *Mental Retardation*, 1966, 4 (6), 28–29.

Porter, R. M. Administrative planning in a new institution. *American Journal of Mental Deficiency*, 1961, 65, 708–712.

Savage, M. J., Rhoda Weltman, and D. E. Zarfas. Short-term care for the mentally retarded. *Mental Retardation*, 1967, 5 (2), 9–14.

Schreiber, M. and S. H. Bromfield. Adolescents who want to help: Some experiences with teen volunteers in a group work setting. *Mental Retardation*, 1966, 4 (6), 13–19.

Scheer, R. M. and W. M. Sharpe. Social group work in day camping with institutionalized delinquent retardates. *The Training School Bulletin*, 1963, 60, 138–147.

————. Group work as a treatment. *Mental Retardation*, 1965, 3 (3), 23–25.

Standifer, F. R. Parents helping parents. *Mental Retardation,* 1964, 2, 304–307.

Tarjan, G. The role of residential care—past, present and future. *Mental Retardation,* 1966, 4 (6), 4–8.

Woody, R. H. and J. J. Billy. Counseling and psychotherapy for the mentally retarded: A survey of opinions and practices. *Mental Retardation,* 1966, 4 (6), 20–23.

Education of the Mentally
Retarded in Residential
Settings

Educational programs for institutionalized mentally retarded persons have come full circle. They began more than 160 years ago and flourished for nearly a century before their objective of elevating human functioning gave way to one of caring for the bodily needs of those mentally retarded whom society could not tolerate in its midst. An amazing number of residential facilities were developed during that period of nearly 100 years, and all of them had education as their goal.

In those early days education did not, in fact could not, objectively differentiate between the several degrees of retardation. As a consequence, the children selected for education were those most obviously in need. Today those children would be referred to as trainable or severely retarded.

By 1900, however, institutions had swung away from education as a major objective and had become increasingly custodial in nature. They reserved education for those few institutionalized individuals who were mildly retarded.

Now the circle is complete. Today's professionals are again concerned with elevating the functional level of all institutionalized retardates. They have disavowed IQ 50 as a cut off point which had served to separate those worthy of education from those not worthy. The arbitrary discrimination which was practiced for more than 60 years against those retardates with IQ's below 50 has given way to efforts to return as many as possible to society.

History

Education for the mentally retarded began in an institutional setting when in 1799 Dr. Jean Itard, a French physician, took issue with his former teacher, Dr. Phillippe Pinel, concerning the prognosis for a young male who had been captured in a wooded area of Aveyron, France. The initial description of the child, Victor, indicated an animal-like creature, devoid of human desires and methods of dealing with the environment (Itard, 1962).

At that time, as today, there was a conflict of professional opinion about the relative influence of heredity and environment in the intellectual and functional development of children. Itard adhered to the environmentalist view (a school of thought which is presently enjoying a cyclical re-emphasis) and held that "The apparent subnormality (was) attributed to the fact that the child had lacked the intercourse with other human beings and that general experience which is an essential part of the training of a normal civilized person (Itard, 1962, p. vii)."

Itard undertook an intensive stimulation program with Victor. He placed him in an institution for the deaf and drew from the field of deaf education. The treatment objectives within that residential setting were similar to those found in institutional programs for lower level retardates today: to develop social skills; to improve and redirect sensory functioning; to improve affective contact with the environment; to improve problem solving ability (". . . to employ the simplest mental operations over a period of time upon the objects of his physical needs, . . . p. 37); and, considered to be of extreme importance by Itard, to develop language and speech. After five years' labor Victor gained in all areas except speech, but he did not achieve a level of functioning considered satisfactory by Itard, i.e., he did not become a normal human being. Fortunately, the French Academy of Science did not agree with Itard's negative view of his work and at their insistence he placed in writing the first report of an effort to improve the functional ability of a severely retarded person through total environmental manipulation—supervised residential living.

Itard's influence on education and residential school programming did not end when he concluded that he had been ineffective as Victor's teacher. His student in medicine, Edouard Seguin, picked up where he left off. As described in detail in Chapter 1, Seguin is credited with the establishment of the first resedential school for the mentally retarded in Paris in 1837, being the father of the movement for the establishment of residential schools in this country, and having developed the first systematic sequential training program for the mentally retarded. Sequin referred to his program of treatment as the Physiological Method because it was theoretically based "upon stimulation of the central nervous system by active involvement of the muscles and senses; in this he moved from stimulation to imitation, then to reflection, and finally to synthesis in purposive activity (Doll, 1967, p. 176)." His procedures bore great similarity to those employed earlier by teachers of the deaf, and as a consequence heavy emphasis was placed upon language development. Talbot (1964) has observed that the present day method of teaching the mentally retarded in a series of approximations and movement by small increments was consistently and successfully applied within Seguin's method.

Seguin was an advocate of both group and individual teaching, but his medical training led naturally to a heavy emphasis upon considering the individual pupil:

> Complete handling of a case included diagnosis, prescription to accord with the diagnosis, and summary of the outcome. Diagnosis was made of general and specific behavior, physical, intellectual, and social. Education materials and procedures were selected upon the basis of examination and observation. And the child's condition at the end of his schooling was made a matter of record. Seguin insisted that idiocy, like a physical disease, was individual, although the instruction might be individual or group. Seguin cautioned against application of any generalization to a specific case of idiocy (Talbot, 1967, p. 187).

Seguin considered a residential institution to be a school and his work, writings, and teachings stimulated the founding of many institutions in Europe and America during the 19th Century. All of these were educationally oriented. His method promised to ameliorate mental retardation. Its objective was to make mentally retarded individuals capable of guiding and directing their own activities and to return them to society. He recommended institutionalization primarily for children deemed capable of profiting from instruction over those years ordinarily assigned to educational experiences. He *did not,* however, consider his method a cure-all for mental retardation. He recognized the need for an institutional extension for those subjects who did not make adequate progress in the school program and for whom lifetime care was considered necessary (Talbot, 1964, p. 71).

European efforts were complimented by the work of his contemporary, Johann Guggenbuhl, who was also a physician. Guggenbuhl established a residential facility (the Abendberg) in Switzerland about 1840 with the intention of curing cretins. He instituted an all encompassing treatment program involving diet, bodily care, medical treatment, and physical exercise but focusing primarily on education as he "went about to develop sensory perceptions, beginning with primitive excitations and progressing from there to more refined and more complex stimuli." He emphasized habit training, exercises in memory, and speech production (Kanner, 1964, p. 24).

Seguin's and Guggenbuhl's words and teachings spread widely between 1840–50 with the resultant rapid opening of institutions in Germany, Austria, Great Britain, the Netherlands, and elsewhere. At the end of this period, however, the work of Guggenbuhl came under attack and the Abendberg closed shortly thereafter.

Institutions as educational facilities continued to mushroom. In England, where Guggenbuhl had had greatest influence, five institutions were functioning by 1870. However, their educational objectives and effectiveness were questionable. Pritchard (1963) has described one such program:

> . . . the instruction given to the children was good only in parts. In the preparatory class they did simple manual work: threading reels, grasping balls, putting nails into holes and pins into pin cushions. All children entered this class when they first came to the school. Some remained there six months, others three years. All, however, when they left the class, started on the formal work of which Itard and Seguin would have disapproved. They were taught to read, to write, and to calculate. But very few, . . . learnt to read and write properly (p. 59).

Interestingly, a governmental committee functioned in England in 1887 to examine the whole question of the education and care of the mentally handicapped—a move that may be likened to the modern day appointment of a committee to do the same by President John F. Kennedy in 1961 (A proposed program for national . . ., 1962). The English committee succeeded primarily in calling the public's attention to the needs of the mentally retarded and insured that they were considered by governmental agencies (Pritchard, 1963).

The establishment of residential facilities for the mentally retarded in the United States was an outgrowth of the interest and work of three individuals: Seguin, Samuel Gridley Howe, and Dr. H. B. Wilbur. In 1846 Howe became chairman of a committee established by the Massachusetts legislature to investigate the number and conditions of the mentally retarded. In 1848 this committee recommended the establishment of an experimental school where "It would be demonstrated that no idiot need be confined or restrained by force; that the young can be trained for industry, order, and self-respect . . . (Kanner, 1964, p. 41)."

The rapid establishment of residential facilities for the mentally retarded in Europe and the United States (see Chapter 1) encouraged experimentation and expansion of specific objectives and methods for the education of the mentally retarded. Guggenbuhl and C. W. Saegert, of Berlin, developed sensory motor approaches and emphasized socio-vocational goals with the ultimate aim of making each child as nearly self-sufficient as possible. Howe added stress upon the teaching of cleanliness and decency with emphasis also on dressing, feeding, ambulation, and the teaching and assignment of household chores. W. E. Fernald developed activities for use in training of very low-grade retardates. As early as 1882 Kentucky developed a vocational training program in which students were placed in educational programs in the morning and job training in the afternoon. Such trained persons frequently became capable of discharge to work for wages (Doll, 1967).

Unfortunately, the sometimes stated and often assumed promise of a cure for mental retardation that was born through 19th Century educational efforts did not approach fruition. Institutional populations increased and, most frequently, included a preponderance of severely damaged individuals. Gradually the concept of the institution as a school was replaced by the concept of the institution as a center for detention and care.

And so, the progressive era in residential education ended about 1900 and the doldrums set in for 60 years.

There were positive developments in the first half of the 20th Century, but they were neither momentous nor widespread. The pioneering progressive leadership provided by such persons as Guggenbuhl, Seguin, Howe, and others was missing. Advances that were made were largely confined to three areas: 1. vocational training and training for institutional living; 2. the development of the residential facility as a training ground for prospective teachers of the mentally retarded with summer course offerings, workshops, and seminars dealing with curriculum and educational methods for the mentally retarded (Survey and study of state institutions . . ., 1963), and 3. some attention to the establishment of special institutional programs for the retarded with particular needs; e.g., the establishment in 1926 of the Wayne County Training School at Northville, Michigan "for the purpose of caring for, educating, and rehabilitating children who show signs of social maladjustment and who are low in intelligence (Kirk and Johnson, 1951, p. 342)."

The period of stagnation began to draw to an end in 1950 when the National Association for Retarded Children and the parents it represented began to demand that the objectives of institutional life be redirected. The recycling was given further momentum by John F. Kennedy and his President's Panel Report on Mental Retardation which in 1962 emphasized the concept of the institution as one of many services which form a "continuum of care" for the mentally retarded. By 1968 the recent attitude of hopelessness had given way to one of hopefulness and experimentation. Even the least capable residents of many institutions are now receiving attention through sensory stimulation programs, the application of operant conditioning techniques, and ward training programs.

Residential facilities have finally begun dropping assumptions and are returning to the central emphasis of Seguin's approach: continual evaluation, revision, and projection of their educational efforts (Talbot, 1967). The movement has just begun, however, and much remains to be done in virtually all institutions.

Population Characteristics

It is impossible to consider current educational programs for the institutionalized retarded without considering the characteristics of the retarded themselves. People are not institutionalized simply because they are mentally retarded. Institutional residents certainly do lack intellectual ability (or at least functional adequacy), but it is invariably other problems which precipitate their institutional placement.

Hobbs (1964) compared institutionalized retardates with non-institutionalized (CA 13-25, IQ 45-78) counterparts who attended public school programs. She found that the factor which discriminated best between the two groups was the incidence of antisocial or immoral behavior. Male residents of the institution "tended to have acts of violence, stealing, arson, unmanageable and destructive behavior occurring most frequently in their records . . . (p. 208)." Problems associated with sex were most prevalent among the females. Maney, Pace, and Morrison (1964) reported similar findings regarding antisocial behavior when they investigated the prevalence of 30 different attributes in institutionalized retardates considered to be habilitable. Among the six most conspicuous factors they also noted trouble getting along with teachers and learning problems in school. In regard to education, Hobbs (1964) noted that the institutionalized persons had fewer educational opportunities than those non-institutionalized and less in the way of professional help. Even the educational backgrounds of their parents differentiated between the groups: the parents of the non-institutionalized population had attained higher educational levels.

It is highly probable that the great majority of retardates placed in residences have had no previous attention from special education or have been provided such programs only after inadequate educational programs had snuffed out their desire to learn. The prolonged failure experiences which too many retardates experience in public schools can only have a negative effect on the self-confidence of retardates and eliminate their willingness to undergo the process known as education.

Institutions cannot prevent poor school attitudes. They do not receive those retardates most capable of benefiting from formal education until the ball has been fumbled, until asocial behavior has been established and school hatred fostered. This is not to say that young retardates are not being admitted to institutions. O'Connor and Hunter (1967) reported that in 12 institutions in nine western states almost 50 per cent of the patients were under 18 years of age and 5 per cent were between 0 and 5 years. Three-fourths of all patients had IQ's below 50 with 25 per cent falling in the 0–19 range. Tarjan (1966) had indicated that 80 per cent of institutionalized retardates have IQ's below 50. Educationally, the latter figure would indicate that a large institution of 2,000 residents would have no more than 400 who were mildly retarded (hereafter referred to as *educable mentally retarded* in accordance with present day educational terminology). They would range in age from early childhood to adulthood. It is clear that the greatest educational need, from the standpoint of numbers, is presented by those institutionalized individuals falling in the moderate and severe ranges of intelligence (hereafter referred to as the *trainable mentally retarded*).

An example of measured intelligence of residents in an institution with a population totaling 1,922 residents is shown in Table 9–1. The educable group of appropriate age for formal education (encompassed by the dotted line) totals only 166 or 8.6 per cent. The trainable group includes 263 or 13.7 per cent of the total population. These are small groups around whom to plan comprehensive sequential school programs.

Jaslow and others (1966) recommend criteria for admission to institutional programs which emphasize physical disability, asocial behavior above CA 8 and, mental level: profound, above CA 5 and severe, above CA 8.

Table 9–1. Measured Intelligence of Residents in
Gracewood State School and Hospital, by Age as of
June 30, 1967*

| | | | | Intelligence Quotient | | | | |
Age	Total	70–80	55–69	40–54	25–39	0–24	>80	Unknown
0-4	8	0	0	0	0	4	0	4
5-9	97	1	1	3	12	66	0	14
10–14	287	7	29	41	33	158	0	19
15–19	535	50	78	98	76	202	0	31
20 years	112	7	20	14	26	43	0	2
21–24	315	16	37	74	77	107	1	3
25–29	232	12	24	49	59	87	1	0
30–34	111	2	12	21	36	39	0	1
35–39	79	4	8	12	31	24	0	0
40–UP	146	8	9	40	51	37	0	1
TOTALS	1,922	107	218	352	401	767	2	75

*Source: Annual Report—Gracewood State School and Hospital, Gracewood, Georgia, June 30, 1967.

Such criteria are apparently in widespread usage today. Tarjan (1966) summarized the commonly found reasons for institutional placement as

(a) the presence of retardation of such profound or severe degree that a hospital setting is necessary for survival; (b) there are severe super-imposed physical, emotional, or behavioral symptoms; (c) if left in the community, the retarded person constitutes a danger to himself or to others; (d) the retarded person cannot be cared for at home or in a foster setting because he is too much of a physical or emotional burden to members of his household; (e) there is no family available to care for the retardate or the home conditions are inadequate; and (f) the necessary community resources are either absent or insufficient (p. 5).

It is significant that educational need is not mentioned in any of the foregoing reasons for institutional placement except as might be inferred in (f). Even there, however, the recent surge in the establishment of community services makes it doubtful if lack of community educational provisions presently accounts for placement of retarded citizens. In regard to the insufficiency of community services, however, there are instances where the retarded are excluded from school and that exclusion serves as the stimulus for institutionalization. Today the moderately and mildly retarded persons entering institutions are those who have severe physical abnormalities, have been rejected by the public schools, or present such antisocial behavior that their home and community will not tolerate them.

The foregoing basic facts regarding residential placement are forcing institutional schools to realize that to be effective they must involve the total institution in education. This broad involvement is occurring although it is often masked by applying names such as recreation therapy, music therapy, behavior shaping. Institutions are beginning to recognize that they exist for one major purpose—the elevation of the functional ability of every subject with whom they come in contact. This realization carries with it the dictum that a lack of potential can no longer be assumed for any patient.

Each resident should be viewed as having potential for growth and development. This potential should be recognized as limited, not only by the individual's presently recognized potential, but also by the lack of scientific knowledge on the part of those working with him. Potential, therefore, should not be viewed as static or as having fixed limits according to types of individuals or present-day ideologies (Standards for State Residential . . ., 1964, p. 3).

The institutional school is also being forced to recognize that it shares a diagnostic and therapeutic role, that the educational population will become increasingly less able, that the few higher level individuals accepted into the institution will be more and more of the "hard-core" variety, and, that education in its narrow sense will decrease in importance. Educational programs are being redirected toward remedying those problems which account for the child's being institutionalized.

Educational Objectives

Institutions for the mentally retarded are presently going through the throes of rebirth as an attempt is made to find their most useful place among the myriad of organizations and services, from the federal to the local levels, which have sprung up in the past 10 years to assist the mentally retarded. Rather than dropping by the wayside as community services are emphasized, residential facilities continue to receive attention at the state level through developmental planning as outlined in state documents such as "Miles to Go" (Connecticut, 1966) and "Arizona's Comprehensive Plan . . ." (Arizona, 1965). Waiting lists of most institutions reflect an upward trend in the reestablishment of such facilities as education and treatment centers rather than facilities for care only. Gradually such institutions are being redefined as organizations dealing with the mentally retarded, in an effort

> to maintain or raise the functional levels of the cognitive, psycho-motor and affective abilities and thereby help these individuals to develop the mechanisms necessary to satisfy their basic psychological, biological, sociological, educational and other needs in a manner that meets general societal approval (Goldbery and Younie, 1968).

The primary goals for the education program in an institution cannot differ therefore from those of all other institutional services—only the means varies. The ultimate goals are to elevate to a status of productive and independent community functioning those persons with such capabilities, and to elevate the functional level of those destined to long-term institutionalization in areas of awareness, appreciation, and contributions to self and the immediate environment.

For return to the community or satisfactory institutional adjustment to occur all attention must be turned to the individual patient and the problems accounting for his presence therein. Tarjan (1966) has indicated these subgoals as being "(a) the alteration of those symptoms in the patient, the family or the community which precipitated admission; (b) the emphasis of the factors which encourage maturation of the patient; (c) the treatment of mental retardation and of the super-imposed handicaps (p. 6)." It is significant that the three key phrases, *alteration* of symptoms, *emphasis* of factors, and *treatment* of mental retardation, all have educational connotations.

Specific statements of educational objectives for educable retardates have been published elsewhere (see "Educating the Retarded Child" by Kirk and Johnson, 1951) and generally differ from those for normal children only in regard to (1) more specific concentration on personality adjustment and the development of social skills and (2) less emphasis on academics. For institutionalized persons the emphasis is more on social adjustment and skill development and the approach is more problem oriented than that normally found in public school classes for the mentally retarded.

The American Association on Mental Deficiency publication "Standards for State Residential Institutions for the Mentally Retarded" (1964) has itemized objectives of education for the educable retarded in residential facilities:

a. Intellectual development and academic proficiency in tool subjects
b. The development of emotional stability
c. The development of good habits of health and personal hygiene
d. The development of personal and social adequacy
e. The development of attitudes, interests, and skills leading to the wholesome use of leisure time
f. The development of attitudes, interests, and skills leading to good citizenship and community responsibility
g. Learning to work for the purpose of earning a living (p. 40).

High level retardates in an institution must be equipped (or reequipped) with the personal ability to live, contribute, and interact effectively with the community environment. Furthermore, they must come to enjoy their own accomplishments or the lasting development of higher level skills, be they social, academic, or work oriented.

The general objectives as earlier stated apply to the trainable mentally retarded. Care must be taken, however, not to assume that these residents are necessarily in permanent institutional placement. For many trainable mentally retarded persons, placement can be temporary. Educational treatment in a residential setting too often fails to recognize that trainable children have needs for self-fulfillment if only at a very reduced level when comparisons are made with normal children. They, too, have needs for acceptance and challenge at their utmost level of capability; they, too, must be viewed as people capable of personal adjustment to the demands of the environment whether it be institutional or community.

The often stated objectives of self-help, language development (including communication), and socialization apply in working with the institutionalized trainable child following programs as outlined in texts such as those by Rosenweigh and Long (1960), Perry (1960) and Frankel, Happ and Smith (1966). The American Association on Mental Deficiency has listed objectives of school programs for the trainable mentally retarded as:

a. The development of self-help skills, safety, social and interpersonal relationships, and speech and language skills necessary to increase their potentials for more independent living.
b. The development of emotional stability.
c. The development of good habits of health and personal hygiene.
d. The development of attitudes, interests and skills leading to a more wholesome use of leisure time.
e. The development of social attitudes and behavior patterns necessary for more adequate group living and participation.
f. The development of work habits, skills and tolerances for work for the purpose of personal satisfaction and usefulness in a sheltered environment. (Standards for state residential . . ., 1964, p. 43).

It is an often repeated criticism of public school programs that they, in some cases, become a baby sitting service, and the danger of such a development is even greater in a residential facility. In the latter, the school day is shorter and more open to interruptions than in a public school, and the shortage of teachers specifically trained to work with the mentally retarded is even more acute. The untrained personnel, employed as a stop-gap measure to keep classes functioning, will in most cases bring with them the attitude of hopelessness toward such children that has historically been displayed by the general society. The limited interrupted program makes positive change even slower and more difficult to observe. At times this results in programs where puzzles, picture-books, and other accoutrements of education are essentials in and of themselves without attention to the specific objectives to be gained through the manipulation of such articles, thereby losing their educational value.

In the case of programs for the trainable mentally retarded it is important to recognize what are not the objectives of education. The classroom does not exist for 1. the emphasis of enjoyment of the moment—there are other departments, such as recreation, with this objective, 2. the release of pressure from the wards and cottages, 3. the allowing for a letter to be written to the home indicating that the child is now being educated, or 4. to increase the number enrolled in educational programs to show that the institution is valiantly working to see that all children receive all possible benefits.

The educational goal for all retarded individuals must be defined in terms of the future. Any objective or activity which will not add to the positive functioning of the subject in adulthood is a waste of time, and there is already too little time in the usual educational program.

To paraphrase, in an institutional vein, Ingram (1960) regarding questions that must be asked about activities for any retarded child in a classroom:

1. Does it promote the mental and physical health and the intellectual capacity of the child?
2. Does it promote better home understanding and potential membership?
3. Does it promote better community (including residential) understanding and living?
4. Does it provide for learning for present future use of leisure time—independently or semi-dependently?
5. Does it provide for the development of desirable work habits, attitudes and knowledge for application outside the classroom?
6. For the educable child, does it increase his ability to apply the tool subjects in a life setting?

Residential Education

There is little recent information about the various residential education programs in the United States to assist in the development of general statements about how such programs are structured and operated. Only two studies have been reported (Younie, 1965; A survey and study . . . 1963), and two are currently being conducted: one by the National Association for Retarded Children and one by a committee of the President's Panel on Mental Retardation. For perspective readers may wish to review information concerning programs of the 1950's (Levine, 1954; Cassell, 1956).

To provide some current information, I conducted a study of education programs in 36 state institutions located in 15 southeastern states. Directors of Education in residential facilities for the retarded were questioned about general administrative considerations, programming for the educable mentally retarded, and programming for the trainable mentally retarded. The questionnaires were returned by 24 (66.6 per cent) of the directors with one superintendent indicating no educational program inasmuch as the institution was aimed specifically at the treatment of the severely and profoundly retarded (Blue, 1968—hereafter referred to as the Southeastern Survey).

STRUCTURE AND OPERATION

The Southeastern Survey indicates that a variety of agencies direct institutions in the various states although usually it is the Department of Institutions or the Department of Mental Health. Two respondents indicated that the Department of Education and the Department of Institutions were jointly responsible, with no one noting a State Department of Education

alone. Interestingly, 7 out of 23 indicated that they do operate their educational programs under the supervision and guidance of the State Department
of Education as a result of legal requirement. This can be contrasted with
Younie's finding of 0 out of 96 nationwide in 1965. All of the remaining
16 indicated that they operate voluntarily in accordance with State Department of Education directives and guidelines in certain specific matters, most
notably certification of teachers, 100 per cent; pupil attendance, 81 per cent;
curriculum, 75 per cent; school day, 62 per cent; and pupil evaluation, 62
per cent.

Within institutions, education is usually programmatically and budgetarily independent rather than being a subdivision of another department.
In the survey reported here, 19 of 22 reported that such was the case with
18 of the 19 operating under a guaranteed yearly budget allotment. Thirteen respondents furnished information regarding the average per-pupil
educational expenditure. These expenditures ranged from $114.43 to
$683.82, with an average of $383.84 for the educable retarded. Twelve
of the 13 respondents reported identical per-pupil costs in the program for
trainable children, and one reported costs to be $100 per year per child
lower. The failure to find increased costs for program for trainable children
is surprising in view of the common finding that the greater the extent of
disability, the greater the costs of education. The present finding may simply reflect the newness of such undertakings, but it may also reflect an
insensitivity to the educational needs of trainable mentally retarded children, e.g., small pupil teacher ratio, classroom attendants, and greater
expendable supply costs.

In relatively large institutional programs a Director of Education is
usually responsible for the overall planning and management of the education program and in all programs one or more principals have charge of
matters relating to instruction. In those rare programs where more than one
principal is employed it is for purposes of specific program management,
i.e., trainable mentally retarded, educable mentally retarded.

It is common to find that the Director of Education also has primary responsibility for program areas which are tangential to formal education.
Younie (1965) reported that directors often have responsibilities in areas
of recreation, assignment of institution jobs, religious education, volunteer
services, and occupational therapy. As institutions for the retarded draw
nearer to a total educational and treatment orientation the responsibility of
the educational leaders will become even greater. Already, "One-half of
the chief education officers consider themselves to be administrators in the
sense that they determine policy (Younie, 1965, p. 452)."

Institutional education programs are organized like public elementary
schools but without grade level designations, i.e., assignment of students is

based on considerations other than academic achievement. The Southeastern Survey determined that 20 of 22 educational directors employ the categories, educable mentally retarded, and trainable mentally retarded, for purposes of educational placement. However, there was not complete agreement about the definition of these terms. Thirteen institutions indicated an adherence to an IQ definition—25 to 50 TMR, 50 to 75 EMR—but in most instances prognostic criteria were also involved. Six institutions reported placement based on prognostic factors only and one considered a combination of IQ and MA. Two other institutions indicated use of the non-educational classification system suggested by the American Association on Mental Deficiency (Heber, 1959). Consistency was demonstrated in the prognostic factors listed: a composite definition of the educable child would indicate that he is one with potential for academic learning, and social and emotional adjustment to the extent that eventual community return and work placement can be expected. The classification of trainability is based on the expectancy that the individual will need supervision throughout his life, but that he can improve in his ability to care for himself and communicate with others along with improvement in social and work skills.

Placement of a child in an educational program has been most frequently based on psychological and medical examination. Educational evaluation employing objective instruments has been carried out in only a few institutions (Younie, 1965). The place of education evaluation in the total institutional picture is apparently changing, however, because 20 of 21 respondents in the Southeastern Survey indicated that such evaluation is a part of the total evaluation process for all children entering the institution. Furthermore, 20 of 23 (87 per cent) respondents indicated that periodic reevaluation is required. The mean requirement interval was 10.5 months. The views of education regarding individual children are also of concern in case staffing, as indicated by 21 of 23 responses, with the educator involved most frequently being a principal, director of education, or supervisor.

The survey asked the educational directors to rank, on a four point scale, the amount of emphasis placed on each program area, e.g., reading, writing, social studies, music, recreation, self-help, and others. Consistency in the emphasis on academic areas was demonstrated in programs for the educable mentally retarded, with all respondents indicating at least some emphasis and 100 per cent indicating moderate or major emphasis on reading and arithmetic, 95 per cent on writing, and 80 per cent on spelling.

Equal consistency was not found concerning academics for the trainable retarded. Responses were about equally divided between no, little, and moderate emphasis on the four academic areas. One respondent indicated major emphasis on these four areas. It is noted, however, that all institutions greatly emphasize self-care and socialization for the trainable mentally retarded.

Generally speaking, classes are structured on a modified self-contained basis in which a pupil is assigned to a specific class for a major block of time with additional time scheduled in other areas of the school program as needed. Institutional school programs vary greatly in the extent of non-academic offerings and may contain none, some, or all of the following: vocational instruction, vocational guidance, home economics, music, physical education, speech therapy, arts and crafts, and occupational therapy. The following is offered as an example of personnel and departments in a rather extensive residential school program for 136 EMR students (CA 7-22) and 118 TMR students (CA 6-20) at Murdoch Center, Butner, North Carolina:

Director of Education	1
Principal	1
EMR teachers	7
TMR teachers	6
Vocational instructors	2
Vocational counselors	4
Home Economics teachers	2
Music teachers	1
Physical Education teachers	1
Librarian	1
Speech therapists	1
Audiologists	1
School Psychologists	1
Special Teachers for Emotionally Disturbed	4
Special Teachers for Orthopedic Handicapped	1
Industrial Arts teacher	1
Printing	1
Arts and Crafts	2

As earlier indicated institutions vary widely in the areas included under the title "education" and frequently

... education encompasses only the academic school program conducted for educable residents. Activity programs, developmental classes for trainable residents, and work study programs may be assigned to departments other than education, and often are conducted by persons having little educational background or direction. In some institutions, education is charged with all functions commonly defined as education and rehabilitation. . . . It is apparent that individual institutions have conducted and will continue to conduct educational programs in relationship to what they perceive as specific needs and according to a philosophy attuned to the social and political elements peculiar to their particular setting (Younie, 1966, p. 374).

A majority of the respondents in the Southeastern Survey reported that the following activities were carried on outside of the school itself: work training, self-care training, adjustment training, and stimulation programs for the profoundly retarded. Only three of 23 respondents noted attention to driver's education and in two of the three instances instruction was carried out by the vocational rehabilitation department. Fifteen of 23 noted provisions for sex education, although formal instruction was employed in only seven institutions. The department of education has responsibility for sex education in eight of the 15 programs.

Even the amount of time devoted to education varies greatly from program to program as dictated by the CA and IQ level of the children. Twenty-one respondents indicated that classes for the primary and intermediate level EMR children ranged from one and a half to seven hours per day for the former and from two to seven hours for the latter. Only 15 institutions reported classes at the secondary level with a range of three to seven hours. In regard to the length of the class day for trainable mentally retarded children 22 indicated classes at the primary level, one to five and a half hours, and at the intermediate level, one and a quarter to five and a half hours. Fifteen conduct classes for the trainable at the secondary level with an hourly range of one to five hours. It is interesting to note that although the class day for trainable children is not, on the average, so long as that for the educable the length of the school year is sometimes longer; 13 respondents in the Southeastern Survey reported that a student may be taken from class during the school day for an extremely large variety of reasons. A listing of the reasons noted by 50 per cent or more of the respondents follows:

1. Limited home visits (82%)
2. Unlimited home visits (50%)
3. Speech therapy (50%)
4. Discipline (68%)
5. Staffing (55%)
6. Clinic visits (91%)
7. Testing (86%)

In spite of the inconsistency from institution to institution in established educational practices, there is a widespread questing for improvement. A modern day drive to evaluate and improve existing services, initiate new programs, and include more children was triggered by the President's Panel

Report in 1962 and has been energized by funds made available through various federal acts since that date. The use of such funds has been largely dictated by local needs and has been left to the imagination and planning of the education staff of individual institutions. In the Southeastern Survey, Directors of Education were asked to rank (1 most important to 7 least important) areas of educational importance which have been improved with such monies. All respondents had received federal funds and they ranked the areas as follows:

1. Inclusion of more children
2. and 3. Instructional materials and equipment (a tie in ranking)
4. Program development
5. Teachers salaries
6. Plant expansion
7. Staff education

In addition, respondents were asked to itemize innovative programs that had been added to previously existing programs as a result of federal funding. The responses, in the order of their frequency, were:

1. The development of preschool programs
2. Program expansion for the multipli-handicapped and/or sensory impaired
3. Program development for the severely and profoundly retarded
4. Educational services for the adult retarded
5. Physical education
6. Language development programming
7. Speech therapy
8. Home economics
9. Sheltered workshops
10. Field trips

The variation of the foregoing responses reflects the different concerns of different institutions, as well they should, for each facility is different from the others in many ways. "Every institution has some unique quality or potential that can be developed for the benefit of the entire field (A proposed program for national . . ., 1962, p. 137)." As a result, a spirit of experimentation must be a part of institutional programming. Residential facilities are in reality natural laboratories for the initiation of innovative ideas. They contain a variety of professional viewpoints and a large pool of resources, equipment, and so forth. This research philosophy, first emphatically expounded by Seguin, has only recently been reasserted. Younie (1966) has pointed out a number of educational questions that lend themselves to investigation in an institutional setting and has indicated that "the newer educational programs in institutions capitalize on the inherent advantages of the institutional structure which permits the formulation of instructional programs and research activities that cannot be organized as effectively in the community (p. 376)."

THE TEACHER AND TEACHING

The success of any educational enterprise is dependent upon the teacher, and no area of teaching is so demanding of ingenuity as the teaching of retarded children in a residential setting. In all programs, heterogeneity of pupils is the rule, and this along with problems related to a fluid population, population characteristics and time demand a superior and well adjusted teacher. She must be imaginative, extremely flexible, and capable of seeing and accepting small gains in pupil performance. Without the latter characteristic no teacher can (or should) long remain in institutional work with the mentally retarded for the sake of her own mental health as well as for the already damaged mental health of her students.

A successful teacher is one who understands and can teach academic subject matter where realistically called for but, does not get "hung up" on academic improvement. Rather, she must recognize that her major goal is to improve each student's specific weaknesses and to capitalize upon his strengths.

Such teaching demands a constant search for new and improved methods of teaching and guidance applicable across a broad spectrum of abilities and problem areas. The teacher must have a therapeutic as well as a developmental and educational focus, and this focus must be strengthened in the future as institutions strive to heed the advice of the President's Panel on Mental Retardation that "Every such institution, including those that care for the seriously retarded, should be basically therapeutic in character and emphasis . . . (A proposed program for national . . ., 1962, p. 137)."

An important first step in the therapeutic management of the institutionalized retardate is to furnish, upon entrance into the school program, an opportunity for immediate success, for his past had undoubtedly been a succession of failures. Even with the high level retardate who is intellectually capable of academic achievement, the first year and perhaps longer may have to be devoted to improving the child's view of himself, his perspective of society (a representative of which is the classroom itself), and his place in that society. Initial activities should, therefore, have social and ego developing as well as academic objectives.

A vital part of classroom activities is the opportunity for personality development and expression which comes through creative activities such as music, painting, drawing, modeling, and drama. In many institutions there are separate departments of music, arts and crafts, etc., but this should be taken as an incentive to bring such activities into the classroom through cooperative planning rather than acting to remove them from the class because "those activities are taken care of down the hall."

Activity centered learning experiences are extremely important to retarded children. They need to be given the opportunity to start off in activities under someone's direct guidance and gradually develop the ability to listen carefully, follow directions, complete a job started, and eventually set the direction they should pursue themselves as independent workers. Use and care of materials for example, including cleaning up after a job, is a skill which can be developed through art activities and which is directly pertinent to eventual job training and placement in adulthood.

The teacher must be imaginative in her planning to allow for repetition. After identifying a specific objective which she wishes to pursue with a given child she must develop a variety of realistic and meaningful experiences which relate to it; experiences which will serve to "stamp in" and insure over learning. The variation of activities will also prove motivational and reduce boredom, a problem that does occur in retarded children and which, perhaps even more unfortunately, can influence the teacher herself.

Through activity centered experiences each child, no matter how limited, can know success and its accompanying enjoyment. The latter is important, for the residential facility is at best an artificial setting and an institutional pall can easily descend throughout the facility including the classroom.

However, the successful classroom does not develop a carnival atmosphere, quite to the contrary, for the aforementioned objective of self direction carried with it the trait of discipline—at first teacher-directed but gradually self-directed. The successful teacher may then be said to be one who exerts cheerful control in a moderately structured setting, a setting that gradually establishes limits of acceptable behavior and enterprise.

Disciplinary problems may arise in the institutional classroom as a result of previous failure experiences in education. Firm management is required, but demands for adherence to rigid rules without understanding generally brings chaos. The rule that the child who is busily engaged in an enjoyable and meaningful learning experience will seldom be a disruptive force applies here as well as in all other classes. In the case of severe behavior problems, however, the usual rules of discipline do not seem to apply and direct forms of correction do not bring results. Generally speaking these children will be, or should be, under psychiatric care within the institution, and the teacher must keep in close contact with the psychiatrist for guidance in the handling of very deviant behavior and the selection of procedures for bringing about improvement. The teacher owes an obligation to herself and to the other children in the classroom, and on occasion direct intervention is necessary. If such is the case, and direct discipline is not psychiatrically desirable, the child should not be a responsibility of the school (except for tutorial help).

Every teacher of the mentally retarded must engaged in child, class, and personal evaluation, or stagnation will occur. This is of particular importance in an institutional setting where the teacher loses contact with normal children and the consideration of sequential developmental schedules. Methods of measurement of pupil growth at these levels are not refined, and there are few demands for proof of change through the usual methods of grade reporting, completion of a particular text by a specific time, and passage from one grade to the next. Graphs and charts should be used wherever possible, both for pupil motivation and for checks on progress, and the teacher must continually evaluate her efforts with each child with a willingness and ability to make changes.

Periodic evaluation of the success of each teacher and of the overall program should be conducted by the principal of the school. Furthermore, it is advisable that program evaluation also involve outside experts in the form of consultative personnel who have the freedom to express honest opinions about the need for program changes.

Institutional Characteristics
Influencing Educational Programming

Invariably, persons looking at the subject of educational programs in institutions use personal experiences with public school day classes for the retarded and literature related to such classes as a frame of reference. Comparisons of the effectiveness of public school and institutional programs are unfair and inappropriate in many ways because of basic differences which exist in population, location, and administration.

Retardates in a residential setting are those whose social, emotional, and physical (seldom intellectual) problems have proved too great for the public school and other community services. They often come from homes where the level of education is low, and education is not prized.

There are also problems and limitations associated with the institutional environment that interfere with the establishment of an educational program that is adequate by community standards. Goldberg and Younie (1968) indicate a number of factors which intervene in the establishment of an institutional education program that is child centered first and society (institution) centered secondarily stating that "it is difficult to implement the child-centered concept in the institution and although it is defended it is not often observed in a viable form. Yet, the need for a balance between individual and societal objectives still exist . . .". Among the factors which Goldberg and Younie note are the following:

1. The tendency to place the institutions organizational needs above those of individuals
2. The inevitability of "dual control"—administrative lines of control vs. the the dictations of the professional staff
3. "Multiple subordination"—the authoritative direction by several individuals or disciplines of one given child, and
4. The inevitable placement of each child into a number of new social situations all conducive to behavioral change either positively or negatively.

There are specific factors of interference which demand and are receiving attention today in program development. These are problems in program continuity, time allocation, reduction in the artificiality of the learning setting, the administrative view of education, and personnel recruitment.

FACTORS IN BUILDING CONTINUITY

The truly effective education program for the retarded is one with built-in continuity. Regardless of the level of children involved, planning should be so thorough that there is step-by-step preparation of each individual as he progresses from his level of functioning at entrance through to successful community or institutional placement in adulthood. Without such continuity it is not only possible but highly probable that success in the elimination of problems secondary to mental retardation will simply give way to the development of new problems. Continuity is extremely difficult to establish for any child in an institutional setting because of a number of factors, one of which is institutional admission policy. It is virtually impossible, for example, to develop a preschool program for the retarded because the children who would benefit most from it are not admitted until they are too old for such a program. This same factor interferes with effective programming at the lower elementary age levels, for the trend is toward the admittance of moderate and high level retardates at age 10 or older, when problems secondary to mental retardation have already become well entrenched.

Sequential programming is influenced also by the recognized need to release as soon as possible every retardate for whom successful community placement can be predicted. So class populations change with entrances and exits determined by non-educational factors. Children who enter the class may present varying types and degrees of educational experience—from no school experience at all, to unsuccessful regular school placement, to unsuccessful special class placement. All of these factors serve to interfere with a program planned in advance, and for a teacher to be successful she must be flexible and capable of shifting instruction within the school year to meet the changing needs of her pupil load. She must accept and adapt to changing pupils and pupil needs as a fact of institutional life. She must also accept the preponderance of severe behavior and educational problems, because as she is successful her success must leave for community life to be replaced by another challenge.

For continuity to exist in the educational life of the institutionalized mentally retarded it must be planned at two levels—within the instituional program, and between the institutional program and that of the community to which the child returns—if the institutional program is effective. The former is a common goal of institutions today, problems herein noted notwithstanding. The latter, however, is a goal of the future because working relationships between residential facilities and community agencies are just now beginning to develop. Both community agencies and the institutions themselves are to blame for the past lack of mutual planning. As David Ray pointed out

> Too many of our state institutions are 'closed shops'. They pay little attention to community services for the retarded, they pay little attention to public school classes, they pay little attention to parent groups, and they even pay little attention to other State institutions. Each of us can learn something from the other fellow. (Survey and study . . ., 1963, p. 19).

Unfortunately, both continuity and comparability fail to exist between residential and public school programs within a given state. This is due in part to the dissimilarities between populations and environment (factors resistant to change by the very nature of institutions), but also results from a lack of common leadership. Invariably public school programs within a given state are subject to rules, regulations, and guidelines set forth by one state agency responsible for establishing and maintaining structured educational programs for exceptional children—the State Department of Education. That agency has had little if any official influence on educational programs in residential settings. Younie (1965) surveyed 115 institutions in the United States and Canada and found that none of the 96 facilities responding were responsible to a State Department of Education. In fact, a very large percentage indicated no interest on the part of state special education consultants in the problems of institutions. Younie did note, however, that 73 per cent of the administrators voluntarily employed state education department guides on specific administrative matters, e.g., teacher qualifications. There is recent evidence of greater involvement of State Departments of Education in institutional education programs. In 1968 the Southeastern Survey found that State Departments of Education administer education programs in seven of 23 institutions, and all of the remaining 16 adhere voluntarily to specific state recommendations.

Not only is there a lack of continuity and comparability between residential school programs and those in public schools, but there are great differences between residential school programs themselves. Younie (1965) commented in this regard that "It is certainly difficult to set program standards without reference points and the professional points of departure for the institutions surveyed are not well defined (p. 459)." Complete freedom in program development and operation is the rule, rather than the exception, but it is a kind of restrictive freedom inasmuch as institutions have no common guidelines for achieving the accepted goals, and many of them are floundering rather than flourishing.

The current minimal collaboration between institutions is due almost entirely to the exchange of ideas at professional meetings, visits, and workshops with invited speakers from other institutions. Efforts toward program evaluation have been instituted by the American Association on Mental Deficiency, and this should reduce differences between residential programs at least in matters of administrative structure and minimal programming standards.

For years institutions for the mentally retarded have been administered by state departments of health, institutions, and even corrections, and this has been used as the explanation for differences between institutional and community programs. State education agencies have apparently felt that they would be intruding if they requested an opportunity to view an institutional program, even when such a request was based only on a desire to learn. They have feared that they might be accused of meddling in the affairs of other state agencies. Such petty bureaucratic jealousies hardly justify what can only be termed the negligence of State Departments of Education in the matter of improving institutional education programs. However, institutions themselves must share the blame. Superintendents of institutions have too seldom sought the assistance of State Departments of Education through invitation. It would behoove both institutions and departments of education to stop contending that they don't have the time to take on new ventures. Within the current philosophy of education as one link in a chain of services, those links must be joined, or the chain will continue to be fragmented.

TIME ALLOCATION TO EDUCATION

In an institution the education program is just one of many services, any or all of which may have active daily contact with a given child. Services such as recreation, physical therapy, occupational therapy, vocational training, religious life, medical treatment, and psychotherapy make demands for a part of the child's day and, in effect, education must get into line.

As new projects and activities are developed in institutions, as they currently are with federal funds (and which are usually quite valuable), time is taken from an already crowded day, and education frequently finds itself interrupted again. For example, an enthusiastic new teacher with a well planned program suddenly realizes that by ones and twos her children are being taken from the class day for a new and exciting train ride, or mass music lesson, or circus visit—activities which often would make excellent adjuncts to education if they occurred after school hours and if the teacher were advised sufficiently in advance to explore their learning properties and plan for preceding and following class sessions.

The unlimited visitation and vacation policies currently in operation in many institutions also interfere with the conduct of a well planned continuously sequential program of education for any resident. The residential education program also has the problem of too many children to handle with its plant and personnel and is forced to operate on a partial day basis for each child. The result of all of these factors is a frequently interrupted school day which seldom exceeds four hours. In short, education is generally viewed as a small part of the institution's treatment program. It is simply one of many services, all of which are viewed as being somewhat equal.

This is quite different from public school programs for the retarded. Here education is viewed as the ultimate agency for preparing children for adulthood. School time is greedily conserved and every school day contains five or more hours which are devoted specifically to education.

The institutional situation is not only different from the community practice, it is also contrary to the philosophy of modern day institutions. According to Thorne (1965):

> The institution is properly thought of as a community with definite objectives and with the capacity to provide life experiences for each of its residents not totally unlike those planned and provided for mentally retarded children outside institutions and residing in the community (p. 58).

If such a philosophy is to be put into practice, then it must be recognized that during the school year attendance of a child in a school program is of utmost importance. The child who knows he may be absent from school for home visits, clinic appointments, the barber shop, will come to view education as unimportant and will be poorly motivated to do well in educational areas. Furthermore, the child who goes home on visits (or is absent repeatedly for other reasons) may never be able to adjust satisfactorily to either his home or the institution.

In a consistent school program a child can develop a "niche" where he feels secure and where he can develop a sense of accomplishment. Regular school attendance is itself a lesson in acceptable adult living—the lesson of responsibility and punctuality. Efforts should be made to develop within every child self responsibility for daily school attendance. Children should be made aware of the time that they are to be in class and the teacher of the group should always be present when the children arrive and remain there with planned instructional programs until the children leave. It is the daily recurrence of important events which makes it possible for many children to learn to tell time, and the beginning and ending of the school day should be two such important events.

THE ADMINISTRATIVE VIEW OF EDUCATION

There are rare well established institutional programs in which a specific block of time is set aside for the education of each child, and nothing is allowed to infringe upon that time. The development of such a program seems highly dependent upon several interacting factors: acceptance of the educational program by the superintendent, the superintendent's philosophy and view of the place of education in the total institutional services picture, the imagination, forcefulness and leadership ability of the person in charge of the educational program, and the extent of the entrenchment of the custodial concept.

"Power structures" develop in all closed communities, and that is what institutions generally are. The institution's leadership sets the philosophy and direction of every service in it. The professionals' training and past experience quite often determine the direction of their leadership, and as a consequence it has been common for institutions to be heavily oriented in one direction and for them to pay minimal attention to other areas. Dybwad (1964) has commented in this regard, "a medical superintendent may greatly improve the medical services, but by the same token the education and rehabilitation facilities and services may be severely neglected (p. 90)." It is difficult to obtain accurate information about how much progress has been made, but guidelines set forth by various state mental retardation planning groups indicate a widespread intention to move away from the one-man or one-profession direction of institutions.

The very historical structuring of institutions presents problems in the movement away from the custodial concept. Older institutions are invariably large, massive structures containing hundreds and often thousands of residents. It is extremely difficult to program for individual residents in such a mass of humanity. It is easier and more expedient to care for each one than it is to see that each one learns to care for himself. Methods for group care have been developed and refined until their very efficiency interferes with change. Dybwad (1964) has commented in this regard that institutions are built of brick and mortar, and an unwieldy, out dated, three-story mass housing monstrosity of a building just continues to sit there as a road block to progress. Compare this with the situation in the public schools, where obstacles such as an out-dated curriculum, inadequate teacher training, and inferior testing programs can be remedied in much shorter time and with much greater ease (p. 99).

The modern day concept of institutional development with its emphasis on small community based installations may do much to eliminate the problems of large institutions. The movement to smaller living units in some of the older and larger facilities is assisting, to a minimal extent, in a re-focusing on the individual, but a more intensive and imaginative effort is clearly in order.

ARTIFICIALITY OF THE SETTING

Even under the best of circumstances the institution is a poor setting for education because of its inherent artificiality. In effect, it must provide substitutes for all dimensions of childhood living and learning, i.e., parental, community contacts, religious experience, and others. In this regard Thorne (1965) has commented

... the institution must continually strive to provide for all children a great multitude of experiences and variety of activities so that no child will be further handicapped because he was institutionalized and thus deprived of an environment which would provide the normal experiences, adventures, and activities that are fundamental to learning and development. The institution must also be a mirror of community living and community problems, because it is expected that many institutionalized persons will eventually be returned to the community (p. 53).

An artificial setting does not lend support to the achieving of educational objectives, and even with the best of planning those "experiences, adventures, and activities" furnished within the institution can be only pale imitations of life on the outside.

In a unit on movement within a community, for example, it is difficult to establish rules for the pedestrian, including use of crosswalks, adherance to stop lights, and responsibilities of the police, without opportunity to observe and practice. In learning about money, it is one thing to learn to identify it and even add sums in a classroom but an entirely different matter to learn about it through use and, perhaps as importantly, misuse: the nickel or dime a week handled by most students in an institution is not sufficient experience on which to build a concept of care and utilization of sums of money. Development in social areas must also suffer, for the retarded are limited in their contacts to others who are themselves retarded—there can be no give and take with individuals of varying intelligence and varying social positions. It is difficult in such an artficial setting for the teacher to adhere to the rules: to teach realistically, to introduce material in a concrete way, to give opportunity for the application of the tool subject and newly developed skills in a life setting, and to develop social skills and adjustment to assist the child to live as a member of a total society.

The limitations of artificiality are certainly recognized by today's institutional teachers and compensatory measures are taken primarily through the use of organized visits to the community surrounding the institution—visits to the post office, a shopping center, a park, and even overnight visits involving a stay in a motel and meals in a restaurant. Care must be exercised, however, that an educational objective is maintained and that such trips do not evolve into mere holiday outings.

Inasmuch as other institutional departments (e.g., recreation) are often involved in the organization and conduct of field trips, close cooperation between those departments and education is demanded. It is in the educational setting that meaningful discussion of what is going to occur can best be conducted to establish a framework for the child's learning on the trip and, likewise, subsequent class discussion. The preplanning, preteaching, logistics, management, and post-teaching are all aspects which demand careful interdepartmental attention and even then can only be viewed as substitutive.

Factors in Personnel Employment

The finding and employment of trained, highly creative teachers is a chronic problem. Institutional settings are not very glamorous places in which to teach, and this coupled with low salaries and other factors have discouraged young teachers from selecting institutional work for a life's career.

Younie (1965) in surveying state institutions found that the reasons given most frequently for difficulty in locating new teaching personnel were (from most to least often given)

1. institution salary scale
2. rural location of institutions
3. lack of local colleges which offer courses leading to public school certification
4. public school competition with personnel
5. lack of suitable living accommodations
6. long work year.

Similar findings, particularly as pertaining to salary scale, were reported after a survey by the National Association for Retarded Children (A survey and study . . ., 1963). Recent evidence obtained in the Southeastern Survey from 23 respondents showed 30 per cent of the institutions indicating a pay scale comparable to that found in public schools; 26 per cent higher; and 44 per cent, a lower pay scale. The salary problem has not been solved.

Younie (1965) reported that the institutions having the easiest time employing trained teachers had a close relationship with local teacher education centers, and such arrangements are becoming more and more prevalent. In recent years there has been an expansion in college and university teacher training programs in the area of mental retardation, and quite frequently these programs make use of institutions for observation and, to a lesser extent, for practice teaching. In a few instances training programs (such as that at Florida State University) require extensive daily practical experience in an institutional setting. Such requirements bring young people into contact with the opportunities open in the institutional field and reduce the trauma once associated with the thought of devoting one's life to work in such places.

Another recent development that is assisting in the solution of the teacher shortage in institutions is the trend toward the establishment of new facilities near metropolitan centers. This allows better living arrangements, educational opportunities for individual staff members, and promise of a richer social life.

Although the teacher shortage is easing to some extent, it is doubtful if current teacher training programs will fill, in the near future, the great need for trained teachers in state institutions—they are not close to meeting the demand even for public school personnel. Institutional education directors therefore are going to have to continue to plan for the retraining of unqualified teachers through in-service training courses taught both by institutional personnel and cooperating college staff members. In reality such training is generally needed (although to a lesser extent), even with teachers who have been through college and university training programs for the education of the mentally retarded, programs which tend to emphasize the needs of the retarded in a public school setting with little attention to factors at play in institutional education.

It is anticipated that in the future education departments in residential facilities will turn to a source of classroom help which is relatively untapped at the present time—the sub-professional, including the volunteer worker. Such individuals can do much to relieve the professional teacher from mundane chores such as simple record keeping, conducting individual children through the activities of daily living, and even tutoring individuals and small groups. Such efforts are needed to allow each classroom teacher to devote the little time she has with each child to areas which require sophisticated teaching skill.

The Effectiveness of Institutional Education Programs

If the effectiveness of education programs in institutions is judged on the basis of reports in the literature to date, the conclusion must be negative. Such reports, however are undoubtedly misleading because no satisfactory solutions to the many and varied research problems have been developed.

One approach to the determination of effectiveness has been the comparing of the status of mentally retarded students enrolled in regular public school classes, special classes, and institutional classes in areas such as academic achievement and adjustment. These studies are largely invalid because they fail to take into account the fact that different programs serve different populations; have different objectives; and differ in continuity, time allocations, settings, philosophical views, and personnel. The lack of valid and reliable measurement devices for use with the retarded is another concern, and this coupled with differing definitions of the designations of educability of populations. Stanton and Cassidy (1964) pointed out in their study that even the sex ratio differed between groups—regular class, boys to girls almost equal; special class, 1.86 male to 1 female; and residential class, 2.61 male to 1 female. They also observed that

> The residential school children were both more keenly interested in school and more afraid to fail. The apparently conflicting elements in this picture can be reconciled in view of the facts that placement in the classroom is highly desirable for the residential school children to whom it is a source of both prestige and diversion, and that lack of competition reduces incentive to function at maximum capacity (p. 12).

A second approach to the determination of effectiveness is to compare a group's achievement, as determined through objective testing, with its expected achievement, as predicted from mental age. Such studies fail to take into account the status of the retarded on other pertinent parameters upon entrance into the institutional program and the objectives established for the students. In most instances, academic objectives are secondary considerations. Furthermore, mental age is an imperfect predictor for normals (Morphett and Washburne, 1931, reported correlations of .50 to .65 for MA and reading), and it is an even poorer predictor for retardates: Boyle (1959) found a correlation of .33 between MA and reading achievement among noninstitutionalized educable children. MA is probably an even poorer predictor for the institutionalized because of the high incidence of multiple involvements.

Efforts have also been made to evaluate academic achievement as a predictor of successful community placement. Eagle (1967) surveyed the literature in regard to prognostic factors and made virtually no mention of educational achievement. In fact Shafter (1957) found that ability to read, write, and tell time were not indicators of either placement success or failure. In contrast, Jackson and Butler (1963) found minimal evidence that academics are somewhat important. They examined 16 environmental and maturational variables as discriminators between successful and nonsuccessful samples. Reading achievement was significant at the .05 level, and arithmetic achievement was significant at the .01 level. Consistent research evidence that academic achievement is positively correlated with successful placement is obviously lacking but it must be noted that the "biases in selecting patients for release probably prevent determining the prognostic benefit of academic skills in clinically selected release populations (Windle, 1962, p. 92)."

A more realistic approach to evaluating the efficacy of institutional programs is to follow up individuals who are discharged from institutions to determine adjustment to community living and work life. Unfortunately, such studies have not generally singled out discharges from the educational program, but rather have considered all individuals who leave the institution. Peters (1958) and Cohen (1960) did evaluate the placement success of former students. Peters compared subjects discharged after educational treatment with subjects discharged without educational treatment in regard to rate of return to the institution. She found a ratio of 64 to 1 against return for the former as opposed to 12.3 to 1 for the latter. Interestingly, the "educated group" who were successful in adjustment in society averaged only 2.9 years in the academic program with an average institutionalization period of 6.2 years. The average achievement grade recorded for this group was 3.2 for girls and 3.3 for boys. Cohen analyzed job failures in a community returned population of 57 students—41 male and 16 female. In about one-third of the cases difficulty in community adjustment was experienced, but with few exceptions students were able to meet the skill and strength demands of the jobs in which they were placed. Seventeen students were returned to the institution with the primary reason given as poor job attitudes.

Current attempts to elevate the functioning of the trainable mentally retarded in institutions through education are so new that little research regarding effectiveness has been reported. That which has appeared has concentrated on growth in social skills (Cain and Levine, 1963) and community return (Peters, 1958). The results of such studies have not demonstrated educational effectiveness. However, these results are questionable inasmuch as the earlier mentioned problems of definition, objectives, instrumentation, and so on, plus the extreme heterogeneity of this specific group makes adequate research difficult to design and conduct.

In view of the manifold problems facing researchers, the determination of the effectiveness of education for the mentally retarded must be an individual matter. Judgment must come from concrete evidence of change derived from pre- and post-treatment evaluations based on the original objectives established for each child.

Recent and Future Developments

As an agency for change, education is playing an increasingly important role in the total picture of institutional services, and the scope of planning in this field is undergoing change. In recent years education has directed its attention to educational concerns in addition to general classroom programming for the educable and trainable mentally retarded. The initiation of speech, hearing, and language development programs has been one concern (see Institutional Speech and Hearing Services). Others have included programming for the multiply handicapped child, efforts to improve the functional ability of the profoundly and severely retarded, adult education, and extension of the institutional program into communities.

The Multiply-Handicapped: In recent years attention has been turned to the plight of those institutionalized individuals who have other handicaps such as blindness, deafness, physical handicaps, and emotional disturbances. Elonen, Polzien, and Zwarensteyn (1967) have reopened an issue (also noted in 1887—Pritchard, 1963) as it pertains to the blind but is applicable to others also:

> many blind children have been—and still are being—unjustly committed to institutions for the mentally defective. In many cases, they are emotionally disturbed children or merely non-stimulated children functioning at a low level, and institutionalization of these children without possibilities for educational and therapeutic programs is not warranted (p. 301).

The authors present evidence of great positive change in a limited sample of blind retarded children in a program involving psychological therapy, speech and language training, physical, occupational and music therapy, remedial reading, and special living conditions. Guess (1967) has also emphasized the need to specifically program for the blind retarded and has described programs in three institutions which emphasize emotional adjustment, social adjustment, and formal academic classroom work aimed primarily at a grasp of the Braille System.

Glovsky and Rigrodsky (1963) have described a program for the deaf retarded ranging in MA from 6–6 to 7–6 within which lesson plans emphasized the association of familiar objects, environment of the institution, clothing, body parts. Although this was primarily a group endeavor, individualized instruction was also utilized as is invariably demanded in any class work with the multiply disabled.

The physically handicapped retarded were a specific concern of Dybwad (1964) who emphasized that many such children "could profit from an intensive residential educational program over a period of one, two, or three years, which would help the youngster sufficiently so that he could return to his home and make a satisfactory adjustment there (p. 84)."

Gottwald (1964) has described a program at the Wayne County Training School for the high level retarded who are emotionally disturbed which emphasizes the team approach to treatment. The school program in such a setting is viewed as an integral part of a total environmental program and academics take second place to personality development and social adjustment.

Efforts toward specific program planning for the multiply handicapped are not presently widespread, but they are increasing. Cawley and Spotts (1967) surveyed 61 institutions for the mentally retarded and found only 25 teachers working specifically with the blind retarded. Of these, only five satisfied state certification requirements and the 25 teachers were dealing with 714 students, an average of almost 29 students per teacher.

It is significant that in the Southeastern Survey seven of 23 respondents noted program improvements or additions for the multiply handicapped as a result of federal funding, but only one noted more than a single class in any specific area and that was for the physically handicapped. Three respondents noted single classes for the visually impaired; two a class for the emotionally disturbed; three a class for the physically handicapped; and, two a class for the deaf.

Evidently programming for specific combinations of disabilities has not reached the level in the United States of that practiced in the Netherlands (Report of the mission to the Netherlands, 1962) where there are two institutions specifically for blind-retarded children ranging from six to 20 years of age; institutional programs which emphasize ultimate return to the community for each resident.

The Severely and Profoundly Mentally Retarded: One of the newest and most exciting innovations in the education of the total group referred to as the mentally retarded is not occurring in classroom settings, but rather is taking place, primarily under the guidance of psychologists, in ward and cottage settings. This education or training program is being aimed at a vast population which has historically taken up the greatest amount of space in institutions—the profoundly and severely retarded. Over the years these individuals have been seriously neglected if not criminally mistreated. They are finally receiving long overdue attention.

Great emphasis is now being placed on three approaches in program development: step-by-step teaching of the basic skills of everyday living, education for attendants, as trainers as well as for care purposes, and the application of operant conditioning techniques and environmental manipulation in the elevation of functional levels.

The literature reveals a great interest in this method of training with application in toilet training (Dayan, 1964), mealtime and general behavior (Edwards and Lilly, 1966; Henriksen and Doughty, 1967; Hamilton and Allen, 1967), dressing and care of clothing (Pursley and Hamilton, 1965) and speech therapy (Pursley and Hamilton, 1965; Girardeau and Spradlin, 1964).

To what extent educators are, or should be, involved in such programs outside of the school setting is questionable, but two observations are certainly relevant: this technique holds promise for classroom application for both educable and trainable children, and educators have, by dint of training experience, much to offer a collaborative effort. In this regard Younie (1966) has commented

> . . . that while institutional educators have performed well in reviewing their philosophy and programs to meet the modern needs of the mildly and moderately retarded they appear to have been less aggressive in charting the directions of those retarded who formerly received care and custody only . . .
> In terms of its meaning to the public schools, education would be hard pressed to broaden its definition to include the severely retarded, the profoundly retarded and seriously disturbed retarded. In the institution, however, it is rather clear that education must be a very adaptable force that can offer service to all groups . . . This program uses professional resources but is not based on the accumulated knowledge of any one professional field. Whatever the reason, it seems apparent that in the area of new programming and research the educator is not as visible as he might be (p. 380).

Education in and for Adulthood: Institutions are no longer bound to an historical application of chronological age in educational planning. The termination of educational opportunities at age 17 or 18, as is practiced in a public school setting, is based on an expectancy of acquisition of certain basic knowledges and is not related to a point in time at which learning terminates.

A common sense view would indicate that the length of schooling in years for the mentally retarded should be a minimal consideration inasmuch as acquisition of knowledge, rather than retention, appears to be the basic problem. This problem dictates a need for a more extended educational period with the ultimate goal being that of education as near to capacity as possible regardless of CA. In regard to the needs and goals of adult education Clarke and Clarke (1965) have commented that

> Adolescents and adults admitted to a mental deficiency institution have, in most cases, been special school pupils and very often school failures. Few

have reached an academic efficiency corresponding to their mental capacity, and nearly all are conscious of their backwardness. Their reactions to their handicaps vary and men often seem more concerned than women. Some are grateful for every opportunity offered to improve, others are discouraged and ambivalent in their attitude, others again are frankly frightened and become neurotically aggressive when again faced with a formal learning situation.

Educational work at this late stage aims not only at supplying academic and social knowledge, but is also a conscious attempt to heal some of the damage the patient has suffered in his past unsuccessful encounters with school and learning (p. 339).

Opportunities for education in an institutional setting are generally organized so that the young adult in full-time work training of placement can attend late afternoon or night classes. Younie (1965) found that 64 per cent of the chief education officers in 96 institutions assumed some responsibility for adult education. Ten of 23 (43 per cent) respondents in the Southeastern Survey indicated that they offer night or after hours education for young adults, and four of the remainder indicated a definite need for such educational offerings.

It is entirely probable that within the institution offering after hours education for young adults there will also be collaborative efforts between those responsible for vocational training and the education department in the form of part-time work, part-time education for young adults. Such collaborative efforts are largely a development of the past 10 years but are rapidly expanding both in quality of programming and in numbers and levels of children served. It has become evident that the retarded cannot wait until CA 16 or older to be imbued with attitudes so necessary for eventual work adjustment or to be introduced to the world of work. The classroom teacher has responsibilities in this area, but unfortunately she is usually ill-prepared for such endeavors. Cooperation and coordination between teachers and personnel skilled in vocational guidance and training can, therefore, produce valuable lessons and activities for the retardate of CA 11 or 12 or even younger, even though the professionals in the area of vocations do not have direct contact with the students until they are older. Younie (1966) has commented that vocational development "is a continuous process which should begin early and be carried out systematically by correlating closely an in-school period of special education and a postschool period of vocational rehabilitation (p. 376)."

Collaborative effort is mandatory if problems of transition from education to work are to be solved for each resident. Rotberg, Cicenia, and Bogatz (1965) have described a five-phase vocational training program in an institution which, although certainly not considered typical, is felt to contain elements of a thorough program which could be instituted in most residential facilities with variations. Within this program each student continues his classwork but adds work in industrial arts, home economics, and specific institutional work areas.

Cooperation between vocational training and education is a present day fact in most institutional programs. The NARC Survey and Study of State Institutions (1963) received 64 per cent "yes" responses to the question "Is there a tie-in between the rehabilitation and education program?" and 69 per cent to the question investigating the prevalence of combined work-training, education programs. In the Southeastern Survey collaborative effort specifically for the classroom is revealed by the finding that 70 per cent of 23 respondents indicated that rehabilitation personnel do work with teachers in planning pre-vocational and vocational education for the educable mentally retarded.

An extension of such efforts to children below the educable range is also clearly in evidence. Younie (1964) has described a program for the trainable mentally retarded which combines education and work-training and leads to placement in production, semi-production, or therapeutic work in adulthood. It is a two-track program, with a child entering at CA 6 to 8, and it emphasizes the development of skills that are transferable to a community setting. Such programs are apparently limited at this time, but they are developing, as well they should in view of the number of residents at this intellectual level. The Southeastern Survey received 35 per cent "yes" responses to an inquiry regarding collaborative efforts in program planning for the trainable mentally retarded.

Community Cooperation: The President's Panel on Mental Retardation seemingly set the stage for increased cooperation between institutions and their surrounding communities when they recommended future development of new institutions of limited capacity (500 beds or less) to be closely associated with community educational, medical, and welfare programs. The Panel emphasized that such cooperation should be a two-way street:

> The internal program of the institution should be developed in cooperation, or at least with a full knowledge of community resources in mind, but the institution itself must have a vital program of its own. When this transpires, the community can draw upon it, and the institution on the appropriate programs in the community, . . . (A proposed program for national . . ., 1962, p. 143).

State planning documents in the area of mental retardation indicate definite planning of small community centered institutions, and Arizona's plan (1965), for example, indicates provisioning in such centers for day-care services including the vocational and educational areas. The community is currently serving the institution educationally in Bridgeport, Connecticut, where mentally retarded children of the Kennedy Center attend public school classes and no educational buildings are located on the institutions grounds (Miles to go, 1966).

Wolfensberger (1964) noted that such cooperation has not, historically, been easy in the U.S. He emphasized, however, the positive aspects, stating that while visiting special education programs in Europe

> I saw instances where local public schools attached teachers to institutions, where institutions residents participated in a number of community programs, and where community residents participated in institutional programs.
>
> In one institution (Monyhull in Birmingham) the entire children's section was handed over to the local education authority. The children continued to live on the institution premises in their old living units, but educators, rather than physicians or nurses, direct the program. In Belfast (Northern Ireland) the institution and the day schools are under the same management committee, and a city hospital cooks the meals for a nearby day school (p. 283).

As institutions are reduced in size, and local politics take into consideration improvement in efficiency and financing, such arrangements will become increasingly prevalent for the sake of both the institutional education program and the local community. The small institution will not have, for example, sufficient high level retardates to institute a thorough educational program, but they will have some. A combined program in a local school system will not only allow for the development of a more effective program and save money, but it will also afford an opportunity to the educable children to keep in contact with a "normal society" in a "normal community"— the very type setting they will hopefully return to as independent citizens in the future. Conversely, the school district surrounding the institution may find too few trainable children for the establishment of its own thorough program, or it may be in need of assistance in educational evaluation, or other areas of need which the institution can assist in fulfilling.

Community-institution cooperation is developing, and hopefully it will become the rule rather than the exception. The extent to which cooperative arrangements are currently in effect between institutional education programs and those in communities is not known, but it is apparently minimal. In the Southeastern Survey only four of 23 directors of education indicated that their institutional education program was serving day students from the surrounding communities—a total of 12 children. Only one of 23 stated that children from the institution were enrolled in educational programs in the public schools—a total of nine. It is anticipated, however, that this trend will become more forceful in the near future.

Programs in Foreign Countries

A discussion of educational services in institutions for the mentally retarded cannot be complete without consideration of such services outside the United States.

The President's Panel on Mental Retardation, appointed by President John F. Kennedy in 1961, became quite interested in the work being done in foreign countries on the subject of mental retardation. The Panel's interest was all-encompassing with attention to residential facilities as only one part of the total, and focus on education in such a setting an even smaller part. Actions and information released by the President's Panel aroused interest on the part of other professionals. As a result in the period since 1962 there has appeared a quantity of literature pertaining to activities on foreign soil. Descriptive information regarding the U.S.S.R., Israel, Australia, Belgium, and many other countries has appeared, but generally speaking, with little attention to descriptions of educational efforts in a residential setting.

One of the best descriptions is that furnished by a delegation from the President's Panel (Report of the mission to the USSR, 1962) and then Dunn and Kirk (1963) regarding work in Russia. The terminology employed by the Russians is not that of English speaking countries nor is their administrative approach to education similar. Oligophrenia is utilized as a generic term with levels indicated as idiot, imbecile, and debile (comparable to dependent, trainable, and educable, respectively). Their administrative approach is through specialized residential schools called *internats* which are operated with attention to a much smaller percentage of the total population as a result of the restricted definition of retardation, i.e., an organic impairment. Dunn and Kirk speculate that the reduced prevalence figure might result from the Russian's ban on use of standardized intelligence tests, reduced cultural deprivation, free prenatal care, legalized abortion, and a lower prematurity rate.

Education of the mentally retarded is operated under centralized authority in Russia, but responsibilities are divided between two agencies. The Ministry of Education has responsibility for the "debile" group, and the program for imbecile children is under the Ministry of Social Welfare.

Educable (debile) children receive an educational program in a combination day and boarding school, operating five and a half days a week, within which the program is viewed as a 24-hour-a-day educational matter. Authorities in Russia report a preference for the residential approach indicating that such students make greater progress than day pupils. Trained teachers are on duty for two shifts daily. They emphasize academics and shop in the morning and social and physical skills in the afternoon and evening. Class size averages around 16, with placement made between the ages of seven and 10.

Diagnosis for placement in such classes lies in the hands of the neurophysiologist and a psychologist, with subsequent placement in many cases in diagnostic classes where diagnostic teaching is carried out by a highly trained "defectologist," speech therapist, and pediatrician. This involves, of course, remedial assistance and in some cases students are returned to the regular grade. Most, however, are assigned to appropriate classes within the internat.

The elementary curriculum, established by the Ministry of Education, includes language arts, speech training, arithmetic, hand work, singing, dramatics, drawing, rhythmics, and physical education and is organized for a self-contained classroom. For the older group, the program is for a self-contained classroom and is departmentalized, including geography, natural science, history, and mechanical drawing. Until 1962 the program for educable children terminated at age 16, but occupational adjustment problems in a number of the students led to an upward extension and currently emphasizes vocational education for those ranging in age from 16 to 18. This program includes sewing, weaving, knitting, book binding, carpentry, metal work, and construction. Academic achievement upon termination averages from fourth to fifth grade level, and job placement is in unskilled and lower semi-skilled jobs.

The program for imbecile children is also organized into internats, divorced from those serving the educable and deals with children ranging in age from four to 16 in groups of approximately 20 children. Two trained teachers work with each group on activities such as washing and dressing themselves, making their beds, physical exercise, and recreation. Specific classroom skill development is emphasized for three and a half hours of the day. The goal of these programs is the return of the individual to his community with enough skills to be capable of adequate adjustment and placement in a sheltered workshop. Those who require continuing institutionalization are transferred to units for older groups.

Teachers for both debile and imbecile children receive instruction in teacher training institutes. Two approaches have been employed in teacher training: summer and five-year-undergraduate training, with the latter having been judged to produce the better teachers. Students in training to become defectologists receive a 50 per cent higher stipend and upon graduation, a 25 per cent higher salary than teachers of normal children.

A delegation from the President's Panel visited the Netherlands (Report of the mission to the Netherlands, 1962) and, as contrasted with programs in Russia, residential education for educable children is seldom employed.

Institutional placement is reserved primarily for those of the imbecile level and below, with the educable receiving educational treatment in community day schools. Educational programming in the institution received very little attention by the visiting delegation's report, but if one can assume that such programs are comparable to the described day school programs, then academics are de-emphasized with the heaviest concentration of work on the development of motor skills and consequent work training.

Curriculum planning in Russia is done by a centralized agency with consequent similarity from program to program, while in the Netherlands curriculum is developed by officials of the individual schools, as in the United States.

As in the Netherlands, residential placement is not viewed with favor in Denmark and Sweden, and such placement occurs only when the needs of the individual cannot be met by the home or community programs. Foster home placement is preferred to institutionalization. Those residential living units which are necessary are kept as small as possible. Academic instruction, speech therapy, physical education, arts and crafts, manual activities, preparation for community living, and pre-vocational training are emphasized at the elementary level and occupational training for the teenagers (Report of the mission to Denmark and Sweden, 1962). The report indicates that for older subjects there is a great occupational orientation as witnessed by the description of one institution in Denmark where 40 out of a total of 160 boys and girls, CA 9 to 16, are privately employed in the surrounding community after school hours and on weekends. Sweden also emphasizes manipulative skills in the residential setting and the authors comment that "the classrooms available in the boarding schools are generally superior to those observed in the day schools (p. 20)."

In spite of other descriptive articles regarding foreign programs such as that by Stephens and Heber (1968) which was international in scope, and by Jordan (1964), descriptive of special education in Latin America, it is virtually impossible to obtain a picture of institutional education programs and their problems as encountered apart from the United States. This is not so strange when one considers the great difficulty in obtaining information from the literature regarding such programs in the United States. Wolfensberger (1964) has reported programming on a comparative basis. Although his comments which were drawn in large measure from institutional visits showed insight, they were almost entirely limited to administrative considerations and sheltered workshop provisions.

The comment by Dunn and Kirk (1963) regarding educational programming in Russia seems pertinent to other foreign countries: "We found little which was excitingly new by way of curriculum or teaching procedures (p. 303)." In fact, little definitive information can be obtained.

Conclusion

The advent of federal funding, increased state support, and an increase in the interest of the general society in the problems of the mentally retarded is encouraging the development of an attitude of experimentation towards institutional programming. This attitude is reflected in new programs involving greater numbers of children and increased numbers of professional personnel. Problems attendant to institutions in the areas of population characteristics and historical institutional characteristics are being attacked in an effort to provide improved settings and opportunities for learning.

It is anticipated that the next decade will see great improvements in the articulation of education programs in institutions with those in local communities and that increased communication will occur between the various programs across the United States. Improved communication and cooperation is mandatory to bring about greater uniformity in educational efforts.

References

Arizona's comprehensive plan to help the mentally retarded. Phoenix, Arizona: Arizona State Department of Health, 1965.

Blue, C. M. A survey of educational programs in institutions for the mentally retarded in the Southeast United States. Unpublished paper, The University of Georgia, 1968.

Boyle, R. How can reading be taught to educable adolescents who have not learned to read? Washington, D.C.: U.S. Office of Education, 1959.

Cain, L. and S. Levine. Effects of community and institutional school programs on trainable mentally retarded children. *CEC Research Monographs, Series B,* 1963.

Cassel, J. T. A survey of the major problems affecting the education of the mentally retarded in residential schools (public and private) and in public day schools. *American Journal of Mental Deficiency,* 1956, 60, 470–487.

Cawley, J. F. and J. V. Spotts. Mental retardation and accompanying sensory defects: Some implications of a survey. Unpublished paper, The University of Connecticut, 1967.

Clarke, A. M. and A. D. B. Clarke. *Mental deficiency—The changing outlook.* (Rev. Ed.) New York: Free Press, 1965.

Cohen, J. An analysis of vocational failures of mental retardates placed in the community after a period of institutionalization. *American Journal of Mental Deficiency,* 1960, 65, 371–375.

Dayan, M. Toilet training retarded children in a state residential institution. *Mental Retardation,* 1964, 2, 116–117.

Doll, E. E. Trends and problems in the education of the mentally retarded: 1800–1940. *American Journal of Mental Deficiency,* 1967, 72, 175–183.

Dunn, L. M. and S. A. Kirk. Impressions of Soviet psycho-educational service and research in mental retardation. *Exceptional Children,* 1963, 29, 299–311.

Dybwad, G. *Challenges in mental retardation.* New York: Columbia University Press, 1964.

Eagle, E. Prognosis and outcome of community placement of institutionalized retardates. *American Journal of Mental Deficiency,* 1967, 72, 232.

Edwards, M. and R. Lilly. Operant conditioning: An application to behavioral problems in groups. *Mental Retardation,* 1966, 4, 18–20.

Elonen, A. S., M. Polzien, and S. B. Zwarensteyn. The 'uncommitted' blind child: Results of intensive training of children formerly committed to institutions for the retarded. *Exceptional Children,* 1967, 33, 301–307.

Frankel, M., F. W. Happ, and M. P. Smith. *Functional teaching of the mentally retarded.* Springfield, Illinois: Charles C. Thomas, 1966.

Girardeau, F. and J. Spradlin. Token rewards in a cottage program. *Mental Retardation,* 1964, 2, 345–351.

Glovsky, L. and S. Rigrodsky. A classroom program for auditorily handicapped mentally deficient children. *Training School Bulletin,* 1963, 60, 56–69.

Goldberg, I., and W. J. Younie. Education as a function of the residential setting. *Mental Retardation,* 1968, in press.

Gottwald, H. L. A special program for educable-emotionally disturbed retarded. *Mental Retardation,* 1964, 2, 353–359.

Guess, D. Mental retardation and blindness: A complex and relatively unexplored dyad. *Exceptional Children,* 1967, 33, 471–479.

Hamilton, J. and P. Allen. Ward programming for severly retarded institutionalized residents. *Mental Retardation,* 1967, 5, 22–24.

Heber, R. F. A manual on terminology and classification in mental retardation. *American Journal of Mental Deficiency,* 1959 (Monograph Supplement).

Henriksen, K. and R. Doughty. Decelerating undesired mealtime behavior in a group of profoundly retarded boys. *American Journal of Mental Deficiency,* 1967, 72, 40–44.

Hobbs, M. A comparison of institutionalized and non-institutionalized mentally retarded. *American Journal of Mental Deficiency,* 1964, 69, 206–210.

Ingram, P. *Education of the slow-learning child.* New York: The Ronald Press, 1960.

Itard, J. M. G. *The wild boy of Aveyron.* New York: Appleton-Century-Crofts, 1962.

Jackson, S. and A. Butler. Prediction of successful community placement of institutionalized retardates. *American Journal of Mental Deficiency,* 1963, 68, 2–17.

Jaslow, R. I., W. L. Kime, and M. Green. Criteria for admission to institutions for the mentally retarded. *Mental Retardation,* 1966, 4, 2–5.

Jordan, J. E. Special education in Latin America. *Phi Delta Kappan,* 1964, 45, 208–213.

Kanner, L. *A history of the care and study of the mentally retarded.* Springfield, Illinois: Charles C. Thomas, 1964.

Kirk, S. and O. Johnson. *Educating the retarded child.* New York: Houghton-Mifflin, 1951.

Levine, S. Educational problems in state institutions for the mentally retarded. *American Journal of Mental Deficiency,* 1954, 58, 403–407.

Maney, A., R. Pace, and D. F. Morrison. A factor analytic study of the need for institutionalization: Problems and populations for program development. *American Journal of Mental Deficiency,* 1964, 69, 372–384.

Miles To Go—Connecticut mental retardation planning project report. Hartford, Conn.: Connecticut State Department of Health, March, 1966.

Morphett, M. and C. Washburne. When should children begin to read? *Elementary School Journal,* 1931, 496–503.

O'Connor, G. and R. M. Hunter. Regional data collection as an aid to institutional administration and program planning. *Mental Retardation,* 1967, 5, 3–6.

Perry, N. *Teaching the mentally retarded child.* New York: Columbia University Press, 1960.

Peters, R. The role of the institution academic school in the rehabilitation of the mentally retarded. *American Journal of Mental Deficiency,* 1958, 63, 506–510.

Pritchard, D. G. *Education and the handicapped—1760–1960.* New York: Humanities Press, 1963.

A proposed program for national action to combat mental retardation. (President's Panel on Mental Retardation). Washington, D.C.: U.S. Government Printing Office, 1962.

Pursley, N. and J. Hamilton. The development of a comprehensive cottage life program. *Mental Retardation,* 1965, 3, 26–29.

Report of the mission to Denmark and Sweden. (Report of the President's Panel on Mental Retardation). Washington, D.C.: U.S. Department of Health, Education, and Welfare, 1962.

Report of the mission to the Netherlands. (Report of the President's Panel on Mental Retardation). Washington, D.C.: U.S. Department of Health, Education, and Welfare, 1962.

Report of the mission to the USSR. (Report of the President's Panel on Mental Retardation). Washington, D.C.: U.S. Department of Health, Education, and Welfare, 1962.

Rosenweig, L. E. and J. Long. *Understanding and teaching the dependent retarded child.* Darien, Connecticut: Educational Publishing Corp., 1960.

Rotberg, J., H. Cicenia and B. Bogatz. A residential school program preparing educable retardates for on-the-job training. *Mental Retardation,* 1965, 3, 10–15.

Schiefelbusch, R. L., R. H. Copeland and J. O. Smith. *Language and mental retardation.* New York: Holt, Rinehart & Winston, Inc., 1967.

Shafter, A. J. Criteria for selecting institutionalized mental defectives for vocational placement. *American Journal of Mental Deficiency,* 1957, 61, 599–616.

Standards for state residential institutions for the mentally retarded. American Journal of Mental Deficiency, 1964, 68, (Monograph Supplement).

Stanton, J. and V. Cassidy. Effectiveness of special classes for educable mentally retarded. *Mental Retardation,* 1964, 2, 8–13.

Stevens, H. A. and R. Heber. An international review of developments in mental retardation. *Mental Retardation,* 1968, 6, 4–23.

A survey and study of state institutions for the mentally retarded. Vol. II. The Committee on Residential Care. New York: National Association for Retarded Children, 1963.

Talbot, M. Edouard Seguin. *American Journal of Mental Deficiency,* 1967, 72, 184–189.

———. *Edouard Seguin: A study of an educational approach to the treatment of mentally defective children.* New York: Bureau of Publications, Teachers College, Columbia University, 1964.

Tarjan, G. The role of residential care—past, present, and future. *Mental Retardation*, 1966, 4, 4–8.

Thorne, G. *Understanding the mentally retarded*. New York: McGraw-Hill, 1965.

Windle, C. Prognosis of mental subnormals. *American Journal of Mental Deficiency*, March, 1962, 66 (Monograph Supplement).

Wolfensberger, W. Some observations on European programs for the mentally retarded. *Mental Retardation*, 1964, 4, 280–285.

Younie, W. J. Approaches to educational therapy in state supported institutions for the mentally retarded. In J. Hellmuth (Ed.) *Educational therapy*. Vol. I. Seattle: Special Child Publications, 1966, pp. 371–388.

————. A survey of the administration of educational programs for the institutionalized mentally retarded. *American Journal of Mental Deficiency*, 1965, 69, 451–461.

————. The work-oriented continuum for the moderately retarded in an institution. *Training School Bulletin*, 1964, 61, 26–33.

Medical Services in Institutions
for the Mentally Retarded

Programs and services for the mentally retarded are undergoing changes, not only in this country, but throughout the world. New approaches are being tried, and traditional activities are being reappraised. One significant change has been the emphasis placed on the development of community programs and services. This has resulted in a redefining of the role of residential facilities. Their role is now being conceived as one of transitional care with the return to the community as the ultimate goal. This concept is altering the character of institutional populations and has resulted in rather radical changes in all the components of institutional programs. Another significant change is the types of residents being admitted to institutions for the retarded. Some very definite trends in admissions are evident. *New admissions are younger.* Recent sampling across the nation indicates: "Over 21 per cent are under five years of age." "New admissions will be in the main 'less than nine years old." "The median age is under eight years." *New admissions are more severely retarded, and there is a reduction in the proportion of mildly retarded.* Various surveys indicate: "In the last few years a definite increase in admissions of persons with extreme impairment." "Future admissions will be in the main the severely retarded." "The median I.Q. for all recent first admissions was 32." (A Manual on Program Development . . . 1962).

The trend for the admission of the younger mentally retarded who is more severely retarded has many implications for the medical service program in institutions.

Components of Medical Services

The medical services program in a residential facility for the mentally retarded includes whatever medical services might be needed by individuals assigned to the facility—diagnostic, preventive, supportive, therapeutic or restorative. For the larger multipurpose institution, a host of medical specialities are required. In it's "Standards for State Residential Institutions for the Mentally Retarded," the American Association on Mental Deficiency suggests the following as components of basic medical services: "A staff of competent fulltime physicians assisted by an appropriate complement of nurses, physical and occupational therapists, dentists, dental hygienists, sanitarians and related personnel." (Monograph Supplement to AJMD, 1964). In contrast the smaller, special purpose, community oriented facility may not require so many full-time medical personnel on the staff but may utilize the services of these specialities from the community as needed or required by the residents. The medical program of the facility should be tailored to the needs of that facility and be in keeping with its total program in treatment and training.

Organization of Medical Services

Institutions for the mentally retarded and the programs in each are generally organized into one of three types: the traditional medical model; the modified medical model; and the interdisciplinary model. The earliest concepts of institutions for the mentally retarded were based on the medical model. The mentally retarded were regarded as "sick," were usually referred to as "patients" and the institutions were called "hospitals." The literature is replete with statements which perceive the retarded as sick: "The biological, economic and sociological bearings of feeble-mindedness have over-shadowed the fact that is fundamentally and essentially a medical question (Fernald 1915, p. 96)." This idea is still prevalent today as can be seen in *Mental Retardation, a Handbook for the Primary Physician* (American Medical Association, 1965) which repeatedly refers to mental retardation as a "disease" or an "illness." Under this concept, the retarded are viewed as a diseased organism, and residential facilities for them are structured on the medical or hospital model. The following are some of the characteristics of the medical model: 1. The facility is administered by a medical staff; the chief administrative officer (the Medical Superintendent) is a physician with a corps of other physicians under him, and a corps of nurses under them. 2. The facility is often referred to as a hospital (e.g., "State Hospital and School"). 3. Living units may be referred to as nursing units or wards. 4. Residents are referred to as patients, and their retardation is identified as being a "disease" that requires a "diagnosis" and "prognosis." 5. Resident care is referred to as nursing care. 6. Case records are referred to as charts, and hospital routines prevail throughout the institution. Other indications of the medical model may be seen in the wearing of uniforms or medical jackets by both professional and non-professional staff; all programs are referred to as "treatment" or "therapy;" all decisions, even those of a non-medical nature such as residents' rights and privileges, visits, discipline, and inclusion in school are ultimately made by the physician; patients are more likely to be physically restricted or settled with drugs than to be counseled or trained; and there is an obsessive abhorrence of any chance or likelihood of injury to the retardate.

The modified medical model in institutions for the mentally retarded is one in which the top administrator may be a physician. Certain programs will be directed by a physician, such as the non-ambulatory service or those for the severely and profoundly retarded. Other services, however, such as the cottage life programs for the moderately and mildly retarded, may be directed by non-medical personnel. Thus, the programs are split between those whose components are largely medical management problems and those whose components are more related to educational or social problems.

The interdisciplinary model features the team approach to the care, treatment, and training of all residents. The administrator may be a physician, educator, or psychologist, and the treatment team which works with all residents regardless of I.Q. or degree of ambulation may include a variety of specialists in addition to medical specialists. These usually include nurses, social workers, psychologists, educators, therapists, nutritionists, and others.

Medical Needs of the Retarded

The medical needs of the mentally retarded might be listed in three categories: the normal medical needs of any individual child or adult, the special medical needs related to handicapping conditions, and the need for periodic reevaluation of the patient's status in relation to his evolving potential and to the array of services necessary for his changing needs (Pearson and Menefee, 1965).

To benefit to the greatest possible degree in any or all service programs in the institution, the resident must be in the best possible physical condition. This calls for frequent careful routine medical examinations to prevent minor medical problems from becoming major complications. For instance, because the more severely retarded person may be unable to communicate, hidden infection (such as otitis media, urinary tract infection, and apical abscess) may escape notice until it is well advanced. Poor dietary and hygenic habits may cause nutritionnal anemia or intestinal parasites. Dental problems, including peridontal disease, are common in the retarded and require special consideration.

If the routine health care is neglected, progress in other areas of development will be less and behavior and performance will be adversely affected. Dr. Robert Jaslow emphasized this point in his statement, "I would say that anytime there is a change in a retarded individual as far as functioning, behavior or health, before I would look at the more complex psychological or emotional or environmental factors, I would first provide a complete physical re-evaluation. The patient who is physically healthy, normal or retarded, is in a better condition to handle changes and stress situations than the patient who is in poor health" (Pearson and Menefee, 1965).

The special medical needs of the mentally retarded relate more to their associated physical and sensory handicaps than to their intellectual deficits. A study of some 25,000 children who were served in mental retardation clinics supported by state maternal and child health programs revealed that at least 75 per cent of those less than six years old had physical handicaps in addition to retardation (Pearson and Menefee, 1965). Dr. Samuel M. Wishik (Georgia Study of Handicapped Children, 1962) reported an average of 2.2 different diagnoses per child in his study of multiple handicapped children. Further, a survey conducted by the Child Development Center, Memphis, Tennessee, found that 47 per cent of the mentally retarded had three additional handicaps and that 90 per cent had at least one additional handicap (Task Force Report on Clinical Services, 1965). In the more severely and profoundly retarded, the percentages of additional sensory and motor handicaps are usually very high. The effects of these additional handicaps can have an even more catastrophic effect on the mentally retarded child than on the child with normal intelligence. Prevention, amelioration, or correction, therefore, become even more imperative. In addition to physical handicaps, associated hearing defects, speech disorder, impairment of vision, seizures and neuromuscular abnormalities are frequently noted in retarded individuals. Careful attention to these conditions can help to overcome barriers to communication with the retarded. Correction of physical defects will prevent the occurrence of deformities which may seriously affect progress in learning self-help skills and total rehabilitation.

The need for continuous medical evaluation and re-evaluation is obvious. No individual, normal or retarded, remains static. As time passes the mentally retarded individual either progresses or falls behind. The role of specific medical programs in the progress or regression should be noted and adjusted. A comprehensive medical appraisal at least annually is essential.

Types of Medical Programming

Type of medical programming in institutions for the mentally retarded will vary with the size of the institution, its geographical location, whether it is multi-purpose or special purpose, and its particular organizational model. Detailed information about the nursing services program of an institution are not included here but are recognized as component parts of the total medical services program. The following services are desirable components of a total medical services program. Some may be provided by the institution itself, and others may be secured from the community in which the facility is located as needs arise. In either case, their availability is mandatory to comprehensive medical care.

Diagnostic and Evaluation Services

PREADMISSION

A complete diagnostic and evaluation workup is desirable in every case before admission to a residential facility. This should be done by an inter-disciplinary team which may be headed by a physican. It may be handled in a community diagnostic and evaluation clinic or by a team in a residential facility as an out-patient service. Temporary admission to the facility may be necessary if the individual lives some distance away, and commuting for the length of time needed for the diagnostic work-up would create a hard-ship on the family. Temporary admission also provides an opportunity for a more lengthly observation by the staff, individually, and in teams. The evaluation normally would include a review of the case history reports submitted by a variety of agencies, an interview with the family, a social, medical, educational, and developmental history, and observations and recommendations by members of the diagnostic and evaluation team. Alternate plans for the care should be projected, depending on factors such as the availability of community services, the waiting list for admission to residential care and the quality and availability of treatment programs within residential facilities. Other considerations include the specific treatment needs of the patient, emotional stability and attitudes of the family, presence of other children in the family, age of the individual and associated handicaps, degree of mental retardation, and the economic status of the parents. Where residential care is the treatment of choice, recommendations for priority classification on the waiting list should be formulated.

ADMISSION

At the time of admission to a residential facility, the information developed during the diagnostic and evaluation (D & E) work-up should be made available to the staff of the institution. It will probably be necessary to up-date certain information, depending on the length of time which has elapsed between the diagnostic and evaluation workup and the time of admission. It is unlikely that it will be necessary to repeat the entire D & E process. Many individuals and families are unnecessarily subjected to repeating the same tests and supplying the same information simply because some profesisonals are unwilling to accept anything but first hand information.

Complete in-depth information is necessary to establish a treatment and training program for the resident that will be of most benefit to him. The following should be considered at the time of admission: a careful and de-tailed family, personal, and developmental history; physical examination in-cluding neurological and developmental assessment; psychological evalua-tions; and perhaps an array of specialized studies including laboratory work, EEG, orthopedic, physical medicine, EENT, and psychiatric. Every resi-dent should be classified by etiology and prognosis, and recommendations should be made for medication, special therapies, and general program goals.

Counseling with Parents

The medical staff has a particular responsibility to impart the information to the parents concerning the treatment and training program planned for their child. To gain their cooperation, they must understand what is planned and how the program will be implemented. Their expectations must be evaluated in terms of realities. Their questions and anxieties must be han-dled with consideration and concern.

Throughout the time the individual is in the institution, the medical staff should be available for counseling with the parents and in cooperation with other disciplines should provde guidance for them in understanding progress, failures, and limitations of the treatment program.

Preventive Medicine and Promotion of Health

Day-to-day medical supervision of all the residents in an institution for the mentally retarded is essential. Adequate medical staff is needed to pro-vide general health supervision which includes attention to related areas such as nutrition and personal hygiene.

A system of daily medical rounds by the staff physicians is usually the best method by which this can be accomplished. The length, intensity, and depth of these daily medical evaluations will depend upon a variety of cir-cumstances. In the non-ambulatory service, for instance, rounds should be made every morning. In the hospital area for the acutely ill rounds may be made several times a day and in some cases even hourly or more frequently depending upon the condition of the individuals under treatment. The nursing staff will generally alert the staff physician to any changes in the condition of individual residents and call for immediate attention if indicated.

The staff making daily medical rounds in the cottages for the ambulatory severely, moderately, and mildly retarded will usually rely on the cottage staff to identify those residents needing medical attention. Competent cottage staff can greatly assist the medical staff in providing services, particularly those related to preventive medicine, such as minor acute illnesses and accidents. During the daily rounds the medical staff will ordinarily review prescribed medications such as anticonvulsants and tranquilizers, particularly those prescribed for extended periods of time. Frequently, modifications will be indicated in the drug regimen, and a system for periodic review is necessary.

Daily medical rounds are very useful as teaching and training experiences for medical students and other staff gaining clinical experience at the institution. The observations provide opportunities for first-hand experience under supervision and are being utilized increasingly by many disciplines as a way of evaluating progress and development in the social and behavioral sciences.

Periodic physical examinations and progress reports on all residents should be scheduled along with routine immunizations and booster immunizations, including those to prevent diphtheria, tetanus, pertussis, measles, smallpox, and polio. Tuberculin skin tests and follow-up x-ray examinations for positive reactors are also recommended particularly in institutions where pre-employment physical examinations are not required for the staff.

In the event of an outbreak of a communicable disease, the institution should have facilities for isolation. Careful attention should be given at all times to sanitation because of its relationship to the spread of certain diseases. Water, milk, and ice machines should be routinely inspected and tested for bacteria. Sanitation in the preparation of food should be carefully attended and regulated.

Emergency medical services should be established with 24-hour, 7-day-a-week coverage by a physician. Staff physicians or medically trained persons should be on call at all times. In addition to such common occurrences as falls, cuts, and bruises, emergency care for incidences of acute trauma should be provided. Many institutions are utilizing interns or senior medical students to provide this service at night and on weekends. Their work is supervised by a staff physician who is readily available should the need arise.

Medical care for cases of severe illness and necessary surgical procedures may be provided by the institution or may be secured from a general hospital in the community. The latter is probably preferable and more economical in the long run because operating room, blood bank, and other specialized services may be required. The availability of emergency ambulance service, private duty nurses, and other ancillary medical personnel are also factors to be considered. In some institutions provisions are being made for pre-operative and post-operative care where staff and facilities allow. These institutions are then contracting for surgical services through community physicians and general hospitals.

A certain percentage of the residents of institutions may require long-term medical and surgical services. Provisions should be made to handle problems of specialized care such as tube feeding, tracheotomy, or complete paralysis. The medical staff supervising services of this type should give particular attention to problems such as nutrition, skin care, sanitation and the prevention of complete physical and mental regression.

Comprehensive medical services in an institution call for the involvement of a variety of specialties: pediatrics; psychiatry including child psychiatry; neurology; electroencephalography; neuro-surgery; orthopedic surgery; physical medicine and rehabilitation; internal medicine; general surgery; anesthesiology; opthalmology; otorhinolaryngology; radiology and pathology. Because it is equally difficult to obtain and to compensate specialists in these fields as staff members of the institution, provision should be made for them to conduct regular clinics where possible in the institution or to be available on a regular basis in the community.

Pediatrics particularly is becoming more important in institutions for the mentally retarded because the trend is for the younger age child to be admitted. Psychiatry, particularly child psychiatry, is assuming an increasingly important role in work with young people who have borderline or mild mental retardation associated with severe personality and behavioral disorders.

Supportive Medical Programs

General medical services for the mentally retarded in an institution should be augmented by a variety of supportive services such as dentistry and ophthalmology along with programs in speech, hearing, and physical therapy.

Full-time dentists, dental hygienists, and dental technicians should provide a program of preventive dentistry including periodic dental checkups for all residents. Checkups should be scheduled so that every resident will be seen at least every six months. The teaching of good dental care and oral hygiene should be a part of this service. Provision should be made for specialized needs such as dentures, crowns, and bridges. Oral surgery and orthodontics will also be required for some residents. These services may be a part of the regular dental program of the institution or may be secured through a specialist in the community.

Ophthalmological services would be desirable for every institution, but is generally one of those services secured from a specialist in the community. Examinations for those residents who seem to be having eye problems, prescription of glasses, periodic reexamination of those already wearing glasses, and repair service for broken glasses are included in this program.

The diagnosis of speech and hearing handicaps and the recommendations for therapy is usually a joint function of the medical and educational program in an institution. These disabilities should be noted during diagnosis and evaluation at the time of admission. The prescription for and the provision of hearing aids greatly enhances the potential for development in cases of hearing impairment. Speech therapy is often indicated for the mentally retarded whose communicative abilities may be greatly increased with proper training.

Nutrition and its role in the physical and mental development of the mentally retarded is closely related to the medical program of an institution. Nutritionists are frequently members of the diagnostic and evaluation team both in the pre-admission and admission processes. They provide an evaluation of the nutritional status of the individual under consideration by obtaining nutrition and dietary histories of the individual and his family. They are able to evaluate the dietary and food habits of the individual and, in consultation with the medical staff, suggest changes as indicated. At appropriate intervals during residency, reevaluation of the dietary habits of all residents should be conducted for the promotion of health and the prevention of debilitating conditions.

The nutritionist should also consult with the families of the residents returning home to help them understand the need for modified diets including the selection and preparation of food in relation to nutritional needs, family income, cultural food patterns, home facilities, and the development of self-feeding skills. Of particular importance in planning the total food service program of the institution is menu planning for those residents with special dietary problems such as phenylketonuria, galactosemia, and other metabolic conditions.

Auxiliary Medical Services

One of the most vital services for adequate diagnostic work by the medical team in an institution is that provided by its laboratories—pathological, clinical, anatomical, x-ray, and EEG laboratory services.

A well stocked, carefully controlled pharmacy under the direction of a registered pharmacist is indicated for most larger institutions. A system for record keeping and control of narcotics, alcohol, and other drugs in accordance with federal and state laws is required. The pharmacy should be under the direction of the medical services program of the institution and regulated in accordance with approved hospital procedures.

The role of physical medicine, including physical therapy and occupational therapy, in rehabilitation of the mentally retarded who have complicating physical handicaps cannot be underestimated. Where possible, the institution should have a complete physical therapy department directed by a qualified physical therapist. A therapy pool and tanks for full body and partial body hydrotherapy are invaluable assets to treatment. The provision of braces, walkers, special chairs, crutches, and other physical rehabilitation equipment can greatly improve ambulation of residents. Muscle reeducation and the prevention of joint contracture as well as daily exercises administered by the physical therapist or technicians under his direction have proven valuable assets in the care and treatment of non-ambulatory residents.

Medical Records

A centralized case record is the key for research in mental retardation. The record should contain a chronological recording of therapy rendered and results obtained by the physician, psychologist, social worker, chaplain, teacher, physical therapist, recreational therapist, nutritionist, consultants, and other members of the interdisciplinary professional team. The record department should be responsible for records from the time of acceptance of the applicant, either as outpatient or inpatient, until the final discharge. Where the physical plant permits, centralized filing of current resident records is ideal; this allows periodic review of records for completeness, consistency, and accuracy. The Director of the Medical Record Department should be a Registered Record Librarian. If the services of a full time Registered Record Librarian cannot be obtained, the services of consultant R.R.L. should be sought.

The record should contain comprehensive reports from the physician made at periodic intervals. Progress notes should be recorded at least once monthly and more often if necessary. The record should contain reports from the psychologist and an annual physical examination by the physician. Social workers, special education teachers, chaplains, nurses, consultants, and other professionals should make periodic reports on the programs in which the patient is involved. Reports of encephalograms, x-rays, laboratory examinations and dietary recommendations should be recorded in accordance with the recommendations of the Joint Commission on Accreditation of Hospitals. A centralized dictating system facilitates recording of these reports.

A master index of all residents should be maintained in the record department. This master index card should include identifying information, unit number, dates of admission, and discharge. A diagnoses and therapy index should be maintained as well as other special files needed for control of records and research purposes. A daily census listing admissions, discharges, and movements of residents such as leaves and trial visits should be compiled and distributed to all departments concerned.

Whenever possible, all reports in the permanent file should be typewritten. Information recorded in the record should be signed by the responsible staff member and the information must be current at all times.

Procedures and record keeping must be suited to the needs of the institution. A centralized record facilitates retrieval of information necessary for research, and unless recorded information can be retrieved, it is practically worthless.

References

Clements, James D. Program Plan for Georgia Retardation Center. The Georgia Department of Public Health, June 1964, revised October, 1965.

———. The Residential Care Facility—Indications for Placement. *Pediatric Clinics of North America*, 1968, 15, 4, 1029–1039.

Decker, Harold A., Edward N. Herberg, Mary S. Haythornthwaite, Lois K. Rupke, and Donald C. Smith. Provision of Health Care for Institutionalized Retarded Children. *American Journal of Mental Deficiency*, 73, 1968, 283–293.

Kugel, Robert B. and Wolf Wolfensberger (Eds.) *Changing Patterns in Residential Services for the Mentally Retarded—A President's Committee on Mental Retardation Monograph:* 1969. January 10, 1969.

A Manual on Program Development in Mental Retardation. *Monograph Supplement to American Journal of Mental Deficiency*, 1962, 66, 4.

Mental Retardation—Improving Resident Care for the Retarded. Proceedings of an American Association on Mental Deficiency Workshop, December, 1965, 20–21.

Pearson, Paul H. The Forgotten Patient: Medical Management of the Multiple Handicapped Retarded. *Public Health Reports*, 1965, 80, 10, 915–918.

Pearson, Paul H. and Allen R. Menefee. Medical and Social Management of the Mentally Retarded. *GP*, 1965, 31, 78–91.

Standards for State Residential Institutions for the Mentally Retarded. *Monograph Supplement to American Journal of Mental Deficiency*, 1964, 68, 4.

Task Force on Clinical Services. Georgia Mental Retardation Planning Project, Georgia Department of Public Health, 1965.

Task Force on Prevention, Clinical Services, and Residential Care. The President's Panel on Mental Retardation, 1962.

Wright, Stanley W., Mario Valente, and Georgie Tarjan. Medical Problems on a Ward of a Hospital for the Mentally Retarded. *American Journal of Diseases of Children*, 104, 1962, 142–148.

Residential Speech and Hearing Services

Since 1960 professionals involved in childhood education and reeducation have become increasingly aware and concerned about language and communication in children. They have recognized that success in life is highly dependent upon learning language in childhood, inasmuch as it forms the basis for eventual academic success and successful interpersonal relationships. Researchers have tried to define language, delineate normal language development, and isolate biological and environmental factors which influence both overt and covert language functioning. Increased attention has been given to deviant children—those whose language structure and usage is atypical when compared with the average child—such as mentally retarded children.

The recognition that defective communication is associated with mental retardation cannot be considered new nor can efforts to ameliorate it. In the early 18th Century, Esquirol based his designation of levels of retardation on the ability to speak. Dr. Jean Itard pioneered treatment when, in 1799, he initiated an institutional program for an extremely retarded 12-year-old child, Victor, who was devoid of speech or other methods of communication. Itard might well be considered the first language therapist in an institutional setting, for his program was heavily oriented toward language learning. Although five objectives were listed by Itard (one of which specified the development of language and speech), attention to speech and language was to be found in virtually all of his teaching activities. The techniques employed by Itard in striving for speech and language development were strikingly similar to the techniques employed today. He emphasized

326

sensory stimulation and discrimination (gross to fine), awareness of speech as a tool for environmental manipulation, imitation, and vocabulary development and concept formation (Itard, 1962).

Itard's direct efforts in speech and language production in mental retardation were limited to one child, but his sphere of influence was much greater due to his writings and the extension of his work through a student, Edward Seguin. Seguin devoted his life to programming for the mentally retarded. He established the first residential school for the retarded in Paris in 1837 (Seguin, 1907) and assisted in the establishment of other residential facilities in Europe and the United States. Seguin developed a systematic instructional program employing procedures which bore a great similarity to those used by early teachers of the deaf, consequently having language development (emphasizing production) as a dominant objective.

In contrast to the great attention directed to speech and language instruction for the mentally retarded during the 19th Century institutional movement, virtually nothing was done during the first half of the 20th Century. During this period, attention was turned away from elevation of functioning of the mentally retarded and was directed toward custodial care. Speech pathologists paid little heed to the needs of the mentally retarded, concerning themselves with only those whose potential for improvement (as indicated by intelligence test scores) seemed greatest.

Students of speech pathology through approximately 1960 (and, it is feared, to some extent today) were introduced to the subject of mental retardation, if at all, only in order that a label could be applied. The following are representative authoritative comments of that era:

> Mental subnormality is still a fact, and, when a child fails to learn to talk because of real mental deficiency, hope is still an illusion and must remain so under the limitations of our present knowledge (Immel, 1947, p. vii).

> The mongol is particularly unresponsive to speech rehabilitation, and its is practically useless to attempt such training. Rehabilitation of speech of the mongol, therefore, should be undertaken only with the clear understanding of everyone concerned that the therapy is experimental, and any possible results will be meager and in proportion to the patient's level of intelligence (West, Ansberry, and Carr, 1957, p. 296).

In 1957 Matthews surveyed the status of mental retardation and its relationship to speech and language training and concluded that

> although speech pathology as a profession may not have actively discouraged speech therapy for the mentally retarded, certainly there has been little encouragement given by the profession to devote attention to communication disorders associated with mental retardation (p. 532).

In view of such attitudes, it is not surprising that very few speech and hearing specialists were employed on the staffs of institutions for the retarded until the latter portion of the 1950's. In 1942 there were only four state schools in the United States with such services (Sircin & Lyons, 1942). A recently completed survey of speech and hearing services in state institutions in the Southeastern United States, with 35 of 36 institutions responding, indicates that such services were established primarily during the 1960's (Sumner, 1968). As indicated in Table 11–1 only one current program dates as far back as 1958.

The newness of therapy programs in institutions is not specific to the relatively new institutions of the South. Lincoln State School in Lincoln, Illinois (established 1865) began speech and hearing services in 1961, and Glennwood State School, Glennwood, Iowa (established 1876) began services in 1957.

Sumner's (1968) finding that speech and hearing services in institutions for the mentally retarded developed during the 1960's is undoubtedly related to the actions of President John F. Kennedy and findings of the multidisciplinary committee he appointed to survey the problems and needs of the mentally retarded. The pessimistic attitude of speech pathologists toward mental retardation was recognized and challenged by the committee report which emphasized the need to eliminate assumptions of hopelessness and engage in definitive study of mental retardation (A proposed program . . . , 1962). Subsequently, a report of the American Association on Mental Deficiency noted that the mentally retarded

should be viewed as having potential for growth and development. This potential should be recognized as limited, not only by the individual's presently recognized potential, but also by the lack of scientific knowledge on the part

Table 11–1. Length of Existence of
Institutional Therapy Services
as of 1968

Duration of Program	No. of Institutions
No. of services	6
1 year or less	3
2 years	5
3 years	3
4 years	2
5 years	5
6 years	5
10 years	1
Established since 1958 but not now in operation	5

of those working with him. Potential, therefore, should not be viewed as static or as having fixed limits according to types of individuals or present-day ideologies (Standards for state residential . . ., 1964, p. 3).

Increased governmental support, first at the national level and then grad-ually at the state level, produced three conditions which were conducive to the establishment of institutional speech and hearing programs:

1. increased availability of professional personnel with a commitment to work with the mentally retarded or speech handicapped;
2. increased emphasis on upgrading of treatment programs for the mentally retarded;
3. increased attention to the need for both basic and applied research.

With the foregoing there came speech and language investigations with the mentally retarded. New efforts evolved to investigate the relative im-portance of environment and early childhood experiences (as opposed to biological endowment) on the development of intellect. Language behavior had been taken as a primary index of intellectual functioning inasmuch as intelligence tests have always been heavily weighted with language factors. Improvement in verbal ability, therefore, came to be considered a step in the improvement of intellectual ability (Schiefelbusch, Copeland, and Smith, 1967). Robinson and Robinson (1965) stated,

> It has long been recognized that a child's use of language is intimately related to his general intelligence. Indeed, if psychologists were suddenly (and against their better judgment) limited to measuring only one aspect of behavior, the majority would probably choose language development as the single best index of intelligence in most children and adults. (p. 439).

The hypothesis that improved functioning in the use of language sym-bols, particularly as it relates to the ability to express these symbols, will improve intellectual functioning is certainly not new. At a time in the history of mental retardation when efforts to elevate their functioning through edu-cation was passé, G. Hudson-Majuen (1902) stated that

> if you deprive a person of speech you deprive him at the same time of his most effective means for mental development and it also follows that if you train and perfect his speech you must greatly improve his mentality (p. 273).

Thus, in the 1960's, the mentally retarded began to be viewed as a lan-guage deficient population which should be studied, and the institution a natural 24-hour-a-day laboratory for that study.

The actions of two professional organizations during the 1960's brought too long delayed acknowledgement of need and respectability to efforts to improve symbolic functioning in the mentally retarded.

American Speech and Hearing Association: The American Speech and Hearing Association became the professional home of workers in the fields of speech pathology and audiology in 1925; its purpose was to

> encourage basic scientific study of the processes of individual human speech and hearing, promote investigation of speech and hearing disorders, and foster improvement of therapeutic procedures with such disorders; to stimulate exchange of information among persons thus engaged, and to disseminate such information. (By-laws of the . . ., 1960, p. ix).

ASHA currently certifies both individuals and training programs, disseminates research findings through three journals, operates a placement bureau (to which superintendents of institutions may turn for speech and hearing personnel), and stimulates advances in speech pathology and audiology. After 1960 the journals of the organization began to reflect a professional interest in the speech problems of the mentally retarded. A significant step was taken in 1968 when the organization recommended that the profession of speech and hearing take a definite responsibility for language evaluation and training for all children (Marge and Irwin, 1968). The report noted that such specialists should be able to evaluate and manage all types of language problems. Of equal importance, particularly from the standpoint of institutional programming, was the recommendation that the specialist

> must be able to function as a consultant to all professionals working with the child. He must be able to supervise the activities of the professional aide. must be a clinician-educator. . . This aspect of his new role includes the ability to engage in teaching as well as in clinical activities (p. 222).

American Association on Mental Deficiency: The AAMD took a significant step toward the development of speech and hearing services in institutions when it published guidelines for the establishment of such services. The guidelines indicated that the principle functions and services should be

   I. Diagnostic
     a. Speech evaluation
     b. Language and communication appraisal
     c. Hearing screening, testing and diagnosis
     d. Hearing aid evaluation program
     e. Diagnostic therapy (differential diagnostic examinations).
  II. Therapeutic Training (Not included in Education and Training Programs)
     a. Speech programming, including speech correction, speech (lip) reading, auditory training, and hearing aid utilization offered individually or in small groups.
     b. Speech training and speech education, individually or in small groups
     c. Language development and speech stimulation offered in group therapy to infirm, non-ambulatory, or nursery living care areas.

    d. Auditory training in relation to problems of instruction, offered on the pre-school, kindergarten, or school classroom level, and in relation to all phases of clinical activity.

    (Standards for state residential . . ., 1964, p. 47).

AAMD also established a specific subsection for persons directly involved with the language, speech, and hearing problems of the mentally retarded.

The foregoing developments indicate that the long held pessimistic attitude toward the potential of mentally retarded individuals for language and speech improvement has diminished. It is now considered an appropriate area of endeavor rather than ethically improper. The new and evolving viewpoint holds that speech and language functioning can be influenced in the mentally retarded and that any improvement is a step in the development of intellectual and social potential. The professional literature has begun to reflect this change. In addition to a large increase in journal articles, three texts have recently been published in the specific area—one, a general consideration of speech and language in mental retardation (Schiefelbusch, *et al.,* 1967) and two containing specific suggestions for treatment (Malloy, 1961; Lillywhite and Bradley, 1969).

The Problem

Recent reviews of the literature make it clear that speech and language problems are much more evident in populations of retarded children than in the general population. This is true regardless of level of deficit or location in institutions or public school classes. There have been a number of such reviews including those by Spradlin (1963), Kirk (1964), Jordan (1967), McCarthy (1964), Spreen (1965), and Webb and Kinde (1967).

SPEECH

Evidence indicates that the lower the IQ and mental age, the greater the probability of speech defect in a mentally retarded child. Spradlin (1963) noted that there is a much higher percentage of speech defectiveness among institutional populations of retarded individuals than among noninstitutionalized, noting incidence figures ranging from 57 to 72 per cent for the former and 8 to 26 per cent for the latter. This probably reflects the greater incidence in institutions of individuals below the educable range of intelligence, with organic impairments, and from poor care, nonstimulating environments.

Schlanger and Gottsleben (1957) reported a comprehensive survey of an institutional population. Well trained and experienced examiners evaluated the status of speech in an entire institutional population (N = 516). They found that 79 per cent of the residents had speech disorders (Table 11–2) and that multiple speech problems were very evident; e.g., virtually all of the subjects with voice and stuttering problems also had some degree of articulation disorder. A more recent survey found virtually the same results. In 1967, 1476 residents of a total population of 1922 (76.8 per cent) were diagnosed as having speech problems in the Gracewood State School and Hospital in Augusta, Georgia (Annual report, 1967). A total of 1116 residents were judged to have moderate to severe problems, with only 806

Table 11–2. Incidence and Types of Speech Defects of the Training School Population ($N = 516$)

Defect	Total*	Total Per Cent
Total of all subjects		79
with defects	408	79
Articulation	400	78
Dyslalia		
1	21	
2	40	
3	83	
4	196	
Dysarthria		
1	31	
2	50	
3	39	
4	55	
Normal (5)	116	22
Voice	240	47
hoarse-husky	60	
aspirate	22	
hypernasal	62	
hyponasal	14	
pitch	40	
sing-song	9	
monotone	15	
rate	73	
volume	33	
Stuttering	89	17
clonic	82	
tonic	51	
secondary reactions	24	

*Total defects exceed N as many subjects have multiple speech defects. The subgroup totals also exceed articulation, voice, and stuttering group totals. For example, many subjects are included under both dyslalia and dysarthria.

(Source: Schlanger & Gottsleben, 1957)

(41.9 per cent) having mild problems or none at all. When 14-year-old children (those years in which speech problems are most manageable) were viewed, 91 per cent were noted to have speech defects.

No examiner has yet identified a specific speech pattern as characteristic of the mentally retarded. On the contrary, speech problems of the retarded do not differ in type, only in degree and incidence, from those of the non-retarded. The findings by Schlanger and Gottsleben (1957), Table 11–2, of 78 per cent articulation problems, 47 per cent voice disorders, and 17 per cent problems in fluency, contrasted with anticipated findings in the general population of 4 per cent, .5 per cent and .7 per cent respectively (Van Riper, 1963). Schaeffer and Shearer (1968) did not record so high an incidence for problems in fluency. They surveyed a total population of 4307 residents of a state school and found 7.6 per cent of the speaking population to demonstrate stuttering symptoms. "No relationships were found between the IQ level and the incidence of stuttering or the severity of stuttering within the group (p. 44)."

Lerman, Powers, and Rigrodsky (1965) analyzed the patterns of stuttering in a small institutional sample. They concluded that the stuttering behavior observed closely resembled that of intellectually average children except for less evidence of avoidance and apprehension of the speech act. Schlanger and Gottsleben (1957), noting the same dissimilarity, suggested that the noncompetitive, permissive attitude of institutional life may diminish the need of stuttering subjects to develop overt means of avoiding stuttering. They also noted that the retardates' "Low standards of self-criticism and lack of insight undoubtedly contributed to this comparatively low incidence of secondary reactions (p. 101)."

Only limited research attention has been given to the question of whether different speech disorders are characteristic of different kinds of retardation. Gottsleben (1955) matched mongoloid retardates with non-mongoloids on sex, CA, and IQ and found that more of the former showed clearcut evidence of stuttering. Zisk and Bialer (1967) surveyed the literature concerning speech and language problems in mongolism and concluded that progress in understanding has been impeded by misconceptions such as "Mongolism causes defective speech."

HEARING

Fulton and Giffin (1967) reported a comprehensive audiological and otological survey of a state institution's population of 2483. Over a four-year period, 92.2 per cent were tested using differing testing techniques in accordance with the subjects' ability to respond. An incidence rate of hearing loss of 27.4 per cent was found. Judgment of loss was made on the hearing of the better ear with 17.7 per cent of the population having mild,

7 per cent moderate, and 2.7 per cent severe losses. The predominant pathology was impacted cerumen with severe impaction in a majority of cases.

Webb and Kinde (1967) pointed out that great variability is found in the results of hearing surveys in institutions due to varying criteria and the fluctuation of loss with both age and IQ:

> If a 15-db screening level was used and two or more frequencies failed before hearing loss was identified, the incidence was 40.5 percent. When the criterion was a 20 db or more loss for one frequency, the incidence was 32 per cent, and when a two frequency loss was required, the incidence was 24 per cent (p. 98).

A reasonable estimate of the incidence of behaviorally significant hearing loss in institutionalized populations would seem to be no less than 25 per cent, with a very large percentage medically treatable. Because so many personal and social deficits encumber residents of institutions, remediable sensory deficiencies should be eliminated.

LANGUAGE

Mentally retarded children develop language late. Developmental deviations are also invariably noted when judgment is based on factors such as vocabulary understanding and use, sentence length, sentence complexity, and verbal fluency.

Comparative studies between institutionalized and non-institutionalized populations are difficult to interpret because of selection factors, examiner bias, and differences in early childhood experiences. Such studies have been conducted, however, and they agree that institutionalized individuals have greater deficits. (Mueller and Weaver, 1964, found evidence to the contrary).

Spreen (1965) concluded, after reviewing evidence in this regard, that

> the studies cited indicate clearly that institutionalized groups are inferior in their language development to defectives living in a home environment, and that the language deficit increases with length of institutionalization . . . (p. 490).

Schlanger (1954) controlled for CA, MA, IQ, and articulation proficiency in making a comparison between institutionalized and retarded children in public school classes. Superior language performance was found among the non-institutionalized children leading the writer to suggest six possible contributing factors:

1. emotional reactions resulting from the destruction of family ties;
2. lack of familial speech models to imitate;

3. almost complete association with sub-normal peers which reduces the desire and need for oral communication;
4. overt actions can be substituted for verbalization much more easily;
5. lack of privacy, resulting in withdrawal behavior;
6. lack of speech motivation due to fewer challenges in the environment.

A seventh factor, the tendency of the institutional environment to reward quiet nonverbal behavior, might be added to the above list and the seven items used as guidelines for the establishment of a total institutional program conducive to language development and oral expressiveness.

The Speech and Hearing Therapist

Work with mentally retarded individuals is undoubtedly the most challenging of all endeavors of speech pathology and audiology. All of those who work to elevate the language function of the retarded can be considered pioneers, but no area is so new and unknown as that of symbolic behavior.

The institutional speech and hearing therapist certainly needs to be an effective teacher. Van Riper (1963) has made note of a large number of personal attributes of any successful therapist including humor, social poise, ingenuity in inventing and adapting techniques, sensitive and discriminating hearing, objective attitude toward their own insecurities, and curiosity. He stressed one attribute which is of paramount importance for the therapist dealing with retarded children—empathy. To truly identify with the retarded individual is extremely difficult (and to many, threatening). Without an effort to empathize, the therapist will find it difficult to anticipate the actions and reactions of children and to motivate desired behaviors. Furthermore, empathy is essential for the therapist to reduce his own communicative behavior to a level where he can make contact with the retarded child and to obtain a response, i.e., to establish communicative rapport. In this regard Schiefelbusch (1965) commented

> if the adult is intent upon teaching the child new sounds, he may present these in a manner which is above the child's levels of comprehension or understanding, or at least above his level of functional performance. In this case, the child may 'withdraw' from participation simply because he is not able to function with confidence or with predictable success. Thus the conventional mode of presentation in the therapy context might be inappropriate . . . . In effect, the adult may simply reinforce inappropriate behaviors (p. 5).

A feeling for or, at the very least, a knowledge of institutional life is a prerequisite for successful functioning in such a setting. This is necessary so that the therapist can establish realistic language and communication goals for each child and establish a common ground for conversation; i.e., questions or comments concerning home life are frequently out of place. At the present time, the major responsibility for the development of knowledge of institutional life remains with institutional pre-service and in-service training programs.

STANDARDS OF THE AMERICAN SPEECH
AND HEARING ASSOCIATION

One function of ASHA is the certification of competency of its members in speech pathology or audiology. Requirements for certification include a Master's degree in the field, sponsored clinical practice, and successful completion of a qualifying examination.

Unfortunately, persons with such credentials are in short supply. In 1962 fewer than 40 speech and hearing specialists certified by ASHA were employed in institutions for the retarded (Copeland, 1962). Fifteen (44 per cent) of the therapists serving in southeastern institutions in 1968 were members of ASHA but only seven (21 per cent) held the Certificate of Clinical Competence. It is doubtlessly true, in view of the shortage of certified personnel, that many programs have been initiated and continued with minimally trained therapists. This is as it must be for the present, or the programs would not exist.

NEED FOR SPECIFIC TRAINING IN MENTAL RETARDATION

Few, if any, training programs in the field of speech pathology and audiology require specific theory or practicum in the field of mental retardation. In consideration of the extremely limited numbers of therapists now available to work in institutions the therapist in attendance at the 1964 Parsons Conference (Institutional speech . . ., 1964) recommended that "previous training and experience in this area should not be a requirement for consideration of new personnel (p. 5)." This factor, although recognizably true, should not prevent the initiation of course work and practicum concerning mental retardation in therapy training programs because 1. the lack of such experience perpetuates the pessimistic attitude of trained therapists; 2. all active therapists need to know about intellectual limitations whether they work specifically with the mentally retarded or not; 3. introduction to the subject would assist in the recruitment of effective therapists for such work.

The 1968 Sumner study found that 23 of the 34 therapists (68 per cent) in institutions in the southeastern United States had had specific coursework in the area of mental retardation although the number that had had such training before employment was not determined. The number of college credit hours earned by the 23 therapists varied from two to 45 semester hours ($\overline{X} = 12.7$, $M = 9$). The remaining 11 reported that they needed such training. Directors of institutional speech and hearing programs were asked to indicate what, if any, training in mental retardation should be required of speech and hearing therapists. Responses were received from the 21 therapists directly responsible for programs and also from eight administrators who did not at that time have programs (Table 11–3).

All respondents felt that some knowledge of mental retardation was essential in the training of speech and hearing therapists to function in an institutional setting although one person (not a speech therapist) felt that such knowledge could be gained in-service. Each of three aspects of college work was given approximately the same weight; 22 respondents felt that coursework in theory was important, 21 methods, and 23 practicum in an institutional setting. In the combining of two aspects of college work, which seems realistic in view of the time demand already placed on therapists in training, the inclusion of theory with practicum was mentioned more than any other (19 of 29).

Knowledge of mental retardation and institutional life are essential for effective functioning of the institutional speech and hearing therapist. Without such knowledge communication with aides, house parents, teachers, and others who are important to a successful program will be greatly impaired. The newly graduated therapist generally approaches her patients as if they were intellectually average. As a result, the vocabulary and sentence complexity she commonly employs, the skills and techniques she has developed, and even her selection of materials are often inappropriate.

Table 11–3. Need of Training in Mental Retardation
for Speech Therapists—as Expressed by
Institutional Administrators

Response Combinations	Therapists (N = 21)	Administrators (N = 8)	Total
Theory-Methods-Practicum	7	3	10
Theory-Methods-Practicum In Service	1	1	2
Theory-Methods	2		2
Methods-Practicum	4		4
Theory-Practicum-In Service		1	1
Theory-Practicum	5	1	6
Theory-Methods-In Service	1		1
Methods	1	1	2
In Service		1	1

Perhaps the inexperienced therapists' expectations for progress are even more inappropriate than the choice of methods. The usual college training program imbues its students with the feeling that the successful therapist is one who achieves a reasonable degree of "normalcy" in speech in a great majority of cases. Although they may not be taught in so many words, they still strive to "cure" speech disorders.

Speech and language work with the mentally retarded demands a reorganization of personal goals because few of their severe speech or language problems will be eliminated completely. The successful therapist is one who can derive a feeling of accomplishment from small improvements in her retarded patients' language functioning.

A more adequate frame of reference for work with the intellectually subnormal should be established in college training programs prior to employment, because the knowledge necessary for a reorientation of goals to occur is difficult to obtain after training.

Objectives

Speech and language abilities in the mentally retarded range from those with no responsiveness to speech and no evidence of the utilization of symbols internally for thought to those highly articulate individuals whose deficiencies in language are revealed primarily through their responses to verbal test items. Those in institutions, however, increasingly tend to range from no responsiveness to minimal, frequently unintelligible, verbalization.

The present limitations of knowledge make it impossible to predict that such individuals can be developed to a normal level in language functioning. Therapists indicate, however, that each subject can be improved to some extent in the understanding of language, the meaningful and understandable production of speech, and the utilization of language as a tool for thought. This, then, must be the overriding objective—the obtaining of as high a level of functioning as possible in each of the three foregoing elements of language utilization for each child.

The role of the successful institutional therapist is many faceted; it includes

1. evaluation of language status in individual children;
2. programming for the great masses of children in institutional populations whose initial need lies in the area of language learning;
3. the evaluation of each child's ability to communicate;
4. institutional programming and specific therapeutic involvement in the improvement of communication skills.

The establishment of specific goals becomes an individual matter for, as Schiefelbusch (1965) noted,

Regardless of its inadequacy, the child's speech has to serve as the starting point; and regardless of the nature of the child's communication responses, they should be regarded as relevant to the eventual goals that the therapist seeks to help the child achieve (p. 5).

Speech therapy has historically operated as a correcting or a reestablishing profession. That is, professionals have functioned to improve a behavior that developed improperly or to bring back a behavior once properly developed but deficient due to acquired causes (e.g., stroke, accident). Recently the profession has begun to work with problems which result in the failure of development—habilitation as well as rehabilitation—as is demanded in the work with the mentally retarded. The objectives of speech and hearing therapy with the mentally retarded should be:

1. to develop in the non-responsive individual an awareness of and a responsiveness to language as it is exhibited through gestures, facial expression, and speech;
2. to improve the child's ability to utilize language symbols as a means for thought;
3. to develop in the child a desire to communicate;
4. to improve the physical capacity of the individual for speech;
5. to establish an environment which is conducive to spoken communication;
6. to obtain from the child efforts toward oral communication;
7. to assist the child in making his oral communication as intelligible as possible.

For these goals to be obtained, each child must be viewed as capable of interpersonal communication. In this regard Schlanger (1958) has commented that

Therapy should concentrate on the reduction of negative interpersonal interaction and attempt to make communication rewarding. Therapy based on sound analysis, drills and the manipulation of articulators would not be feasible. A speech-in-use idea with pleasant and meaningful associations presented 'non-directively' is likely to prove more successful than direct practice in the production of speech sounds (p. 298).

Indeed, the primary aim of the speech staff should be to establish within the institutional setting a milieu that is conducive to increased language functioning, including oral communication. For gains to be made, communication must become rewarding for each child. The intellectually average child with a speech problem will cease efforts to improve if he does not receive positive feedback. The needs of the retarded child for encouragement and feedback are even greater.

The therapist can furnish feedback only when she is with the child. It is imperative that the entire staff recognize the importance of encouraging each child to use language. Speech can not be an incidental or infrequent tool; so its improvement must be a joint effort of the entire staff, assisted and directed by the speech and hearing personnel. Van Riper's (1963) statement in regard to speech therapy with the retarded is equally applicable to all disciplines from whom children learn in an institutional setting: "We emphasize tool speech, not display speech. We try to create the same conditions of interaction which produce speech in the normal infant: love and mutual sharing of activity and imitation (p. 111)."

Improved communicative ability in institutionalized mentally retarded children is followed by improved reactions to the environment and less anxiety and asocial behavior (Schneider & Vallon, 1955; Weiss and Horton, 1966). Inasmuch as the entire staff stands to gain from the development of communication skills in the residents, staff members should be made an active part of the developmental process.

Program Operation

Because of the newness of efforts and the lack of collaboration between institutions, there is little available information concerning the extent or the structure and functioning of speech, language, and hearing programs in institutions. The only collaborative effort we know was the gathering of 12 institutional speech and hearing therapists in 1964 for an exchange of program information (Institutional speech . . ., 1964). It was noted at that time that

> there is very little clinical activity in the state institutions around the country by comparison with more traditional speech and hearing settings and the activity which is taking place needs coordinating with other similar programs (p. 7).

Three questionnaire studies of speech and hearing services in state institutions for the mentally retarded have been conducted. The staff of the Parsons State Hospital and Training Center Speech and Hearing Department received responses from 75 institutions (70.7 per cent of those contacted) in the United States of which 41 (54.6 per cent) employed at least one staff member in speech and hearing. (A report on the speech . . ., 1964). Two years later Leach, Rolland, and Lloyd 1966) found 163 full-time and 42 part-time therapists employed in 110 state institutions. A more recent survey conducted by Sumner (the Southeastern Survey) involved questionnaire contact with 36 state institutional programs (100 per cent response) in the Southeastern United States and telephone contact with the superintendents of 35 of those institutions (97.2 per cent responses). Programs were reported for 21 of the 36 institutions (58.3 per cent) although two of them were dependent upon part-time personnel. Thirty-four (nine part-time and 25 full-time) therapists were employed by the 21 institutions, divided as follows:

1 therapist	15 institutions
2 therapists	3 institutions
3 therapists	1 institution
5 therapists	2 institutions

There were 49,451 residents in the 36 institutions surveyed in 1968, 1454 for each of the 34 part-time and full-time therapists. The American Association on Mental Deficiency recommended one therapist for each 400 residents (Standards for the state residential . . ., 1964).

ADMINISTRATIVE LOCATION

The administrative location of professional services varies widely, although telephone interviews with 21 superintendents who had programs, plus eight others who had had programs previously, indicated a definite preference for location within departments of education or education and training. Specific responses in the Southeastern Survey were as follows:

Education, or education and training	18
Clinical services	4
Hospital improvement projects	3
Vocational rehabilitation	1
Medicine	1
Human development	1
Psychology	1

The American Association on Mental Deficiency has suggested the placement of speech and hearing therapy services in education or medical and health service. Whether speech and hearing is a part of another department or a separate department, it "should maintain itself as an individual profession within the administrative framework. Since SPAR (speech pathology, audiology, and research) represents a multidisciplined area of specialization, effective communication with other departments and services is highly essential (Standards for state residential . . ., 1964, p. 48)."

Leach (1964) strongly recommended that speech and hearing services be an independent department. He argued that locating these services within another department assumes that the department is capable of supervising and directing activities in speech and hearing. The persons directly knowledgeable are therefore robbed of decision-making powers concerning their own programs. He further stated that the acceptance of a prescription role (as in medicine) by speech and hearing impairs the image of the personnel themselves as well as in the eyes of other institutional staff.

QUALIFICATIONS OF THERAPISTS

The 34 speech and hearing therapists serving the 21 southeastern institutional programs reported highest degrees and college majors as follows:

Degree	*No.*	*Major*	*No.*
Non-degree	1	Speech Pathology	28
Bachelors	16	Audiology	2
Masters	16	Deaf Education	2
Ph.D.	1	Education	1
		Theater	1

Fifteen (44 per cent) of the therapists serving in southeastern institutions for the mentally retarded in 1968 were members of the American Speech and Hearing Association, and only seven (21 per cent) of them held the Certificate of Clinical Competence in Speech Pathology and Audiology. Results in the southeast cannot be taken as a national indicator, however, because Leach, Rolland, and Lloyd (1966) reported that 45.3 per cent of 205 therapists employed nationally held certification in 1966.

RESPONSIBILITIES

Assuming that the number of therapists is a valid indicator of program scope, it appears that hearing problems of the mentally retarded are receiving scant attention in institutions in the Southeastern United States. Thirty of the 34 respondents in the Survey noted speech therapy as their area of primary employment—only one noted audiology and two, deaf education. One person indicated primary responsibility in language development. Leach, et al. (1966) noted more concern for hearing on a national level— 52 of the 205 (25.3 per cent) respondents noted hearing as their primary area of work.

As institutional workers become more aware of the need for attention to the speech and language problems of the retarded the demands on speech and hearing personnel will increase. The work of such individuals in an institutional setting cannot be viewed as strictly a matter of clinical functioning. In the Southeastern Survey, it was found that 16 of the 21 institutions with speech therapy services utilized a therapist on the diagnostic team, and 18 had a speech therapist as a consultant to the total educational program. All respondents indicated a need for service in such capacities. Twelve of the 21 programs were involved in the in-service training of house parents, attendants, and aides. Therapy cases were followed into the school for teacher assistance in 20 of 21 instances, but only nine noted such efforts in the cottage or ward setting.

Programming for language development is becoming an increasingly important aspect of institutional work with the retarded, and speech and hearing therapists can and should serve as leaders. Language training programs were conducted in 24 of the 36 institutions in the southeast in 1968—including 19 of 21 institutions with therapists. Therapists were directly involved in 17 of the 19 programs, but the arrangement for involvement was not consistent from institution to institution; a number of approaches are employed. In five institutions therapists and teachers conducted language programs but independently of each other. Therapists were responsible for the specific conduct of language improvement sessions in six programs, but they were expected to follow up by serving as consultants to teachers who furthered the work in the classroom. Therapists were responsible for language improvement programs in three instances where there was no contact with teaching personnel. In three other programs the teacher was responsible with consultant help furnished by the therapist. The two remaining programs were conducted by teachers with no involvement on the part of speech therapists.

In spite of the demands on institutional therapists to broaden their base of operations, their work has remained largely clinical in nature. The 34 therapists serving in southeastern institutions in 1968 indicated that they devoted almost three times as much time to speech therapy as to diagnosis, with consultation, in-service training, and research taking minimal time (Table 11-4).

The numbers of children seen by individual full-time therapists responding to the Southeastern Survey varied greatly. The weekly caseloads ranged from eight to 97 persons for the 24 informants providing useful information ($\overline{X} = 38.6$). A total of 929 persons received services per week with the majority—628—being seen for group therapy. Interestingly, five of the 24 therapists indicated no attention to group work, whereas only two specified no individual therapy. Obviously, a very small percentage of the retardates in institutions in the Southeastern United States in 1968 were receiving direct attention from speech and hearing therapists.

The Parsons Conference (Institutional speech. . ., 1964) commented, in regard to time allocated for clinical functioning, that

Table 11–4. Time Allocation of Therapists in State Institutions in the S. E. United States

	N	R(%)	$\overline{X}$(%)	M(%)
Full-Time Therapists (*N* = 25)				
Diagnosis	22	2–70	17.3	12.5
Speech Therapy	23	13–90	55.1	62
Hearing	17	1–75	18.7	12
Administration	11	2–25	12	10
Consultation	18	2–25	8	9
Research	5	1–33	14.2	4
Other	8	2–60	20	12.5
Part-Time Therapists (*N* = 9)				
Diagnosis	5	17–75	33	25
Speech Therapy	5	25–100	58	50
Hearing	2	20–100	60	
Administration	3	1·5–75	38	25
Consultation	1	5	5	
Research	1	5	5	
Other	1	100	100	

no more than 55 per cent of a clinican's working time be spent in actual treatment and/or evaluation of clients. While it is realized this recommendation may be vigorously opposed in some settings, an administrative demand for a greater time commitment will, in effect, greatly diminish the growth and development of the speech and hearing program (p. 5).

An example of weekly time allocation per therapist which agrees with the foregoing is that of the Parsons State Hospital and Training Center where, in 1964, there were eight professionals serving a total population of 675 residents

Therapy	20 hours
Reporting	4 hours
Staffing and Conferences	2 hours
Experimental work	8 hours
Evaluations and Seminars	4 hours
Training	4 hours

REFERRAL AND CASE SELECTION

An institution for the mentally retarded is an extremely complex administrative structure involving many professional disciplines and departments. In part, the effectiveness of any of the departments involved in the treatment, education, or reeducation of mentally retarded children depends upon the sources, policies, and procedures of referral. Similarly, policies determining case selection are of great interest.

The Southeastern Survey requested information concerning the system employed for case referral in each program. Responses were as follows:

Take referrals from any source within the institution	10
Take referrals from limited sources (e.g., education, medicine)	5
Screen all new children	2
Screen all children	2
Take referrals from a specific referral committee	2

There were obvious differences in policies for referral. The same was true for criteria employed to determine which cases were seen for diagnosis or therapy. Respondents reported using 1. motivation and present potential, six; 2. source of referral, six; 3. IQ (or IQ plus other factors), five; 4. greatest need, two; and 5. all cases seen (new institutions), two.

Unfortunately it could not be determined what the terms *greatest need* and *present potential* meant operationally. These terms seemed to vary from one institution to the next and perhaps from therapist to therapist within institutions. Suspecting that potential might be a determining factor in the selection of cases, source of referral was investigated as an indicator of potential. That is, children referred from vocational rehabilitation or education might logically be expected to have greater potential than children referred from a nonambulatory ward or from a cottage. Only eight of the 21 therapy programs gave preference to persons referred by vocational rehabilitation, and 10 of 21 gave preference to persons referred by the schools. There was some feeling expressed that "all children should be treated equally." Interestingly, those programs utilized prognosis in case selection, but they apparently did not accept source of referral as a prognostic factor.

PERSONNEL CONSIDERATIONS

There were almost as many vacancies for speech and hearing therapists in institutions in the Southeastern United States in 1968 as there were therapists employed. Seventeen institutions indicated that they had open positions (31 total). Furthermore, 26 respondents reported definite plans to increase the number of positions. A number of replies commented on the difficulty of hiring therapists. Others noted that salaries of public school therapists were often higher than those of state institutions. Remoteness of location was also noted as a deterent to attracting speech therapists to institutional employment.

A large number of southeastern institutions have tried to alleviate the problem of a shortage of trained personnel through the use of volunteer workers. Ten of 21 institutions with therapists did make use of such persons. In addition, two other respondents (without therapy services) indicated the use of volunteers for work in speech. Several therapists stated approval of the foster grandparent plan, but they did not know such persons were used in speech and language training.

Affiliation of college and university speech and hearing training programs with institutions might well assist in the alleviation of personnel shortage. In 1968, 15 of 21 southeastern institutions with speech services had such an affiliation. One superintendent noted that "by virtue of our affiliation with a university and the people who rotate through our training program we are pretty well able to keep our positions filled as the vacancies occur." In 1964, 35 of 75 institutions nationally were involved to some extent in the training of college students, institutional professional personnel, or nonprofessional personnel (A report on the speech and . . ., 1964).

PLANT

Public programs in speech pathology and audiology have often begun in make-shift quarters with homemade equipment and materials. Such has been the case in the majority of public school programs, and institutions are undoubtedly no different. They have had their beginnings frequently in one room which served as an office, therapy center, speech diagnostic area, and audiological test setting. A successful program, however, soon gains acceptance, and the need for appropriate space becomes obvious.

Plant needs vary according to institutional population, present and anticipated staff, and the over-all expectations of functions (present and future) of the speech and hearing program. Fulton (1967) considered these factors when he presented a formula for the determination of both personnel and plant needs in an institutional setting.

Information from 75 institutions in 1964 indicated that only three speech and hearing programs were housed in a building designed specifically for that purpose. Forty-two informants indicated that the number of rooms devoted exclusively to speech and hearing services ranged from 0 to 18 ($X = 3.3$) (A report on the speech and . . ., 1964). In 1966, 60 program respondents (142 contacted) indicated an average of 945.65 sq. ft. devoted to speech and hearing services, with 26 of the programs having sound treated rooms available for audiometric testing and other noise-free needs (Leach, *et al.,* 1966).

Figure 11–1 is a floor plan of the area devoted to speech and hearing services in the newly constructed Georgia Retardation Center in Atlanta,

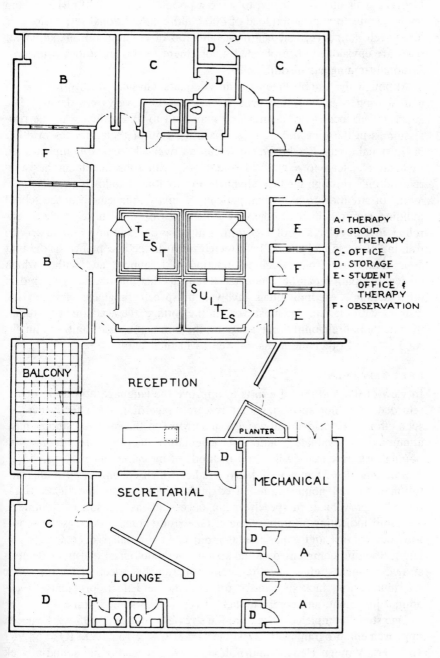

Figure 11–1. Speech and Hearing Suite, Georgia Retardation Center.

Georgia. This unit is designed to serve a population of 1,000 residents and an anticipated day program load of 400 children. Additional responsibilities for speech, language, and hearing evaluation of children on an outpatient basis are envisioned. The planned involvement of this institution with professional training can also be noted.

Although the establishment of an adequate physical facility for speech and hearing is an absolute need it can present a very real danger. The geographical location of such a unit may tend to fix the image of the professionals in the unit and decrease the utilization of their services in other institutional areas. Establishment within an over-all medical complex may, for example, lead to a medical orientation with subsequent emphasis on referral only through medical channels and treatment following the medical model of attention to individual patients. Similarly, placement in the school building may result in the delivery of services only to those residents enrolled in a regular school program. Emphasis in planning and in-service training of personnel should be directed towards the acceptance of the unit as a home base from which to function in treatment and within which clinical evaluation can be conducted to add to that information gathered in other settings. All individuals involved in speech, language, and hearing training with the retarded must work in the cottage, the academic classroom, the vocational rehabilitation classroom, the non-ambulatory unit, the lunchroom, and all other life areas, as well as in their clinic.

EFFECTIVENESS

In view of the newness of efforts to improve the language utilization of the retarded, it is not surprising that research regarding the effectiveness of such efforts has yielded equivocal results. Most of the reported studies have attempted to evaluate traditional articulation therapy procedures with populations, research design, and methods of measurement varying widely.

Spradlin (1963) reviewed twelve studies which encompassed both institutionalized and noninstitutionalized populations. Seven investigations reported improvement in speech or language skills as a result of treatment, with four indicating no improvement. One study noted a decrease in scores for both control and experimental groups but a smaller decrease for the latter. Spradlin commented on the serious methodological questions demonstrated in such studies including contamination by selection factors, poor instrumentation, lack of control for Hawthorne Effect, problems of examiner judgment, and complete lack of controls in some instances.

One study, completed since Spradlin's review, involved a 35-week speech improvement program with 27 subjects ($\overline{X}$ CA = 13.11. X IQ = 54.96) (Shubert, Vanden Heuvel, and Fulton, 1966). A traditional sound-a-week approach was followed using pictures, stories, rhymes, and review of sounds in isolation and in words. A control group of equal CA and IQ was established. Articulation gain was made by both groups, but no significant difference was found. Subjectively, it was felt that the experimental subjects "showed greater awareness of language and communication and expressed themselves more freely within the group structure (p. 277)." The authors noted a need for replication using fewer sounds and greater opportunity for the subjects to develop expressive skills.

Effectiveness of treatment with the mentally retarded can be determined objectively only when the goals of therapy have been clearly identified, adequate treatment procedures employed, and appropriate instruments designed. These items have not been satisfactorily accounted for in completed research, and those studies "which report no differences are hardly of sufficient precision that one could say that therapy has no effect (Spradlin, 1963, p. 542)".

When the gross speech and language problems of a majority of retarded persons in institutions are considered, changing articulation patterns seems relatively unimportant. The subjective findings of virtually all research seems to be more relevant inasmuch as experimental subjects are invariably noted as showing an increased interest in communicating and willingness to do so. Researchers are not currently equipped to pinpoint change numerically in the retarded child's "functional range of communication and his readiness and willingness to participate more actively in communication experiences (Schielfelbusch, 1965, p. 7)"—the major goals of the therapeutic process. Neither are they equipped to detect changes in intelligibility which may occur independently of improvement in articulation skills.

The Present and the Future?

The functioning of most speech and hearing professionals in institutions for the mentally retarded in the United States is currently based on a medical model. Services are rendered in a clinic which is geographically apart from where children daily live and function. Children considered to need therapy are brought to the therapist, one or more (seldom exceeding four) at a time by an aide, attendant, or a high level older-age patient. The therapist applies her skill, returning the children to other parts of the institution at the end of a 30-minute period. This scene is enacted for a limited number of children from one to three times each week. Enacted, that is, when the children aren't gone on a field trip, to the doctor, the dentist, home for a visit, or a myriad of other situations that inevitably make demands on children's time in institutional life.

Similarly, children are taken to a medical clinic where a physician treats an ailment through the administration of an antibiotic, the application of an ointment, or other means. If daily medication or other management is necessary, it is administered by individuals ancillary to medicine who have been trained to follow every prescription rigidly. The physician, therefore, can know that the effects of his treatment will be carried beyond the four walls of the clinic room.

The speech therapist who applies her skill within a clinic setting cannot assume that her treatment will be supplemented outside the clinic. On the contrary, the aides, attendants, house parents, teachers, and others who come into daily contact with a given speech defective or language deficient child generally reinforce what the therapist has attempted to negate, i.e., minimal communicative function or a defective speech pattern. Deviant language behavior is perpetuated by well meaning institutional workers who pride themselves on getting to know their children to such an extent that they can demonstrate understanding of what little the child means even though he does not use language appropriately. As the child produces gestures, other minimal attempts at communication, or incorrect patterns of speech such persons reward the child with understanding and with fulfillment of his wishes—reinforcing the inadequate language behavior. Institution workers may imitate the child, feeling that they are helping him by conversing on his level, but in reality they reinforce those very speech patterns that the therapist is attempting to eradicate.

Therapists in institutions presently do very little to bring others actively into the therapeutic process. What little is done is done through conferences rather than demonstrations and involves teachers to the exclusion of persons more intimately involved with communication for purposes of everyday living. Such separation from the on-going institutional routine is well established and is becoming more and more obvious as the professional staffs of institutions grow. Professional separatism is hard to defend under any circumstance, but in the case of medicine concern lies with the cleanliness of the various areas of the institution and the physical care of the patient, not the elevation of behavioral functioning. Recently institutions have been medically oriented so that today the physician can reinforce his concerns about cleanliness and patient care in the minds of the other staff members by a rare appearance in a cottage where a few well chosen remarks bring lasting effect.

What might occur if language and communication skill development was emphasized as much as cleanliness and health in the minds of institutional workers? A conceivably effective method of doing this would be for the clinic to serve as a home base for the institution's speech and hearing personnel, but the majority of the day-to-day contact with residents (excepting some aspects of diagnosis) would take place in living areas and school classrooms. Such an arrangement will be followed by the cry that routine is being disrupted (that routine established to maintain cleanliness, bodily care, and historically acceptable class work). To be effective, however, steps must be taken to break down barriers of well established routines.

The therapist who works in the ward setting can come to know the day-to-day problems of that setting and can in turn become known. She can, through work by the non-ambulatory child's bed or in a corner of the cottage with three of four children demonstrate elements of proper handling for language growth to cottage life workers. Similarly, contact with psychologists, physicians, and nurses in such settings will do more to encourage them to attend to the development of language skills in children than will contact around a conference table. They may come to reward the actual daily handlers of children for improvement in language spheres. Gradually, the assistance that the therapist can offer should become more eagerly sought.

Both demonstration work by institutional speech and hearing therapists and other approaches are necessary because it is obvious that the number of children in need in institutions exceeds by thousands the number currently receiving services through the medical model approach. Hope that increased numbers of speech and hearing professionals will be added to institutional staffs in the near future to give direct attention to all of those in need is ill founded because it would take hundreds more than are currently being trained. Furthermore, the therapists who do become available will be bid for at increasingly higher financial levels, and even more pessimistically, those in training are not being actively encouraged to consider working with the retarded.

Investigations into varying approaches must be made which may result in more children, per therapist, receiving attention with equal or greater results than are currently obtained. Many other questions concerning the treatment of speech, language, and hearing problems of mentally retarded persons also await investigation. The present low level of knowledge in this area is reflected in the many questions which Schlanger (1967) has posed:

1. Does the therapist working with the retarded need special characteristics or training?
2. On what criteria should mentally retarded subjects be selected for therapy? Where and how?
3. What are the best preliminary approaches to therapy?
4. What therapy procedures should be used?
5. What is success in therapy with the retarded, and how is it measured?
6. Are there nontraditional therapy methods that should be explored? (p. 143)

Institutions are ideally suited to working experimentally with the mentally retarded. No other setting offers the possibility of 24-hour-a-day control over a speech and language environment with the pooling of disciplines which are needed for effective diagnosis and treatment planning.

Leach (1965) has described an institutional program where research is an essential part of the service offered to each child. An experimental clinic

> establishes rigorous demands upon the treatment administered which insists upon both more information and a better quality of information. Since the majority of a clinician's time is spent in treatment of a communication difficulty, then it seems logical to view treatment as the most potent and lucrative source for information which will improve treatment . . . In this situation, all treatment becomes experimental treatment and a line of distinction between what is research and what is service or clinical is difficult, if not impossible, to find (p. 3).

Leach emphasized that the basic element of such an approach was the gathering of vital information to be fed back into the treatment program. Three basic principles of experimental treatment in a service program were offered:

1. Clinical hypotheses must be determined by the staff from the communication handicaps which the children present. Clinical functioning does not allow complete freedom in the selection of questions for investigation.
2. There must be a well formulated treatment plan before the initiation of actual treatment, and it must be followed without change during a treatment session. Only in this way can procedures be fully evaluated. Once a session is completed a progress report is made, and then change in treatment can be made.
3. Measurement devices must be established for the detection of change. It is important to remember, however, that critical attention must be given to the detection of small gains as indicators of success.

Institutions have only begun to serve as centers for treatment research. Rigrodsky and Steer (1961) conducted a study in which a stimulation approach to speech improvement, generated by Mowrer's autistic language development theory, was contrasted with a traditional approach. Peins (1967) structured therapy sessions around conversation, discussion, and role playing. A significant contribution to the treatment of speech and language problems in the mentally retarded has been made in recent years by institutional workers (primarily psychologists) through the application of operant techniques. This approach (discussed fully by Watson elsewhere in this book) is proving useful with even the lowest level retardates for improvement in speech and language skills such as rudimentary vocabulary or even the ability to imitate. As can be seen in the studies cited by Watson, the development of reception, internalization, and response to language is an integral part of operant programming even when the primary objective is toilet training, dressing, or other self-care functions. Steps in operant programming and their place in speech pathology have been outlined by Brookshire (1967), but unfortunately the literature reflects only limited attention to it by institutional speech and hearing therapists.

Shubert and Fulton (1966) were concerned with the problem of insufficient daily attention to the speech and language development of the institutionalized mentally retarded. They conducted a three-phase program in attendant training:

> The first provided a means whereby the attendant staff would be guided and instructed in ways and methods of working with the mentally retarded, particularly in terms of communication. The second phase demonstrated how the attendants could apply the knowledge they had acquired to aid and to build communicative skills in the mentally retarded child. The third phase of the program was to improve inter-group relationships (p. 27).

Lecture and discussion were employed, but in the second phase ways of stimulating children in speech reception and expression were demonstrated —a most vital part of any educational program for institutional staff members.

Closed circuit television was employed by Lombardi and Poole (1968) to work with both educable and trainable children in an articulated sound approach to speech improvement. One sound was introduced each week through story telling, and there was much repetition. Twenty sounds were presented during one year. The classroom teacher, aided by a speech therapist, was responsible for follow through in the classroom. Closed circuit television has also been used at Gracewood State School and Hospital, Augusta, Georgia for the training of aides and attendants in the area of speech and language.

One possible approach to the alleviation of the personnel shortage which has received little attention in institutions is the use of personnel with differing levels of training. The specifics of numbers of levels, training requirements at each level, responsibilities, and so on will best be determined through program operation, but beginning with a three level effort is suggested: 1. Program direction would come from professional personnel holding certification of clinical competence issued by the American Speech and Hearing Association. Such individuals would be responsible for program administration and supervision of other personnel. Direct services to children would include diagnosis, therapy planning, and therapeutic services for a limited number of children. 2. Sub-professional, collegetrained individuals, with a background in child growth and development and basic considerations in speech pathology and audiology, would compose the second level. Their responsibilities would include individual and group work with children who present primary deviations in language development and with those who are minimally speech impaired. Their work would be conducted in life settings rather than in a clinic. 3. Level three would be comprised of volunteer assistants who would receive pre-service and in-service training in speech and language stimulation with the mentally retarded. These individuals would carry out stimulation procedures in the living areas which are planned by the professional and sub-professional personnel.

The suitability of the foregoing plan and of others would best be determined with a collaborative effort between institutions to avoid duplication of effort and to insure coverage of a number of approaches. It is hoped that the future will bring closer collaboration between the staffs of institutions, for they share many common problems, problems which demand shared solutions if progress is to be made in institutional speech and language programming.

References

A proposed program for national action to combat mental retardation. (President's Panel on Mental Retardation). Washington, D. C.: U.S. Government Printing Office, 1962.

A report on the speech and hearing programs for all 106 state institutions for the mentally retarded. *Parsons Demonstration Project, Report # 4,* Parsons State Hospital and Training Center, Parsons, Kansas, 1964.

Annual report (Fiscal Year 1967). Gracewood State School and Hospital, Gracewood, Georgia, 1967.

Brookshire, R. H. Speech pathology and the experimental analysis of behavior. *Journal of Speech and Hearing Disorders,* 1967, 32, 215–227.

By-laws of the American Speech and Hearing Association. *In Directory of the American Speech and Hearing Association.* Washington, D. C., 1960.

Copeland, R. Therapy considerations for the institutionalized mentally retarded. *The Training School Bulletin,* 1962, 59, 53–58.

Fulton, R. T. Speech and hearing programs for the mentally retarded: A model for personnel and facility justification. *Mental Retardation,* 1967, 5, 27–32.

Fulton, R. T. and C. S. Giffin. Audiological-otological considerations with the mentally retarded. *Mental Retardation.* 1967, 5, 26–31.

Gottsleben, R. H. The incidence of stuttering in a group of mongoloids. *The Training School Bulletin,* 1955, 5, 209–217.

Hudson-Majuen, G. Speech as a factor in the diagnosis and prognosis of backwardness in children. *Journal of psycho-aesthenics,* 1902, 6, 81. Cited in D. T. Leberfeld, Speech therapy and the mentally retarded child. *The Training School Bulletin,* 1957, 273–274.

Immel, R. K. Forward. In S. M. Stinchfield and E. H. Young, *Children with delayed or defective speech.* Stanford, Calif.: Stanford University Press, 1947.

Institutional speech and hearing programs for the mentally retarded: A conference report. (Project of the National Institute of Mental Health, Grant #5—R–11 MH01127 and the State of Kansas). Parsons State Hospital and Training Center, Parsons, Kansas, 1964.

Itard, J. M. G. *The wild boy of Aveyron.* New York: Appleton-Century-Crofts, 1962.

Jordan, T. E. Language and mental retardation: A review of the literature. In R. L. Schiefelbusch, R. H. Copeland, and J. O. Smith (Eds.), *Language and mental retardation.* New York: Holt, Rinehart, & Winston, 1967.

Kirk, S. A. Research and education. In H. A. Stevens, and R. Heber (Eds.), *Mental retardation: A review of research.* Chicago: University of Chicago Press, 1964.

Leach, E. An experimental speech and hearing clinic for mentally retarded children. (Parsons Demonstration Project, Report #31), Parsons State Hospital and Training Center, Parsons, Kansas, 1965.

—————. The speech and hearing program. In *Institutional speech and hearing programs for the mentally retarded:* A conference report. (Project of the National Institute of Mental Health), Parsons State Hospital and Training Center, Parsons, Kansas, 1964.

Leach, E., J. Rolland and L. Loyd. A report on the speech and hearing programs for 142 state institutions for the mentally retarded. (Parsons Demonstration Project, Report #67). Parsons State Hospital and Training Center, Parsons, Kansas, 1966.

Lerman, J. W., G. R. Powers and S. Rigrodsky. Stuttering patterns observed in a sample of mentally retarded individuals. *The Training School Bulletin,* 1965, 62, 27–32.

Lillywhite, H. S. and D. P. Bradley. *Communication problems in mental retardation.* New York: Harper & Row, 1969.

Lombardi, T. P. and R. G. Poole. Utilization of videosonic equipment with mentally retarded. *Mental Retardation,* 1968, 6, 7–9.

Malloy, J. S. *Teaching the retarded child to talk.* New York: John Day, 1961.

Marge, M. and J. V. Irwin. The role of the profession of speech pathology and audiology in the management of language problems. *ASHA,* 1968, 10, 221–222.

Matthews, J. Speech problems of the mentally retarded. In L. E. Travis (Ed.), *Handbook of speech pathology.* New York: Appleton-Century-Crofts, 1957.

McCarthy, J. J. Research on the linguistic problems of the mentally retarded. *Mental Retardation Abstracts,* 1964, 1, 5–27.

Mueller, M. W. and S. J. Weaver. Psycholinguistic abilities of institutionalized trainable mental retardates. *American Journal of Mental Deficiency,* 1964, 68, 775–783.

Peins, M. Client-centered communication therapy for mentally retarded delinquents. *Journal of Speech and Hearing Disorders,* 1967, 32, 154–161.

Rigrodsky, S. and M. D. Steer. Mowrer's theory applied to speech habilitation of the mentally retarded. *Journal of Speech and Hearing Disorders,* 1961, 26, 237–243.

Robinson, H. R. and N. M. Robinson. *The mentally retarded child.* New York: McGraw-Hill, 1965.

Schaeffer, M. L. and W. M. Shearer. A survey of mentally retarded stutterers. *Mental Retardation,* 1968, 6, 44.

Schiefelbusch, R. L. A discussion of language treatment methods for mentally retarded children. *Mental Retardation,* 1965, 4, 4–7.

Schiefelbusch, R. L., R. H. Copeland and J. O. Smith (Eds.), *Language and mental retardation.* New York: Holt, Rinehart, & Winston, 1967.

Schlanger, B. B. Environmental influences on the verbal output of mentally retarded children. *Journal of Speech and Hearing Disorders,* 1954, 19, 339–343.

————. Issues for speech and language training of the mentally retarded. In R. L. Schiefelbusch, R. H. Copeland, and J. O. Smith (Eds.), *Language and mental retardation.* New York: Holt, Rinehart, & Winston, 1967.

————. Speech therapy with mentally retarded children. *Journal of Speech and Hearing Disorders,* 1958, 23, 248–301.

Schlanger, B. B. and R. H. Gottsleben. Analysis of speech defects among the institutionalized mentally retarded. *Journal of Speech and Hearing Disorders,* 1957, 22, 98–103.

Schneider, B. and J. Vallon. The results of a speech therapy program for the mentally retarded children. A *American Journal of Mental Deficiency,* 1955, 59, 417–424.

Seguin, E. *Idiocy and its treatment.* New York: Columbia U. Teacher's College Foundation Reprint, 1907.

Shubert, O. W. and R. T. Fulton, An in-service training program on communication. *Mental Retardation,* 1966, 4, 27–28.

Shubert, O. W., C. M. Vanden Heuvel and R. T. Fulton. Effects of speech improvement on articulatory skills in institutionalized retardates. *American Journal of Mental Deficiency,* 1966, 71, 274–278.

Sircin, J., and W. F. Lyons. Treatment of speech defects in a state school. *Psychiatric Quarterly,* 1942, 16, 333–340.

Spradlin, J. E. Language and communication of mental defectives. In N. R. Ellis (Ed.), *Handbook of mental deficiency.* New York: McGraw-Hill, 1963.

Spreen, O. Language functions in mental retardation: A review I. Language development, types of retardation, and intelligence level. *American Journal of Mental Deficiency,* 1965, 69, 482–494.

Standards for state residential institutions for the mentally retarded. *American Journal of Mental Deficiency,* 1964, 68, (Mongr. Suppl.).

Sumner, F. G. Speech therapy services in institutions for the mentally retarded in the Southeastern United States. Unpublished paper, The University of Georgia, 1968.

Van Riper, C. *Speech correction, principles, and methods.* (4th ed.) Englewood Cliffs, N. J.: Prentice-Hall, 1963.

Webb, C. E. and S. Kinde. Speech, language, and hearing of the mentally retarded. In A. A. Baumeister (Ed.), *Mental Retardation.* Chicago: Aldine Publishing Co., 1967.

Weiss, A. and M. M. Horton. Investigation concerning the effectiveness of classroom teacher oriented language development program for severely mentally retarded children. Unpublished paper, Whitten Village, Clinton, S. C., 1966.

West, R., M. Ansberry and A. Carr. *The rehabilitation of speech.* New York: Harper & Bros., 1957.

Zisk, T. K. and I. Bialer. Speech and language problems in mongolism: A review of the literature. *Journal of Speech and Hearing Disorders,* 1967, 32, 228–241.

Adjunctive Therapy in Residential Institutions for the Mentally Retarded

Education and training, recreation and training, cottage and ward life, and therapies and activities are some of the departments that come under the heading "adjunctive therapy activities." "Standards for State Residential Institutions for the Mentally Retarded (1964)" drawn up by the American Association on Mental Deficiency lists the following services under subsection II, Therapies and Activities:

Volunteer services
Library services
Music therapy
Industrial therapy
Occupational therapy
Physical therapy
Recreational therapy

Even though the American Association on Mental Deficiency has recommended general standards, many institutions have their own organization of services. Some of the services often assigned to adjunctive therapy in different institutions are: recreational therapy, music therapy, occupational therapy, vocational training and placement, volunteer services, chaplaincy, industrial therapy, library services, physical therapy, and others.

The basic purposes and goals of the department of adjunctive therapy are "to plan and administer a comprehensive schedule of activities, suited to the individual and group needs of the residents, and contribute to their maximum growth and development (AAMD, 1964)." Purpose of this department are extensive and varied:

1. To offer leisure time activities
2. To aid physical, social, moral, emotional, and mental growth
3. To provide outlets for hostility and aggression
4. To offer activities that aid physical health
5. To promote discipline
6. To provide diversional therapy
7. To offer avocational activities
8. To offer opportunities for residents to be of service

Accomplishing these goals depends upon an integrated adjunctive therapy program and the interaction of that program with those of other departments of the institution.

The director of a department of adjunctive therapy coordinates the department's various programs; he should possess a graduate degree in one of the areas of his responsibility, have some training in administration, and have a minimum of two years experience in an institution for the mentally retarded before being placed in a director's position.

Among the many responsibilities of the director the more important are: (a) supervising all members of the department; (b) preparing budgets and reports; (c) evaluating the effectiveness of the program; (d) meeting with various community organizations, parent-teacher associations, and other community groups interested in the care and treatment of the mentally retarded; (e) keeping records to ascertain the progress of residents; (f) assisting in recruiting qualified personnel for available job openings; (g) coordinating and supervising in-service training for employees; (h) developing policies and procedures for various adjunctive therapy programs for the habilitation of the mentally retarded residents within the institution; and, (i) obtaining research funds and grants that will promote acceleration of programs to meet the growing needs of adjunctive therapy.

Recreational Therapy

Recreation can be therapeutic. Hedonistic activities are not the ultimate goal of recreational therapy, although it is true that all recreation must be fun to be successful. The recreation therapist should gear the program to the particular disability of the individual. If the primary handicap is intellectual retardation, the therapist should program activities that are at or slightly above the level of the resident and his interests, aiming to broaden his interest, stimulate his motivation, create learning experiences, and provide an oultet for emotions.

If the retarded resident has a physical handicap, the therapist must select activities that will enable the patient to substitute a stronger function for the disabled one. At the same time, a program of activities must be directed toward the physical handicap to give that function an opportunity to develop maximally. For example, during a swimming session recreation workers can include special muscle exercise for coordination, conditioning, and tone.

Some of the guidelines for a recreation worker in initiating an activity follow:

1. He must enjoy, lead, and *participate* to be successful.
2. He should keep trying to identify interest of the participant.
3. He must plan the activities to be used during each recreational period.
4. He should adapt activities to meet the limits of the person. When the person excels, the leader should reward him by telling him that he did well.
5. He should initiate group activities even when the residents are not good participants, because a great majority of retarded people need *social acceptance.*

The recreation curriculum of the State Department of Public Welfare, Division of Mental Hygiene, Southern Wisconsin Colony and Training School (1963) states that

> many people approach the problem of recreation for the mentally retarded, believing that the retarded child responds to play material and activity within their comprehension much the same as do normal children of the same mental age. Such is definitely not the case. A retarded child with a chronological age of eighteen, but with a mental age of four, differs considerably from the normal four year old. The predominant interests, urges, desires, and wants he experiences are much the same, but he has a different set of expectations to meet; he has a much larger body to maneuver. The interaction of his social environment and his physical status also govern his play tastes. The normal individual finds play and recreation an ideal way to express his fundamental drives and desires. The mentally retarded child may have the same desires and drives of the normal child, but be thwarted or suppressed by his environment (p. 3).

Many variables influence the recreation program of an institution. The following questions indicate areas in which the institution's administrative philosophy may affect the recreational program.

1. Is it possible to have activities including both sexes?
2. What facilities may recreation use?
3. Do any residents have the freedom of the grounds?
4. Does the institution have a habilitation program?
5. What hours are the residents in specific wards or buildings for recreation?
6. What is the ratio of recreation workers to residents?
7. Is responsibility for the physical education program for residents included in special education or within the scope of recreation?
8. Are there any restrictions on the mixing of residents of different intellectual levels?
9. During what hours can recreation be employed?
10. Can the physically ill receive recreation?
11. May residents attend off campus activities?

Some of the recreational activities that have been used for the retarded are day camping (Gingland and Grould, 1962), overnight camping, intramural softball, league softball, intramural basketball, volleyball, movies, picnics, simple games, arts and crafts, stage entertainment, quiet games (Carlson and Gingland, 1961), social dances, cheer leading, bus rides, parades, attendance at fairs, visits to state and national parks, playground, fishing, trips to sporting events, swimming, miniature golf, institution carnivals, pony rides, field days, gymnastics, track, scouting (Boy Scouts of America), weight lifting, trampoline, bicycle clubs, kite flying, ping pong, shuffleboard, billiards, TV watching, story telling, reading by workers, touch football, skating, crib play, water play, bowling, canteen time, model building, clubs, trips to the zoo, trip to horse shows, physical exercise (Hayden, 1964), active group games, and many others.

Nursing service or cottage and ward life employees can influence the success of a recreation program (Chapman, 1964). The recreation person should strive to include the ward personnel in the program, asking them for assistance and advice. A simple survey filled out by ward employees such as the one that follows can aid in insuring their cooperation.

1. Do you know that you can call on adjunctive therapy (recreation) for books, records, and toys?
2. Does your building have toys, television, games, radios, and books that are usable?
3. Please list any and all recreation supplies that you feel are needed in your building.
4. Could you use volunteers for short play periods to relieve employees for other duties?

5. What is the best time during the day for recreation workers to come to your building?

Occupational Therapy

Occupational therapy has been recognized only recently to be part of the treatment program for the mentally retarded. It is not just a leisure time activity; when properly utilized it will meet certain well defined therapeutic goals. Occupational therapy for the mentally retarded is the use of activities to help recovery from a disability and to aid the development of an individual's strengths. Some institutions have included occupational therapy within the clinical or medical division while others have placed occupational therapy under the administrative direction of the human development division. Occupational therapy should be considered a medical adjunct because of the nature of the training required to become a registered occupational therapist (Kilburn, 1967). However, the occupational therapist has to be highly versatile in all areas of human growth and development. A sharp distinction should not be made between the services rendered to the retardate on prescription and the service rendered on referral from personnel in non-medical disciplines.

Diagnosing a problem area and prescribing an experience that will help alleviate the problem is one of the functions of occupational therapy. Occupational therapists are also responsible for identifying the retardate's strengths and offering a planned program that will develop them. For example, a child who is hyperactive may come to the therapist for experiences that require a certain amount of sitting. The therapist discovers that the child can discriminate between sizes and colors even though he may not know the names of all the colors. By diverting the non-purposeful movement to purposeful movement such as sorting different color skeins of wool or thread for the therapist, the retardate can be programmed to sit and work for increasingly long times.

With the increasing admission of non-ambulatory retardates to the institution, occupational therapists are faced with meeting the needs of individuals who have severe physical problems. An adapted social living skills program can be very beneficial in goal setting for non-ambulatory retardates (Willard and Spachman, 1963). For example, if the patient will respond to the presence of the therapist and has the physical ability to put his hand to his mouth, the therapist may try to teach self-feeding or partial self-feeding (Arnold, 1962).

Whether a resident is mildly retarded or severely retarded, the therapist can be guided by three simple and universally understood suggestions: be patient; use simple step-by-step instructions; repeat instructions frequently.

Crafts, art, physical activity, and sensory stimulation can be used with retarded individuals in a goal-oriented program. However, the more severe the retardation the less useful craft activities are.

The patient with physical problems may be involved in both the occupational therapy and physical therapy departments for the same primary purpose, and cooperation is necessary for the two departments to complement each other's services.

Unfortunately there are not enough registered therapists to meet the needs of the retarded who can benefit from this service. An institution having difficulty in securing the services of a trained therapist may rely on the American Occupational Therapy Association and the schools that offer this specialized training. If a qualified therapist cannot be found an occupational therapy consultant should be sought. He can also be of assistance to a service that includes a full-time registered therapist. The consultant can aid in evaluation of residents, organizing a new department, evaluating standard programs, organizing new programs (such as research projects), training therapist aides.

Music Therapy

Music therapy is a relatively new program for the mentally retarded. The typical music program is a leisure-time activity, but according to Bialer (1967) "procedures involving musical instruments, songs, rhythm, and musical games may also be subsumed under two categories. They may be recreational (i.e., used for fun, relaxation, profitable use of leisure time, or entertainment), or they may be therapeutic (i.e., designed to treat pathological behavior that may or may not be amenable to other forms of therapy) (p. 142)."

Music is often an effective therapeutic agent. Brown (1964–65) has stated: "It is regarded as one of the most valuable communicative arts. Music provides a natural means for the expression of feelings, moods, and innate desires for self-expression" (p. 1).

Whether the retardate is enrolled in the special education program or is included in the ward or cottage program, he should be evaluated by the music therapist as to his musical interests, understanding of written music, performance with musical instruments and participation.

In any event, it is of the utmost importance to reach him as soon as we possibly can in order to help him identify with his environment and begin finding it a pleasant place in which to live. Failure to do so can increase his measure of frustration and add to our difficulty in helping him to grow. Music can help to accomplish this purpose and is often a first means of creating in the child a pleasurable reaction to an outside stimulus. It is often the beginning of a social relationship upon which other things may grow (Gingland and Styles, 1965, p. 6).

Music therapy should be conducted in all resident buildings for all residents who wish to participate as well as for those for whom music therapy has been prescribed. Group singing, piano, or autoharp, rhythm instruments, musical games, music listening, dances, drawing and coloring to music are commonly employed in music programs.

A number of considerations should be taken into account when planning a music program for the individual resident:

1. Some retardates who do not have fluent speech can enjoy a singing session.
2. Some come to feel that they are a part of a group by listening to group singing.
3. Some who cannot hear can "feel" the music.
4. Some will find an avenue of self-expression through folk dancing, modern dances, and tap dancing as well as ballet and creative dancing.
5. Some may require the therapist's friendship before they will participate in a music activity, and others may respond to the therapist because of music.

There are usually residential retardates who cannot benefit from the efforts of special education, and there are those who are on the waiting list for special education (Scheerenberger, 1965). However, the majority of residents can find some area of music therapy in which they can participate and enjoy a certain degree of accomplishment.

The following section indicates some of the music activities that are appropriate for certain general groups of retarded individuals.

Severely retarded ambulatory women:

These women sing best with records. They enjoy nursery songs and some of the most familiar tunes ("Daisy," "Yankee Doodle," etc.). Musical chairs is a good activity for them although this requires considerable supervision. They do fairly well at bouncing balls to music, usually one ball to be thrown from leader to resident and back again. They are especially fond of looking at books (Little Golden Books, perhaps) and enjoy being read to during music listening periods. They have difficulty using rhythm instruments. Dancing is a desirable activity if the residents are constantly encouraged to dance and not sit down.

High severe to low moderately retarded women:

All of the activities listed above are appropriate for these women. They sing better with the record player unless they know the song exceptionally well. Action songs are very good because many of these individuals enjoy moving around and mimicking the leader. They are quite familiar with many folk songs and spirituals and enjoy singing with autoharp.

Severely and moderately retarded geriatric women and men:

These residents have more physical disabilities than younger residents and do best in simple activities. It is good for them to get up at least once in each music session, whether it be for a simple action song, bouncing balls, or marching in time to music. They like to clap while they are singing and enjoy film strips. They are not overly enthusiastic about rhythm instruments but like playing with the melody bells. Most of them know the old favorites and folk songs.

Moderately to mildly retarded young and middle age women and men:

Many in this category consider music to be "kid stuff." A few elementary modern dance exercises add to the program. More complicated music stories and film strips are good for them. They do quite well with simple folk and popular dancing and generally enjoy this very much.

Retarded pre-adolescent boys and girls:

Both the boys and girls enjoy the same activities found in any kindergarten or first grade music program. Follow the leader and bouncing balls are popular. The little boys especially like being airplanes and trains. The little girls like the rhythm instruments. Film strips are not very good because these children cannot sit still for long. They do not do too well with folk dancing but like to march to the music and pretend to be instruments. (Each one must be shown what to do and which instrument to be.)

Moderately to mildly retarded adolescents:

This is a group who usually enjoy any and everything in the activity program. They love stories about trains and quite a few train songs ("Little Red Caboose," "Puff and Toot," "I've Been Workin' on the Railroad," etc.). They may learn to recognize various instruments of the orchestra by the instrument charts and like to try to recognize them by sound. They sing fairly well and learn new songs quickly. Action songs are popular as well as folk songs and dances. They like the rhythm instruments (choosing their own) and playing tunes on the melody bells.

Severely retarded ambulatory men:

These men sing almost exclusively with the record player and not very much even then. They like the rhythm instruments and watching film strips with records. The activity of bouncing balls is fun for them, and they also like to color pictures and look at books while listening to music.

Severely to moderately retarded non-ambulatory women and men:

The music program is usually conducted in the dormitory area. This should be a room that can be used for film strips. These residents usually enjoy virtually everything that has to do with music and they are very rhythmic. They usually do not sing very well, but they do try. The rhythm instruments are popular, and they like to bounce balls, although they obviously experience difficulty in this activity. They also like coloring pictures while listening to music.

High severe to low moderately retarded men:

These men enjoy singing to the records and do fairly well with the rhythm instruments. They like folk songs and lively spirituals. Film strips usually are not very good. While these patients are not very interested in being read to, they like to look at books while listening to music. Very rhythmic records and songs are best.

Profoundly and severely retarded non-ambulatory:

This group has been an area of frustration for many people in the field of retardation for many years. What can you do for a person who cannot walk, talk, see well, or grasp with his hands? Van de Wall and Liepmann (1936) in their book, *Music in Institutions,* offer the idea that the nursing care group can find satisfaction in musical rhythm, shouting to music, and being a member of a social group. If this be true, it is the responsibility of the music person to include as many of these patients as possible in a music stimulation situation (Cotter and Toombs, 1966).

Industrial Therapy

Industrial therapy is work involving therapeutic goals. For many years most institutions for the retarded have had programs of job placement on the campus. Originally, the residents were placed on jobs to assist in the total operation of the institution because of a shortage of employees. As industrial therapy appeared on the institutional scene and therapists were employed to work with the job placement program, the idea of a goal-oriented program of work therapy began to develop. Many institutions adopted the idea that work can offer diversion from the daily routine, support the individual resident in striving for achievement, minimize discipline problems that originate from inactivity, offer an opportunity for socialization, give the resident an opportunity to feel useful, offer an opportunity to work off aggression, and offer the resident an opportunity to prove himself as a candidate for specific vocational training and placement outside the institution.

Placement on jobs within the institution is an important part of industrial therapy. These work areas include nursing service, dietary, laundry, yard service, garbage truck, carpenter shop, paint shop, heat plant, supply, beauty shop, barber shop, farm, dairy, housekeeping, sewing service, messenger service, ambulance service, and others.

For an industrial therapy program to function in the best interest of the resident, the program must be organized to evaluate the resident's vocational aptitudes before placement, offer the resident a chance to learn specific skills on the job, give added responsibilities on the job when they are earned, keep progress reports that will aid programming for the resident, schedule specific times of follow-up and counseling with the resident and supervising employee on the job.

Job placement is the foundation for many industrial therapy programs, but training in nonacademic, special situations can be part of the program's framework. For example, radio repair, auto repair, simple carpentry, car washing, and horticulture are some of the experiences that do not necessarily have to be classified as job placements (Watson and Burlingame, 1960). Following is a progress report written by a volunteer concerning a supporting program to industrial therapy.

The Landscape Gardening Program covers, in the main, a gardening program and a resident produced newsheet.

The program has two basic interrelated goals. A prime objective is to prepare previously nonmotivated residents for jobs either on or off the hospital grounds by encouraging good work skills and habits and encouraging social interaction. Also, very important is a gardening program that gives beauty to the hospital grounds, and, at the same time, instructs the residents in the basics of gardening.

To carry out these objectives, the program works as a follow-up to the remotivation program. The seventeen residents we work with are of all age levels and varying degrees of retardation, and all have been through remotivation sessions. Three of these seventeen work fulltime and the others at scheduled times during the week.

The formation of the Garden Club and the publication of their news sheet help to supplement the garden program. By working on the news sheet, it is hoped that the residents will take a more active interest in other people and happenings around them. We believe that the participation of these residents both in the production of the paper and the activities of the Club have helped them to adjust to hospital life and helped instill in them a genuine dislike for inactivity.

Many of the boys have made outstanding accomplishments in the last few months. Four boys are now working on the hospital grounds. Two residents are working in the Toilet Training Project, one is working in the occupational workshop, and one is working in a resident dining room. One resident begins work in a residential building this week. With the arrival of fall, three boys were placed in the school program.

The program has been partially successful this first year. We have worked with the blind, geriatric, non-ambulatory residents and residents who have only minor physical defects. Though the latter residents have shown a more dramatic improvement than the rest, every resident has appeared to have benefitted from the program. They are more alert to their surroundings, friendlier with fellow residents, and have an extraordinary dedication to their job tasks. The geriatric residents benefitted from the outdoor activity to a degree high above the rest which leads to a suggestion for a comprehensive outdoor program for these residents (Jardine, 1965).

A program of this type gives the resident a chance to develop skills and attitudes that will have carry-over value when he reports to his regular job placement.

There is a trend at the present time for State Vocational Rehabilitation agencies to become more involved in the programs for the retarded in the institution. This trend has been aided by the U.S. Department of Health, Education, and Welfare through grants made under the public rehabilitation program (HEW, 1968, p. 63). In some institutions, responsibility for training and job placement of all residents who are potentially capable of returning to society is included under Vocational Rehabilitation. The industrial therapy program can be an aid to this endeavor by offering the job placements on the grounds of the institution as evaluation areas and by referring possible candidates to Vocational Rehabilitation. For residents of much lower mental capacities who do not qualify for the services of Vocational Rehabilitation, the industrial therapist will continue to be an important part of the adjunctive therapy team.

Volunteer Services

The key to an efficient volunteer program in an institution for the mentally retarded is the volunteer coordinator who should be a full-time staff member. The coordinator plays several different roles—sometimes recruiter, teacher, volunteer representative, public relations representative, or publicity assistant. The coordinator as recruiter must be familiar with the surrounding community and the resources in the community that can be contacted for volunteers. The recruiting program must be pursued continuously because of changing needs of an institution and the problem of volunteer turnover. The coordinator as teacher is the initial educator in disseminating information on mental retardation to the prospective individual volunteer or group. Furthermore, he is a member of the orientation team for new volunteers. As volunteer representative, he is responsible for bringing suggestions and grievances of volunteers to the attention of the administration, and he is responsible for record keeping of volunteer time. As a public relations representative, he has an excellent opportunity to inform the community groups with whom he comes into contact about services and programs for the mentally retarded and services mentally retarded people can render to society. He is also responsible for communicating the appreciation of the institution to volunteers who have aided the institution. The volunteer coordinator is constantly concerned with staff acceptance of volunteers and the coordination of tours. As a publicity assistant, the coordinator initiates the information that is disseminated to the news media concerning volunteer services rendered to the institution, and in some instances, disseminates information concerning progress achieved by the institution (American Psychiatric Association, 1964).

Regular volunteers can be of great assistance in jobs such as: escort service for residents who are not capable of independent travel on the grounds of the institution; recreation aides, canteen assistants; reading for residents; rolling wheelchair patients for change of environment; physical therapist aides; cosmetology for high level girls; music therapist aides, music teachers; occupational therapy assistants; garden therapy; writing letters for residents; receptionists; aiding new residents during their adjustment period; teacher aides; scout leaders; library services; art teachers; and many others. One aid in placing the regular volunteer is the volunteer's application which all volunteers should complete.

If the volunteer feels that he cannot be regular in attendance, he should not be placed in a program where the institution will expect him to meet a schedule. For example, the irregular volunteer may enjoy adopting a friend. He would then feel that as a volunteer he offers a great service to a resident who does not have visitors, does not receive letters or special season cards, does not receive spending money for occasional treats from someone on the "outside," and does not have the chance for a home visit. Of course, a home visit with a volunteer would depend on the social worker's report of the volunteer and the resident.

The irregular volunteer or volunteer group can also conduct parties, seasonal pageants, movie and slide activities, and ward and stage entertainment.

Community organizations can enrich the lives of the residents by donating money, facilities, equipment, supplies, clothing, tickets to community events, and others. Church groups that accept the institutionalized retarded in their church services and activities are meeting a need, particularly for some high level retardates. Some of the organizations that have become interested in institutional programs are:

Councils for Retarded Children and Adults
Parent-Guardian Associations
Churches
Schools
American Red Cross
Federated Women's Clubs
Federated Garden Clubs
Federated Jaycettes
American Federation of Musicians
Home Demonstration Clubs
Friendship Clubs
Civitan Clubs and Auxiliary
Lion's Clubs
Kiwanis Clubs
Optimist Clubs
Sertoma Clubs
Welcome Wagon Clubs
Scout Troops
Dental Auxiliary
Service Men's Auxiliary
Business and Professional Clubs
Trade and Labor Councils
Masonic Lodge
Citizens Band Radio Clubs
Community Theatre
Shrine
College Fraternities and Sororities
Employees of Companies
Eastern Star Orders
P.B.X. Clubs
American Women in Radio and TV
Ladies of Charity
Junior League
New Century Clubs
Parent-Teacher Associations
United Church Women
American Legion and Auxiliary
Elks Clubs
Gideons International
Art Leagues
Merchants

Hairdressers and Cosmetologists
Chambers of Commerce
Ceramic Societies
Senior Citizens

Volunteers who serve an institution for the retarded are essential when they possess skill that employees do not have, fill a void in a needed position that the institution cannot obtain, give residents a chance for contact with the "outside," enrich programs with new ideas, support employees who are involved in a progressive program, offer leisure-time activities for residents, and inform their neighbors and friends about the nature of retardation and solicit their support.

Appendix: Organizations and Agencies

American Association for Health, Physical Education and Recreation, Project on Recreation and Fitness for the Mentally Retarded, 1201 16th Street, N. W., Washington, D. C.

American Association on Mental Deficiency, 5201 Connecticut Avenue, N. W., Washington, D. C.

American Association for Volunteer Services Coordinators, A.P.A. Mental Hospital Services, 1700 18th Street, N. W., Washington, D. C.

American Occupational Therapy Association, 250 West 57th Street, New York, New York.

National Association for Music Therapy, Inc., P.O. Box 61, Lawrence, Kansas.

National Association for Retarded Children, 386 Park Avenue, South, New York, New York.

National Association of Recreational Therapists, American Recreation Society, Inc., Room 622 Bond Building, 1404 New York Avenue, N. W., Washington, D. C.

National Recreation Association, 8 West 8th Street, New York, New York.

National Rehabilitation Association, 1522 K Street, N. W., Room 430, Washington, D. C.

References

AAMD. Standards for state residential institutions for the mentally retarded. *American Journal of Mental Deficiency,* Monograph Supplement, 1964.

Arnold, Carol B. Feeding Suggestions for the Severely Retarded Child In the
Arnold, C. B. Feeding suggestions for the severely retarded child in the institution. *The American Journal of Occupational Therapy,* Nov.-Dec., 1962,

Bialer, I. Psychotherapy and other adjustment techniques with the mentally retarded. In A. A. Baumeister (Ed.), *Mental retardation—Appraisal, Education, and rehabilitation.* Chicago: Aldine Publishing Company, 1967, 138–173.

Carlson, B. W. and D. R. Gingland. *Play Activities for the Retarded Child,* Abington Press, 1961.

Cotter, V. W. and W. S. Toombs. A procedure for determining the music preferences of mental retardates. *Journal of Music Therapy,* June, 1966.

Gingland, D. and K. Grould. *Day camping for the mentally retarded.* National Association for Retarded Children, 1962.

Gingland, D. and W. Stiles. *Music activities for retarded children.* Abingdon Press, New York-Nashville. 1965.

Hayden, F. J. *Physical fitness for the mentally retarded.* Metropolitan Toronto Association for Retarded Children, Ontario, Canada, 1964.

Jardine, J. E., VISTA Volunteer. Landscape Gardening Progress Report. Clover Bottom Hospital and School. Dec., 1965.

Kilburn, V. T. Highlights of the Curriculum Study Conference: Part 1. *American Journal of Occupational Therapy,* March-April, 1967, 102–105.

Mental Hospital Service of the American Psychiatric Association. The Development of Standards and Training Curriculum for Volunteer Services Coordinators, Washington, D. C., Feb., 1964.

Mental Retardation Activities of the U. S. Department of Health, Education and Welfare. Washington, D. C.: U. S. Government Printing Office, Jan., 1968, 63–64.

President's Committee on Mental Retardation, MR67, Washington, D. C.: U. S. Government Printing Office, 1967.

Recreation Curriculum. State Department of Public Welfare, Division of Mental Hygiene, Southern Wisconsin Colony and Training School, 1963.

Scheerenberger, R. C. A census of public and private residential facilities for the mentally retarded in the United States and Canada. In Directory of residential facilities for the mentally retarded. Willimantic, Conn.: *American Association on Mental Deficiency,* 1965.

SREB, Recreation Committee. *Recreation for the Mentally Retarded: A Handbook for Ward Personnel.* Atlanta: Southern Regional Education Board, 1964.

U. S. Department of Health, Education, and Welfare. *Preparation of Mentally Retarded Youth for Gainful Employment.* Washington, D. C.: U. S. Government Printing Office, 1961.

U. S. Department of Health, Education, and Welfare. Special Programs in Vocational Rehabilitation of the Mentally Retarded, 1963.

Van de Wall, W. and C. Liepmann. *Music in Institutions,* Russell Sage Foundation, New York, 1936.

Watson, D. P. and A. W. Burlingame. *Therapy Through Horticulture,* The Macmillan Company, 1960.

Willard, H. S. and C. S. Spachman. *Occupational Therapy,* J. B. Lippincott Company, 1963.

Psychological Services in
the Institution

Psychological services in an institution for the retarded are usually provided by a clinical psychologist. Diversity of function and training combine
to make the clinical psychologist's role in the institution a potentially valuable but difficult one to define. As with most professions, an appreciation
of the activities of the clinical psychologist can best be gleaned by offering
a brief survey of its development and delineating some aspects of its current
practice.

Ebbinghaus has said of psychology, in general, that its past is long
but its history is short. Clinical psychology has both a longer past and a
shorter history with perhaps a nebulous present. An arbitrary but reasonable approach to clinical psychology's history is provided by Watson
(1953), who identifies two traditions with little overlap that may be regarded as the original sources of clinical psychology. The work of Galton,
Cattell, Binet and Terman may be characterized as the roots of a psychometric tradition, with a rigorous commitment to quantification and measurement while that of James and Hall may be regarded as the roots of
a dynamic tradition, with an equally firm commitment to those aspects of
human behavior and personality which more nearly fit the concepts of
common discourse and seem elusive to efforts of measurement. This bi-
furcation stands at the historical base of clinical psychology, and the
history of the interplay of these orientations represents much of the history
of clinical psychology. At different periods one or the other approach

may be seen as ascendant, but throughout both have been present and both remain important concerns for contemporary psychology.

The condition of the mentally retarded has exerted a greater attraction for workers in the psychometric tradition than for the more dynamic psychologists. Indeed the obvious presence of intellectually deficient children in the French schools provided the impetus for Binet to develop the device which has been the mainstay of the psychometric tradition, i.e., the intelligence test.

Commissioned in 1904 by the French Minister of Public Information to "direct a study of the measures to be taken showing the benefits of instruction for defective children" (as quoted by Kanner, 1964), Binet, in collaboration with Simon, produced his intelligence scale in 1905. Through a series of subsequent revisions, the Binet Scale has remained a significant instrument for psychology in general and mental retardation in particular. As Kanner points out, the Binet Scale served to modify the concept of mental deficiency as an all or nothing phenomenon by indicating the wide range of gradations between "normal" intelligence and the profoundly retarded.

Binet's work was enthusiastically introduced into this country by Henry Goddard in 1908. Ironically, it was the same Goddard who subsequently stifled the psychological attention to retardation promised by his enthusiastic endorsement of the Binet Scale. In 1912, Goddard introduced Martin Kallikak Jr., son of an early colonist. The genealogical chart of Kallikak's descendants (mostly retarded) assumed a prominent role in the eugenics movement of the 20's and 30's, a movement which virtually eliminated mental retardation as a concern of psychology. In Goddard's words, "Mental retardation is hereditary . . . segregation through colonization seems to be the . . . ideal method (of treatment)," (as quoted by Kanner, 1964).

The impact of this attitude upon psychological services to the retarded was to reduce them to a minimum. Psychologists during the 20's and 30's served to identify the retarded and consign them to a classroom or residence. They came upon these children in the child guidance centers of the period and intellectual assessment constituted their single service to them. During this period critical attention and attempts at refinement were directed at intelligence testing and occupied a central position in the psychometric tradition. The continuity of IQ and the effects of environment and heredity upon intelligence were the issues of controversy for clinical psychology at this time.

Within the institution for the retarded there was also a marked emphasis upon intelligence testing, but as Hackenbush's (1940) survey revealed, many of those doing this testing were not psychologists and many of those described as psychologists were only poorly qualified. Such inadequate psychological service in institutions for the retarded becomes a consistent theme in any history of these institutions.

The dynamic tradition was at this time assimilating the work of Freud, Murray, and Rorschach and was thereby moving further from a concern for the retarded. A fascination for the complexity of relationships between ego, id, and superego and various other personality constructs did not extend itself to the effects of diminished intelligence upon personality.

The second world war began the 40's and did much to modify clinical psychology. Military needs expanded both the range of competence and the number of clinical psychologists. After the war three times as many military psychologists engaged in clinical work as had done so before it (Andrews & Deese, 1948). More importantly, a greater degree of consensus existed as to the qualifications and training of a clinical psychologist.

Post-war interest in the formulation of clinical psychology culminated in the work of the 1947 Shakow Committee. From this committee came the official effort to fuse the two traditions. Shakow described the clinical psychologist as one enabled by training both to apply psychological principles to daily human problems and to contribute to the theoretical development of these principles. The 1949 Boulder Conference conferred official endorsement upon this concept of the scientist-professional, and an explicit model for training was established. The model attempted to bind the experimental to the clinical, and its success involved an inevitable state of tension between these two poles.

While some uniformity concerning the goals and function of clinical psychology has been achieved, there remains a considerable amount of amibiguity regarding its roles and professional identity. A profession uncertain of its identity and subject to constant revision may be expected to display considerable concern for the training of its future members. This has been true of clinical psychology whose graduate programs have for a score of years been in a state of flux.

A survey of some current attitudes toward the training of clinical psychologists is useful in describing a general notion of present trends and emphases within the profession. Some would see the psychologist's role as solely that of a therapist (R. R. Holt, Report on a Conference on an Ideal Program for Psychotherapists, 1963). Others take the opposite pole and opt for an exclusively experimental orientation. A third view would retain the Shakow model but broaden it to include such activities as community consultation and direction of lay personnel (Cook, 1965). Further, attention is directed toward defining the function of the subdoctoral professionals in psychology. The questions of supervision, delineation of areas of specialization, techniques of training, and subsequent utilization for this group continue to generate considerable controversy (Arnhoff & Jenkins, 1969). As Bloom (1969) sums up the situation,

> There seems to be little question that graduate training in clinical psychology . . . is undergoing serious re-examination aimed toward reorganization of training activities and a reconceptualization of the goals of training.

Perhaps the major signficance of the foregoing review is the evidence of the constant change and revision that characterizes both the past and current status of clinical psychology.

Returning to the psychologist in the state hospital for the retarded, (we left him chiefly concerned with intelligence testing in the 30's), we find little of the attitude, suggested above, which encourages change and improvement. A recent survey (Baumeister, 1967) revealed that 64 per cent of the administrators of state institutions polled regard intelligence testing as the chief service rendered by the psychological staff. Silverstein (1963) reports that 50 per cent of the psychologist's time in an average institution is devoted to testing. A survey of clinical psychologists in general (Goldschmidt, *et al.*, 1969) reported that approximately one per cent of the average clinician's time is spent in administering objective tests such as intelligence scales. Making allowances for the different needs of varying populations, it is nonetheless clear that the emphasis found in institutions is generally atypical of that found in clinical practice.

Perhaps as a consequence of this discrepancy, most competent psychologists do not find institutional work attractive. At any rate, existing conditions reported in the Baumeister (1967) survey do not remotely approximate the AAMD standards for psychological services in institutions (1964). These standards recommend a chief psychologist of Ph.D. level for each institution. Only 66 per cent of the institutions have a psychologist with a Ph.D. The standards also suggest one psychologist for each 200 admission referrals. The actual ratio is 376:1, including MA psychologists and those involved in strictly administrative work. For purposes of contrast, it is also interesting to note, as the standards state, "it is also assumed that institutions have . . . an obligation to contribute to advances in new scientific information through research." Unfortunately, this directive has largely been ignored; fewer than one-fourth of the administrators surveyed granted a position of first or second priority to research.

While focusing on the obvious failure to meet the AAMD standards, some mitigating circumstances should be mentioned. Administrators are often without sufficient funds for minimal services. Moreover, they are most frequently medical men who do not have the training to appreciate the research efforts of psychologists. The point to be made here is simply that psychological services are most often inadequate, a situation which probably derives from the disparity between the administrator's perception of the psychologist as a test administrator and the profession's own conception of its role as scientists-professionals. While clinical psychologists may be uncertain of their present functions, they are adamant against repeating the errors of the past. Yet institutions in general seem content with the image of the psychologist developed in the 30's. The result is an anachronistic emphasis on intelligence testing within institutions and a pronounced tendency for fully qualified psychologists to shun institutional work.

It is important to note that the institution, as such, need not be aversive for the psychologist. There exists in this setting potentials for research and service matching almost any other positions available to psychologists. Opportunity for research into the effects of enforced confinement upon individuals, the behavior of groups, the effects of intellectual inadequacy upon personality, the interaction of clearly defined authority with intelligence, conformity or other motivational variables, are all immediately accessible to the institutional psychologist. In fact, simply the presence of a readily available population of subjects renders the institution an attractive location for almost any area of psychological research. Furthermore, the degree of control with regard to environmental manipulation available in such an institution should present considerable appeal to scientists whose basic orientation is a behavioral one. Finally, there are few areas in which the basicly humanitarian concerns of the clinician could be more deeply engaged than in an institution for the retarded. That the appeal of these attractions has not been entirely ignored is demonstrated by the research and efforts reported later in this chapter. The point made here is that the response of the psychologist, for reasons later related, has not been proporionate to this appeal.

Clearly a disparity exists between the role of psychology both in terms of its practice and of its perception by administrators and by most extra-institutional psychologists. It is appropriate to consider briefly the potentials of psychological services in the institution and to indicate more efficient means for providing these services.

Exemplifying a trend throughout general clinical psychology, Gardner (1967) advocates a shift of focus for the institutional psychologist from attention to individual patients to that of a consultant's role. Psychologists are trained to observe, assess, and implement change in behavior. Contemporary attitudes recognize the relevance of basic psychological concepts to areas outside academic psychology. Thus, a psychologist cognizant of motivational principles may render assistance to the speech or occupational therapist, the special educator, or the recreational supervisor. Learning theory has its application in more effective ward management as well as individual behavior modification. Knowledge of the principles of learning and motivation might be usefully employed in structuring extra-institutional employment placement for residents. Awareness of the effects of institutional life upon the retardate personality is necessary for effectively working in this setting and assisting in the patient's rehabilitation. The psychologist's role is potentially diverse. To needlessly restrict it to intelligence testing represents a waste of resources and a disservice to the patients.

As Sternlicht (1966a) points out, most clinical programs treat mental retardation in a cursory fashion. Some few graduate programs offer a Ph.D. specialty in clinical psychology of mental retardation, but these are decidedly in the minority. For most other programs a single survey course is optional and sufficient for graduation. The institution of University Affiliated Centers for Mental Retardation may provide some impetus to change this situation and stimulate greater interest among graduate students for working with the retarded.

In developing a program of training that includes adequate emphasis upon the retardate, attention should be given to those aspects other than intelligence which distinguish this population. Relevant here is the work of Cromwell (1963) and Zigler (1966), which concerns itself with personality and motivational variables of retardates. This kind of information should be provided for all students in a doctoral clinical psychology program. More specific information regarding medical etiology and the neurological significance of retardation, as well as regular exposure to retardates through practica and research, should be demanded of doctoral students with a defined interest in retardation. Because this latter group may be expected to constitute a small proportion of doctoral students, even under conditions of expanded interest in retardation, the current concern for training subdoctoral personnel becomes relevant.

As demonstrated by statistics cited earlier (Baumeister, 1967), most psychologists in institutions are at the Masters level. Assuming the continuance of current trends, Arnoff and Jenkins (1969) estimate that in the next 10 years 25,000 Ph.D's (not all of whom are in clinical) and 37,500 terminal Masters degrees will be granted. Thus the Masters level psychologist will continue to be numerically dominant, and a realistic response to this situation might entail training some of these people specifically as institutional psychologists. Some areas of general clinical training might be discarded, such as dynamically oriented therapy and diagnosis, while others having more pertinence to institutional work, such as behavior modification and environmental management, might be emphasized. Since it is typically an MA psychologist who works in an institution, it seems appropriate that training at this level be more tailored to the role of an institutional psychologist. A possible consequence of such programs might be an individual more certain of his role and hence more capable of fully exploiting psychology's potential for service to the institution.

Clinical Functions in the Institution

In the following sections the actual work of the psychologist in an institution will be explored. Primary emphasis is placed on reviewing their various functions, but some suggestions and critical assessments are made.

ASSESSMENT FUNCTIONS

The chief service of an institutional psychologist has been that of an evaluator of intelligence. Baumeister (1969) has rather picturesquely characterized this role as that of a "Binet jockey," while Silverstein (1963) more prosaicly states that the Stanford-Binet Intelligence Scale and the Wechsler Intelligence Scale for Children are the most frequently used tests in institutions. Furthermore, among the ten most commonly used tests five were for intelligence.

The importance attributed to intellectual evaluation results partially from the fact that deficiency in intelligence is by definition the primary characteristic of the mentally retarded. Furthermore, intellectual assessment receives emphasis because the institutional classification of patients into a particular level of intellectual functioning is often of primary concern for fiscal and administrative purposes. Finally, as Baumeister (1967) points out, many administrators have little confidence in the psychologist's ability to do anything but intelligence testing.

Considerable attention in the recent mental retardation literature has been directed toward intelligence tests (Allen and Jones, 1967; Baumeister, 1964; Gunzburg, 1965a; Hutt and Gibby, 1965; Robinson and Robinson, 1965). The majority of this literature has been concerned primarily with describing standard tests of intelligence and relating them to the retarded population. Others, particularly Allen and Jones (1967), have been concerned with special tests for evaluation of retardates. Little research, however, has been undertaken to assess the suitability of standardized intelligence tests for this population. In the most relevant work Baumeister (1964) has reviewed the use of the WISC with retardates. He concludes that the WISC is suitable for the higher level patients and serves well as a predictor of school achievement.

Bijou (1966) has proposed a somewhat different assessment of retardation. Rather than view retardation as a state of deficient intelligence as defined by a standard test, Bijou would describe the retardate as one with a limited repertoire of behavior. Retardation is discussed in terms of abnormal anatomical structure and functioning, inadequate reinforcement, consequences of contingent aversive stimulation, and reinforcement of aversive behavior. Bijou proposes that such a functional analysis of retardation avoids hypothetical mental constructs and leads to the identification of observable conditions that produce retarded behavior.

Not surprisingly, personality evaluation of the institutionalized retardate has received considerably less attention than intellectual assessment. In fact, there has been a pronounced tendency to ignore personality variables while emphasizing intellectual deficits as the only distinguishing factor of retardation. In his survey, Silverstein (1963) found that fewer than one-tenth of the institutional psychologists cited personality evaluation as one of the most common reasons for testing referral. In addition, fewer than one-tenth of the respondents thought that an increase in personality testing had occurred over the past five years. Correspondingly, slightly more than one-tenth anticipated an increase over the next five years. Perhaps most important is that almost one-quarter of the respondents saw improvement in personality evaluation as the greatest need in testing of institutionalized retardates.

Within the past decade, personality characteristics of retardates have received increasing attention. Cromwell (1963) has interpreted retardate functioning in terms of Rotter's (1954) social learning theory. Zigler (1966) has presented his research findings relating the effects of social deprivation, institutionalization, and "other-directedness" to the behavior of retardates, while Butterfield (1967a) has reviewed research investigating the effects of different environments on retardate personality.

The theoretical positions of the preceding authors have stressed heavily the importance of personality variables in the retardate. Empirical support for these positions may be found in Beier's 1964 article. He discusses behavioral disturbances in the retardate and reaches a number of conclusions. Major or minor behavioral disturbances can and do occur concomitantly with mental retardation. In fact, these disturbances occur more frequently in the retarded than in the general population. Furthermore, after the degrée of intellectual deficiency, the most compelling reason for institutionalization of the retarded is the manifestation of behavioral disturbances. In view of these facts, it would appear that the place of personality evaluation in institutionalized retardates should be reconsidered.

Personality evaluation within the institution can serve several purposes. Initial ward placement might be determined not only by degree of intellectual deficiency but also with respect to personality variables. Personality attributes might well influence placement in educational programs within the institution. Implementation of therapeutic programs, both traditional psychotherapy and behavior modification, could be facilitated by personality evaluations. Vocational placement should also be based on personality factors.

Cromwell (1967) has examined techniques of personality evaluation that are useful with retardates. Discarding the traditional techniques of projective and objective personality tests as inappropriate for the retardate population, Cromwell recommends the following techniques as more relevant: obtaining objective reports of behavior from different individuals, observing the patient in various natural settings, and attending to his attitude toward test-taking and his actual behavior during the test session. In contrast to this view, Silverstein's (1963) survey indicates that projective tests, particularly the Rorschach, are frequently employed in testing situations within the institution. One quarter of Silverstein's respondents also thought that an increase in projective testing had occurred over the past five years. A followup survey would be useful in determining if Silverstein's 1963 findings still pertain today. Baumeister's (1967) survey indicates that institutional superintendents rated projective testing and objective personality testing as important functions of psychologists working in institutions for the retarded. The projective testing received a slightly higher rating in terms of importance. Thus, despite Cromwell's contentions regarding the inappropriateness of projective testing with retardates, there appears to be a continued reliance upon such techniques in institutions.

TRADITIONAL THERAPEUTIC FUNCTIONS[1]

Although psychotherapeutic procedures with retardates have received considerable recent attention, actual application of the techniques has been somewhat less frequent. One reason for the infrequency of psychotherapy with retardates is the notion of incurability of mental retardation (Robinson and Robinson, 1965). Closely related is the belief that retardates are not suited for psychotherapy because of inabilities to verbalize and achieve insight (Sarason, 1953). Perhaps the most compelling argument against traditional psychotherapy has been voiced by Gardner (1967) who points out that this technique requires considerable time, personnel, and energy. Consequently, Gardner questions whether such a luxury as traditional psychotherapy can be afforded.

Survey findings would appear to support Gardner's contention that personnel and time are not available for traditional therapy in an institutional setting. Silverstein's (1963) survey of 120 institutions reveals that the ratio of patients to psychologists (Ph.D. or M.A.) is 376:1. Such data would

---

1. Traditional therapy is defined here as a face-to-face situation in which a trained therapist helps individuals with their emotional problems. Verbal techniques are the primary therapeutic tools.

appear to indicate that therapy in the traditional sense in an institutional setting would not be a realistic or efficient method of facilitating emotional or behavioral adjustment.

Despite the above considerations, traditional therapy has been practiced to some extent in institutional settings. Woody and Billy (1966) surveyed doctoral level Fellows in the Section on Psychology of the American Association on Mental Deficiency regarding psychotherapy with retardates. The survey indicated that psychologists working with the retarded felt that counseling and psychotherapy could be of "some value" in facilitating the retardate's institutional adjustment, peer group relations, return to the home, and return to the community in an active role. Further, the 64 respondents indicated that they "often" used counseling and psychotherapy to aid retardates in the above-mentioned areas. Baumeister (1967) reports that institutional superintendents rated the psychotherapeutic functions of psychologists as second in importance to testing responsibilities. Ninety-six per cent of the superintendents indicated that psychologists should engage in some psychotherapy. However, therapy in the Baumeister article was not defined and was probably interpreted by superintendents in a broader context than the definition of traditional psychotherapy employed here.

A number of review articles have appeared which discuss psychotherapeutic procedures with retardates (Bialer, 1967; Gunzburg, 1965b; Robinson and Robinson, 1965; Sternlicht, 1966b). In the Woody and Billy (1966) survey, the following approaches to counseling and therapy with retardates were employed by the 64 psychologists in the ensuing order (most frequent to least frequent): Eclectic, client-centered, learning theory, ego psychology, psychoanalytic, individual psychology, rational, conditioning, and psycho-drama. However, the percentage of the respondents who practiced psychotherapy in an institutional setting was not presented in the report.

Several published studies employing various psychotherapeutic approaches with institutionalized retardates have reported improvement in emotional and behavioral adjustment. Successful therapeutic attempts have been reported with individual and group nondirective therapy (Mehlman, 1953; Mundy, 1957; O'Connor and Yonge, 1955; Yonge and O'Connor, 1954); directive therapy (Appel and Martin, 1957; Snyder and Sechrest, 1959; Wilcox and Guthrie, 1957); play therapy (Maisner, 1950; Mehlman, 1953); and depth psychotherapy (Chidester and Menninger, 1936; Jorsweick, 1958). Some studies have also reported increased IQ scores following therapy (Chidester and Menninger, 1936; Mundy, 1957; Yonge and O'Connor, 1954).

Beier (1964) has pointed out that although the majority of published articles report that retardates benefit from psychotherapy, the degree of success is moderate and often poorly defined. A subjective determination of improvement is frequently reported and inadequately explained. Appropriate controls are also frequently absent. Because they are costly in terms of time and their results are often ambiguous, traditional approaches to psychotherapy have left much to be desired, particularly in their application to institutionalized retardates.

BEHAVIOR MODIFICATION

The therapeutic model that has recently received considerable attention with institutionalized retardates is behavior modification or operant conditioning. Baumeister (1967) has suggested that the adoption of such a model is necessary for the institutional psychologist to be considered significant in the treatment of mental retardation. In a later article, Baumeister (1969) indicates that the operant conditioning approach has been accepted as the dominant therapeutic technique with retardates. Gardner (1968) states that behavior modification programs are now prominent in institutions and are accepted as the primary therapeutic tool.

Behavior modification is viewed by the present authors as the most useful technique now available to institutional psychologists. However, a detailed account of the application of these principles to the institutionalized retarded will not be discussed here since a review of such techniques is presented by Watson (see Chapter 7). Watson appropriately focuses on the use of behavior modification with severely and profoundly retarded individuals, probably the most prevalent institutionalized population. Here we mention only briefly two applications of reinforcement principles to other populations of institutionalized retardates.

Malpass (1967) has discussed the use of programmed instructions with retardates. Birnbrauer, *et al.*, (1964) have employed programmed instructions with the institutional retarded in an attempt to increase word acquisition. The results indicate that moderately retarded children can incorporate up to six new words in each session. Reinforcements were trinkets, gold stars, and other material objects. Hunt, Fitzhugh, and Fitzhugh (1968) have used reinforcement procedures to improve the personal appearance of 12 retardates who anticipated discharge within one year. Subjects received points for appropriate appearance while performing various jobs on the hospital grounds. The points could be exchanged for tobacco, toiletries, and other sundries. Relative to baseline and extinction, both continuous and intermittent reinforcement resulted in an increment in the percentage of subjects presenting an appropriate appearance.

Although numerous behavior modification programs in institutions have reported phenomenal success, a note of caution has appropriately been issued by Baumeister (1969). Operant conditioning is currently the fad in institutional programming. However, to justfy the enthusiasm surrounding these techniques, operant principles must be shown to be different from and more effective or efficient than "conventional" techniques. Operant principles must also be demonstrated on purely empirical grounds and must be proven effective in producing relatively permanent behavior changes outside a highly controlled experimental environment. An objective analysis of the current status of behavior modification in terms of methodology, effectiveness, and efficiency would appear warranted. Finally, exception must be taken to the author who simply relabels familiar conditions and trite thoughts with the terms of an operant vocabulary. From such pseudo-science only pseudo-advances are made.

IN-SERVICE TRAINING

The ratio of patients to psychologists reported by both Baumeister (1967) and Silverstein (1963) in institutional surveys limits the direct service that the psychological staff can render retardates. The realization of the shortage of professional manpower has led to the institutional psychologist serving as a consultant, trainer, and supervisor to other residential personnel. Attendant-level staff has already been recognized as the mainstay of most institutional settings (Savino, Kennedy, and Brody, 1968). The success of any therapeutic program is dependent on the ward personnel who have continuous contact with patients. By training and supervising these staff members through in-service programs in such areas as behavioral management techniques, the effectiveness and efficiency of treatment programs and patient care can be greatly enhanced.

In-service training can also help overcome communication barriers between professional and nonprofessional personnel. Shotwell, Dingman, and Tarjan (1960) have found attendants and professional personnel often hold opposing views on patient care. Peck and Cleland (1966) have indicated that cultural differences, status anxiety, prejudices, and attitude discrepancies contribute to the communication gap between professional and nonprofessional staff. Contact between the two groups is facilitated through in-service training. Expression of ideas and attitudes can more easily occur. Problems experienced by attendants, both with patients and institutional policies, can be resolved. In short, by improving communication between staff members the institution can move more rapidly toward established goals.

An increasing reliance on in-service training programs has been reported in the literature. In 1949, Pero found that 31 of 74 institutions that replied had such programs; in 1964 Parnicky and Ziegler found 102 of 108 institutions that responded had in-service training programs. Butterfield (1967b) has noted that the Southern Regional Educational Board (SREB) project to facilitate training of attendants in state mental retardation institutions is another indication of increased interest in in-service training. A cursory review of the literature also indicates the prevalence of residential in-service training programs (e.g., Daly, 1963; Graves, 1958; Harrison, 1963; Johnson and Ferryman, 1969; Shubert and Fulton, 1966).

Watson (see Chapter 7) has discussed the shaping and maintaining of the behavior of institutional personnel. The establishment of reinforcement for personnel as well as the development of stimulus control over their behavior is discussed in detail. As a result, the issue will not be pursued here except for stating that Watson's program provides an excellent guide for teaching psychological principles and actual behavior modification techniques to institutional personnel.

UTILIZING SUB-PROFESSIONALS IN PSYCHOLOGY

Voicing a concern which is heard throughout the mental health field, the American Psychological Association devoted an official position paper (Smith and Hobbs, 1966) to decry the growing shortage of professionals. This shortage is especially acute in mental retardation. Alleviation of this condition may be provided from a number of directions, one of which entails the utilization of sub-professionals in psychological services.

Savino, *et al.,* (1968) have suggested that economically deprived as well as volunteer groups might be integrated into a program of psychological services. Exemplifying this approach is a two year associate degree program initiated by St. Mary's Junior College in Minneapolis. Here the aim is to produce a specialist in retardation who will work with the psychologist and other professionals in clinical or institutional settings.

Goodman and Arnold (1967), reporting on a demonstration project in this area, focus on the benefits to the sub-professional worker. The workers were from low income urban minorities, and the author suggests, "Hopefully their functioning here came to imply something more than a low paying job. A source of gratification and individual fulfillment may emerge as well as improved care for the mentally retarded." Ludkte (1968) details more specifically the role of sub-professionals working in an institution with a psychologist. He suggests the employment of these people in such roles as test administrators who leave the interpretation to the psychologist, or as technicians trained in operant conditioning and employed in shaping adaptive behavior.

PARENT COUNSELING

Another function of a psychologist in an institution is counseling parents of retarded individuals. Such counseling may involve initial inquiry concerning institutional placement, actual placement, parental role after placement, or genetic counseling. In the initial contact between the parents of a retarded child and the institution, the psychologist should be available for consultation regarding placement. Wolfensberger (1967a) has offered a set of guidelines for professionals to follow in the counseling of parents considering institutional placement of a retardate. The guidelines essentially stress the welfare of the retarded individual, the family, and society in determining placement.

Both during the initial inquiry about placement and the actual placement, the institutional psychologist can play a primary role by dealing with parental feelings. As Dittman (1962) has written, parents usually have mixed feelings about institutionalizing a child. Guilt feelings frequently arise from the mere thought of placing a child in an institution, and relatives often express opinions which complicate the parent's decision. In such a counseling situation the institutional psychologist can assist the parents in understanding and accepting their feelings, and the available alternatives can be clearly defined by the counselor. Perhaps most important, the psychologist can listen, accept, and understand the feelings expressed by the parents.

The psychologist may also play a role in the communication between the parent and institution after the child has been institutionalized. Mason (1953) has recommended home visits by institutional personnel, parental visitation to the institution, and counseling of parents. He suggests that institutional personnel work with parent groups. Such contact with parents would allow the psychologist and others further opportunity to deal with parental feelings regarding both retardation and institutionalization. Furthermore, an educational program could be initiated for the parent groups. Such a program might include causes of mental retardation, frequency and prevalance, meaning and implications of mental retardation, professional interest in the retarded, organized parental interest, and future of the retarded.

Genetic counseling offers the institutional psychologist an additional role in parental consultation. In instances where parents wish to know the cause of their child's retardation and the possibility of successive occurrences of retardation in their next child, the psychologist can be of major assistance. Because retardation is occasionally associated with chromosomal anomalies, some understanding of genetics would appear essential for a psychologist working with the retarded. Kaplan (1969) has recently published an article concerning mental retardation which results from chromosomal anomalies. Each relevant syndrome is discussed in terms of the particular chromosomes involved; the frequency, prevalence, degree of retardation, behavioral manifestations, and physical characteristics associated with these syndromes are also delineated. Other information sources are also available (Clarke, 1962; Roberts, 1963; Shaw, 1963).

Wolfensberger (1967a) has emphasized the importance of both genetic knowledge and therapeutic skills for counseling. Through the psychologist's acquaintance with genetics, adequate factual information can be communicated in an appropriate therapeutic environment. Wolfensberger also points out that the role of the counselor is not to dictate whether parents should have additional children, but the counselor should provide the factual information concerning the probabilities of having another retarded child, help the parents clarify their feelings, and then leave the final decision to the parents.

Research in the Institution

AAMD standards (1964) state that the institution has an obligation to stimulate and participate in research activities. Further, the Shakow Commission interprets the clinical psychologist's role as that of a researcher as well as psychometrician, evaluator, and therapist. Unless the administrator views his institution strictly as a residential center for the continued care of the retarded, he will attempt to aid the residents in acquiring skills and achieving some degree of independence. The provision of a wide range of services oriented toward maximizing the development of the retardate's limited capacities becomes paramount to this end. It is through research and continued evaluation of ongoing programs that the most effective services can be implemented. For example, the psychologist can assess his effectiveness as a behavior modifier only through research into the changes occurring in the retarded child's behavior.

At the beginning of this decade the importance of research in the institutional setting was emphasized by President Kennedy's Panel on Mental Retardation which recommended that

> . . . high priority should be given to developing research centers on mental retardation at strategically located universities and at institutions for the retarded
> . . . Continued critical evaluation of the institution's program itself requires personnel with a research point of view. It is important, therefore, when the size of the institution and the quality and experience of the staff justify it, that research in some form be a part of the institution program (Tarjan, 1964).

As reported earlier, however, a glance at the statistics would seem to indicate that institutional superintendents have largely ignored this recommendation. Baumeister's (1967) survey of 120 institutions for the mentally retarded has revealed that research is considered by institutional superintendents to be the least important contribution of the psychologist. In another survey (Wolfensberger, 1965) 51 per cent of administrators surveyed said they had done all they could to encourage psychological research. However, only 50 to 60 per cent were even willing to make subjects available during inconvenient hours. Further, no experimental research had been executed in the preceding three years in 61 per cent of the surveyed institutions. It is thus apparent that most superintendents will not enthusiastically commit their resources to extensive research programs.

A reciprocal attitude characterizes many research-oriented psychologists. Frequently their major objection to working in the institutional setting centers around problems with administrators. Many administrators are reluctant to alter their well established, traditional routines to implement research programs. This is especially true when the program involves entire wards and extensive staff participation. Attendants are typically opposed to taking on additional duties, such as keeping behavioral records or having to respond consistently to certain behaviors, which research programs often entail. Because ward personnel rarely receive extra pay for the increase in work load, the motivation to cooperate with the researcher is understandably low. Other complaints which have also been voiced frequently by researchers include failure of subjects to arrive on time, difficulty in getting subjects released from routines, and limited times during the day when subjects are made available (Wolfensberger, 1965).

In the Wolfensberger (1965) survey some means to remedy the difficulties were suggested. Both administrators and researchers agreed that better research conditions could be brought about by improving the latter's social and communicative skills. A program of education aimed at informing the administrators of the purpose and benefits of psychological research would also be helpful here. Finally, in terms of the obstacles relating to cooperation of attendants and participation of subjects in research projects, the sub-professional personnel earlier described might be used to advantage. For example, they might assist in transporting subjects to the research site or they might assume some of the tasks that would otherwise have fallen to the attendants.

Much of the difficulty encountered between researchers and administrators can be attributed to one basic problem: state institutions for the retarded lack clearly defined policies governing the conduct of research by staff and outside investigators. Wolfensberger (1967b) suggests each institution have a written document stating its research orientation and some basic rules to govern the activities of anyone interested in doing research. Such a policy should include the priority that research would be given, whether research should focus on a certain problem or discipline, and the availability of space for carrying out investigations. In those institutions with favorable research climates, the appointment of a research coordinator, who would interpret policies, supervise the research, and assist the researcher in removing obstacles, would be strongly recommended. Wolfensberger goes on to suggest that staff members interested in research should submit a written proposal including purpose, detailed methodology, demands on the institution, and publication plans. A research committee would review the proposal and evaluate the research project periodically.

Outside researchers should be subject to the same rules as staff members, but areas of possible differential treatment might be stated in the research policy. Some superintendents favor exclusion of outside research when an institution has its own program (Tarjan, 1964). Such an attitude, however, leads to the isolation of an institution from outside contacts and limits the contribution of large institutions to research, one of the major arguments offered in defense of such institutions' existence. If facilitation of research continues to be a strong argument for the existence of large institutions, then administrators should be acutely aware that research demands must not be handled in a negative, indifferent, or inconsistent manner (Wolfensberger, 1967b).

In view of the foregoing, it is important that the attractiveness of the institution for research be emphasized. From the point of view of convenience, the institution as a research setting is unparalleled. It offers a sizable pool of residents having specific characteristics or disorders. The subject population remains fairly stable as a result of low discharge rates and it is thus conducive to longitudinal and repeated measurement studies. Ready availability of case records provides masses of data for selecting populations with required characteristics. Computer storage and retrieval should make this source even more attractive to the researcher, especially because information on noninstitutionalized retardates is not nearly so extensive or easily accessible. Institutions afford interdisciplinary stimulation with staffs composed of specialists in education, medicine, social services, speech and hearing, vocational counseling, and other disciplines.

Institution administrators may find several advantages to encouraging research, not the least of which is securing grants from state and federal sources. To some, the recognition afforded their institution by publications facilitates the recruiting of personnel and attracting of more funds. By offering facilities for research, university affiliation can be attained, leading to increased stimulation of the staff and improved institutional services (Wolfensberger, 1965).

Program Evaluation

Whether programs concern education, rehabilitation, in-service training, or behavior management and modification, it is obviously important for the psychologist working in an institution to have feedback to assess the efficacy of ongoing programs. To justify the continuance of a new, experimental program, the psychologist must be able to demonstrate its desired effect to the staff, superintendent, and often state and federal officials. Because funding is almost always a concern, those controlling the purse strings want empirical evidence that their money is not being wasted. Because the psychologist seeking to direct his efforts toward research is not always warmly received, the success of his program must be assessed and communicated.

Methods of assessment of different programs vary widely and often are only vaguely specified. Typically, the methods used are indirect and subject to numerous confoundings. More often than not, staff members acquire a general impression of a program's progress and communicate it to administrators, and this is where the assessment ends. Many institutions, however, employ some form of behavior check list, often their own, to evaluate their programs. For example, before the initiation of a behavior modification program, staff members may take a baseline measurement of existing behaviors to be compared to the checklist completed after implementation of the program.

A more typical method of assessment is the outcome study, which involves some form of follow up of persons completing an institutional program and receiving discharge (Rosen, 1967). Such studies may serve either predictive, evaluative, or descriptive functions. When concern is with prediction, interest lies in obtaining prognostic indexes so that a retardate's future chance of success in a program can be determined. Evaluation is concerned with assessing the impact of the institution's program upon its participants in terms of later community adjustments. A difficulty in evaluative studies lies in generating an appropriate control group. In most institutional programs participants are chosen in accordance with definite criteria, e.g., verbal ability or motor skills. Subsequent contrasts between such participants who have been discharged from the institution and other former patients cannot be interpreted as reflecting the effects of the specific program. Those factors which led to inclusion in the program may be sufficient alone to account for any difference in extra-institutional adaptation between the two groups. Another difficulty here is that evaluation of such programs can only be accomplished in a gross fashion. For example, evaluation of a rehabilitative program is almost always accomplished by the gross method of tabulating number of people employed, wages earned, jobs handled, and hours worked. This information tells nothing about the efficacy of particular training techniques, only of the success of the overall program.

Outcome studies also may have descriptive value, and possibly provide normative data about the adjustment of a particular group (Rosen, 1967). After a retardate has been outside the institution for several months, he may be interviewed at home several times a year. Checklists, vocational questionnaires, and attitude questionnaires can contribute to a complete picture of the retardate's personal, social, and vocational adjustment. Descriptions of an individual's adjustment can be easily made by checking the presence or absence of marriages, births, drivers' licenses, accidents, legal problems, job stability, social club affiliation, church attendance, hobbies, job absenteeism, promotions, and salary changes. Such data may then be formulated as norms against which patients discharged later may be compared and by which their adjustment may be assessed.

Sources of Funding

For the institutional psychologist to free himself from the Binet kit and embark on any training, research, or behavioral engineering program, he must first have funds available. The support available to the psychologist can come either through the institution or directly to the individual researcher from federal, state, local, or private sources. Private foundations, the most generous being the Joseph P. Kennedy, Jr. Foundation, award sums of money to individuals or organizations showing promising programs in raising the level of functioning of retarded children. Local charities, such as Community Chest or United Fund, often make funds available to institutions, but these are usually earmarked for physical improvements such as new buildings, gardens, or playgrounds. State legislatures traditionally have been the major source of institutional funds, but most institutions have found this money sufficient only for maintaining residential care at a very low level.

It is only in the past decade that the federal government has played an active role in the funding of various programs for the retarded. The impetus provided by the Kennedy and Johnson administrations continues to make otherwise nonexistent sources of funds available to institutions. As a result, the federal government is by far the major source of project funding today. Whereas state funds usually support applied research and rehabilitation programs, federal funding is the primary source for basic research.

The Department of Health, Education, and Welfare[2] has increased appropriations for mental retardation programs from $293 million in 1965 to $508 million in 1969. An increase to $585 million is projected for 1970. These funds are provided for preventive services, basic and supportive services, training of personnel, research construction, and income maintenance. The Division of Mental Retardation maintains a staffing grant program for institutions to provide part of the initial cost of professional and technical

---

2. The following information was obtained from *Mental Retardation Activities* of the U. S. Department of Health, Education, and Welfare (1969).

personnel ($8 million in 1969). The Division also supports two programs directed at improving the quality of state institutional care and treatment for the retarded: the Hospital Improvement and Hospital In-service Training Programs.

The Rehabilitation Service Administration administers the Hospital Improvement Program, designed to assist state institutions for the retarded, improve their care, treatment, and rehabilitation services. The program specifically focuses on the demonstration of improved methods of service and care, rather than research exploration or the development of new knowledge. Maximum yearly support is $100,000, and individual projects are normally approved for no more than a five-year period. The majority of these projects are directed toward the severely and profoundly retarded and emphasize personal development through self-care (toileting, feeding, dressing), socialization training, medical diagnosis and treatment, and speech training. By the end of 1968, 91 projects in 87 state institutions for the retarded had received awards, representing 52 per cent of the institutions eligible to receive such funds. Preliminary feedback reports are quite encouraging and are lending an attitude of optimism and increasing staff and community involvement in treating and rehabilitating the retarded.

Various agencies under the Department of Health, Education, and Welfare stress different programs in the field of mental retardation. The National Institute of Mental Health has for the past decade supported a broad range of research and training projects in mental retardation. Currently, the NIMH research effort is concentrated in three areas: studies of learning processes in the retarded; analyses of the effects of cultural and social deprivation; studies of behavioral and biological aspects of retardation.

The National Institute of Child Health and Development (NICHD), under the National Institute of Health, concentrates on recruiting research workers from all fields to work in mental retardation. In 1968, 13 grants provided training for 60 trainees, which increased to 18, with the programs serving 124 trainees in 1969. Current legislation favors institutions having or planning Mental Retardation Research Centers. In addition, NICHD supports independent investigators but encourages an interdisciplinary approach.

Psychologists can thus expect continued federal support for their various institutional activities, with research and behavior management programs having more likelihood of support. The National Institute of Health continues to be the largest source of research and training funding ($37 million in 1969, $38 million in 1970), with additional support from the Office of Education ($11 million in 1969, $12 million in 1970) and the Social Rehabilitation Service ($24 million in 1969, $30 million in 1970). With continued governmental support and increased community involvement, the institution's job of understanding, treating, and rehabilitating the mentally retarded will be considerably facilitated.

A Concluding Note

The wide range of topics discussed in this chapter reflects the corresponding breadth of psychology's potential contribution to the institution. As indicated in the preceding section, funds are presently available to support both research and service improvements. Thus, the present moment constitutes a uniquely significant one in the history of institutions. Both the scientific and financial resources necessary to advance institutional care beyond a primarily custodial service to the retarded are immediately accessible to directors and administrators. A positive response to this opportunity promises to change the character of institutions.

Institutions currently have the chance to become remediation centers for individuals whose intellectual and behavioral deficits render them incapable of adequate adjustment in the larger society. A definite commitment to this goal would obviously increase the social value of institutions and render them a more attractive setting for all professionals, including psychologists. Such an opportunity justifies a mood of optimism but also demands a note of caution. The attention to mental retardation currently lavished by both federal funding agencies and many psychologists cannot be expected to prevail indefinitely. Hence, it behooves those concerned to resolve immediately to exploit the opportunities now available.

References

Allen, R. M. and R. W. Jones. Perceptual, conceptual, and psycholinguistic evaluation of the mentally retarded child. In A. A. Baumeister (Ed.), *Mental retardation: Appraisal, education and rehabilitation*. Chicago: Aldine, 1967, 39–65.

The American Association on Mental Deficiency. Standards for State Residential Institutions for the Mentally Retarded. *American Journal of Mental Deficiency*, Monograph Supplement, 1964, 68, 4.

Andrews, T. G., and M. Deese. Military utilization of psychologists during World War II. *American Psychologist*, 1948, 3, 533–538.

Appel, E. and C. H. Martin. Group counseling for social adjustment. *American Journal of Mental Deficiency*, 1957, 62, 517–520.

Arnoff, F. N., and I. Jenkins. Subdoctoral education in psychology: A study of issues and attitudes. *American Psychologist*, 1969, 24, 430–443.

Baumeister, A. A. Use of the WISC with mental retardates: A review. *American Journal of Mental Deficiency*, 1964, 69, 183–194.

————. A survey of the role of psychologists in public institutions for the mentally retarded. *Mental Retardation*, 1967, 5, 2–5.

————. More ado about operant conditioning—or nothing. *Mental Retardation*, 1969, 7, 49–51.

Beier, D. C. Behavioral disturbances in the mentally retarded. In H. A. Stevens and R. Heber (Eds.), *Mental retardation*. Chicago: University of Chicago Press, 1964, 453–487.

Bialer, I. Psychotherapy and other adjustment techniques with the mentally retarded. In A. A. Baumeister (Ed.), *Mental retardation: Appraisal, education and rehabilitation*. Chicago: Aldine, 1967, 138–180.

Bijou, S. W. A functional analysis of retarded development. In N. R. Ellis (Ed.), *International review of research in mental retardation*. Vol. 1. New York: Academic Press, 1966, 1–19.

Birnbrauer, J. S., S. W. Bijou, M. M. Wolf, J. D. Kidder, and C. M. Tague. A programmed instruction classroom for educable retardates. (Mimeographed Report) Seattle: University of Washington, 1964.

Bloom, B. Training the psychologist for a role in community change. Unpublished manuscript, 1969.

Butterfield, E. C. The role of environmental factors in the treatment of institutionalized mental retardates. In A. A. Baumeister (Ed.), *Mental retardation: Appraisal, education and rehabilitation*. Chicago: Aldine, 1967, 120–137. (a)

————. The characteristics, selection, and training of institution personnel. In A. A. Baumeister (Ed.), *Mental retardation: appraisal, education and rehabilitation*. Chicago: Aldine, 1967, 305–328. (b)

Chidester, L. and K. A. Menninger. The application of psychoanalytic methods to the study of mental retardation. *American Journal of Orthopsychiatry*, 1936, 6, 616–625.

Clarke, C. A. *Genetics for the clinician*. Philadelphia: F. A. Davis, 1962.

Cook S. W. The scientist-professional: Can psychology carry it off? *The Canadian Psychologist*, 1965, 6, 93–109.

Cromwell, R. L. A social learning approach to mental retardation. In N. R. Ellis (Ed.), *Handbook of mental deficiency*. New York: McGraw-Hill, 1963, 41–91.

————. Personality evaluation. In A. A. Baumeister (Ed.), *Mental retardation: Appraisal, education and rehabilitation*. Chicago: Aldine, 1967, 66–85.

Daly, W. C. Some keys to training personnel in a residential school. *Mental Retardation*, 1963, 1, 97–99, 125–127.

Dittman, L. L. The family of the child in an institution. *American Journal of Mental Deficiency*, 1962, 66, 759–765.

Gardner, J. M. The behavior modification model. *Mental Retardation*, 1968, 6, 54–55.

Gardner, W. I. What should be the psychologist's role? *Mental Retardation*, 1967, 5, 29–31.

Goldschmidt, M. L., D. D. Stein, H. N. Wesissman, and I. Sorrels. A survey of the training and practices of clinical psychologists. *The Clinical Psychologist*, 1969, 22, 89–94.

Goodman, L., and I. Arnold. Training and utilization of non-professional personnel in services for the retarded. *Mental Retardation*, 1967, 5, 11–14.

Graves, W. S. The psychological development of the mentally retarded child: A training course for attendants. *American Journal of Mental Deficiency*, 1958, 62, 912–915.

Gunzburg, H. C. Psychological assessment in mental deficiency. In A. M.

Clarke and A. D. Clarke (Eds.), *Mental deficiency: The changing outlook.* New York: Free Press, 1965, 283–327. (a)

————. Psychotherapy with the feebleminded. In Ann M. Clarke and A. D. Clarke (Eds.), *Mental deficiency: The changing outlook.* New York: Free Press. 1965, 417–446. (b)

Hackenbush, F. Responsibility of the American Association on Mental Deficiency for developing uniform psychological practices in schools for mental defectives. *American Journal of Mental Deficiency,* 1940–41, 45, 233–237.

Harrison, J. H. Discussion of the article on in-service training. *Mental Retardation,* 1963, 1, 16–17.

Holt, R. R. Report of a conference on an ideal program for psychotherapists, 1963 (mimeo). Unpublished Manuscript, 1963.

Hunt, J. G., L. C. Fitzhugh, and Kathleen B. Fitzhugh. Teaching "exit-ward" patients appropriate personal appearance behaviors by using reinforcement techniques. *American Journal of Mental Deficiency,* 1968, 73, 41–45.

Hutt, M. L. and Gibby, R. G. *The Mentally retarded child: development, education, and treatment.* Boston: Allyn and Bacon, 1965.

Johnson, Doleen, and Zilpha C. Ferryman. Inservice training for non-professional personnel in a mental retardation center. *Mental Retardation,* 1969, 7, 10–13.

Jorswieck, E. Analysis of a twelve-year-old child with defective intelligence. *Prax. Kinderpsychol. Kinderpsychiat.,* 1958, 7, 251–254. Cited in Robinson, H. B., & Robinson, N. M. *The mentally retarded child.* New York: McGraw-Hill, 1965.

Kanner, L. *A history of the care and study of the mentally retarded.* Springfield: Charles C. Thomas,1964.

Kaplan, A. R. The use of cytogenetical data in heredity counseling. *American Journal of Mental Deficiency,* 1969, 73, 636–653.

Ludkte, R. Bridging the gap between the professional and the resident. *Mental Retardation,* 1968, 6, 35–38.

Maisner, E. A. Contributions of playtherapy techniques to total rehabilitative design in an institution for high-grade mentally deficient and borderline children. *American Journal of Mental Deficiency,* 1950, 55, 235–250.

Malpass, L. F. Programmed instruction for retarded children. In A. A. Baumeister (Ed.), *Mental retardation: Appraisal, education and rehabilitation.* Chicago: Aldine, 1967, 212–231.

Mason, L. F. Developing and maintaining good parental relationships. *American Journal of Mental Deficiency,* 1953, 57, 394–396.

Mehlman, B. Group playtherapy with mentally retarded children. *Journal of Abnormal and Social Psychology,* 1953, 48, 53–60.

Mundy, L. Therapy with physically and mentally handicapped children in a mental deficiency hospital. *Journal of Clinical Psychology,* 1957, 13, 3–9.

O'Connor, N., and K. A. Yonge. Methods of evaluating the group psychotherapy of unstable defective delinquents. *Journal of Genetic Psychology,* 1955, 87, 89–101.

Parnicky, J. J., and R. C. Ziegler. Attendant training—a national survey. *Mental Retardation,* 1964, 2, 76–82.

Peck, R. F., and C. C. Cleland. Intra-institutional problems: Organization and personality. *Mental Retardation,* 1966, 4, 7–11.

Pero, J. F. Policies in the operation of an institution for the mentally deficient as they are influenced by its location. *American Journal of Mental Deficiency,*

1949, 54, 166–171.

Roberts, J. A. *An introduction to medical genetics.* London: Oxford University, 1963.

Robinson, H. B., and Nancy M. Robinson. *The mentally retarded child.* New York: McGraw-Hill, 1965.

Rosen, M. Rehabilitation, research, and follow-up within the institutional setting. *Mental Retardation,* 1967, 5, 7–11.

Rotter, J. B. *Social learning and clinical psychology.* Englewood Cliffs, N. J.: Prentice-Hall, 1954.

Sarason, S. B. *Psychological problems in mental deficiency.* New York: Harper & Row, 1953.

Savino, M. T., R. C. Kennedy, and S. A. Brody. Using the nonprofessional in mental retardation. *Mental Retardation,* 1968, 6, 4–9.

Shaw, M. W. Genetic counseling. In M. Fishbein (Ed.), *Birth defects.* Philadelphia: J. B. Lippincott, 1963, 311–318.

Shotwell, A. M., F. Dingman, and G. Tarjan. Need for improved criteria in evaluating job performance of state hospital employees. *American Journal of Mental Deficiency,* 1960, 65, 208–213.

Shubert, O. W., and R. T. Fulton. An inservice training program on communication. *Mental Retardation,* 1966, 4, 27–28.

Silverstein, A. B. Psychological testing practices in state institutions for the mentally retarded. *American Journal of Mental Deficiency,* 1963, 68, 440–445.

Smith, M., and N. Hobbs. The community and the community health center. *American Psychologist,* 1966, 21, 499–509.

Snyder, R., and L. Sechrest. An experimental study of directive group therapy with defective delinquents. *American Journal of Mental Deficiency,* 1959, 64, 117–123.

Sternlicht, M. The clinical psychology internship. *Mental Retardation,* 1966, 4, 39–41. (a)

————. Psychotherapeutic procedures with the retarded. In N. R. Ellis (Ed.), *International review of research in mental retardation.* Vol. 2. New York: Academic Press, 1966, 279–354. (b)

Tarjan, G. Facilitation of research through administration. In *Role of the residential institution in mental retardation research.* Report of the Conference sponsored by the National Association for Retarded Children, Philadelphia, 1964, 28–38.

Watson, R. A brief history of clinical psychology. *Psychological Bulletin,* 1953, 50, 321–346.

Wilcox, G. T. and G. M. Guthrie. Changes in adjustment of institutionalized female defectives following group psychotherapy. *Journal of Clinical Psychology,* 1957, 13, 9–13.

Wolfensberger, W. Administrative obstacles to behavioral research as perceived by administrators and research psychologists. *Mental Retardation,* 1965, 3, 7–12.

————. Counseling the parents of retarded. In A. A. Baumeister (Ed.), *Mental retardation: Appraisal, education, and rehabilitation.* Chicago: Aldine, 1967, 329–400. (a)

————. Research policies and problems in residential institutions. *Mental Retardation,* 1967, 5, 12–16. (b)

Woody, R. H. and J. J. Billy. Counseling and psychotherapy for the mentally retarded: A survey of opinions and practices. *Mental Retardation,* 1966, 4, 20–23.

Yonge, K. A. and N. O'Connor. Measurable effects of group psychotherapy with defective delinquents. *Journal of Mental Science,* 1954, 100, 944–952.

Zigler, E. Research on personality structure in the retardate. In N. R. Ellis (Ed.), *International review of research in mental retardation.* Vol. 1. New York: Academic Press, 1966, 77–108.

Name Index

Adamson, W. C., 253
Allen, P., 219, 220, 304
Allen, R. M., 379
Andrews, T., 375
Ansberry, M., 327
Appel, E., 382
Appley, M., 207
Ardey, R., 156
Arnhoff, F., 376, 378
Arnold, C. B., 361
Arnold, I., 385
Ayllon, T., 214
Azrin, W., 214, 215, 216, 217, 221

Backus, F. F., 5
Badt, M. I., 150
Baer, D., 213, 229
Bailer, I., 159
Bailey, J. K., 52
Barnard, C. I., 145
Barnett, C. C., 37, 153
Baroff, G., 217, 218
Barr, M. W., 9, 12
Bass, B. M., 144
Baumeister, A. A., 25, 119, 192, 209, 226,
    376, 378, 379, 381, 382, 383, 384,
    387
Bayres, K., 42
Begab, M. J., 255, 262
Belknap, I., 139, 157
Bell, R. Q., 188

Bennis, W. G., 37, 51
Bensberg, G. I., 37, 146, 153, 201, 209,
    210, 234
Beier, D. C., 380, 382
Bernard, K., 209
Bereiter, C., 125
Best, H., 4, 5, 7, 8, 22
Bialer, I., 333, 362, 382
Bijou, S. W., 379, 380, 383
Billy, J. J., 262, 382
Binet, A., 373, 374
Birnbrauer, J. S., 210, 383
Blake, R. R., 50, 51
Blatt, B., 24
Bloom, B., 376
Bogatz, B., 305
Bowlby, J., 164
Boyle, R., 300
Bradley, D. P., 331
Brody, S. A., 384, 385
Bromfield, S. H., 268
Brookshire, R. H., 353
Brown, H. E., 362
Brown, L. N., 258
Bryson, D. W., 119
Burlingame, A. W., 366
Burlingham, D. T., 165
Burns, W., 37, 51
Butler, A. W., 11, 301
Butterfield, E. C., 25, 26, 34, 119, 133,
    164, 167, 177, 178, 188, 197, 198,
    256, 380, 384

Cain, L., 301
Carlson, B. W., 360
Carr, A., 327
Casse, R. M., 53
Cassel, R., 201, 209, 210
Cassidy, V., 300
Cattell, R. B., 373
Cawley, J. F., 303
Chandler, C. S., 139
Chapman, F. M., 360
Chidester, L., 382
Chinitz, B., 154
Cicenia, H., 305
Clarke, A. D. B., 150, 304
Clarke, A. M., 150, 304
Clarke, C., 386
Cleland, C. C., 15, 34, 140, 143, 145, 146,
    149, 150, 152, 155, 159, 384
Clevenger, L., 227
Clothier, R. C., 145
Coe, R. M., 123, 139
Cofer, C., 207
Cohen, H., 232, 233
Colwell, C., 201, 209, 210, 221
Cook, S., 375
Copeland, R. H., 329, 331, 336
Corte, E., 209
Covert, C., 61
Cramer, M., 119, 120
Cromwell, R. L., 378, 380, 381

Daly, W. C., 385
Daniels, D. N., 157
Davenport, C., 11
Davis, S. P., 14
Doubros, S. G., 262
Dayan, M., 30, 36, 201, 304
de Grazia, S., 144, 152, 153
DeMeyer, M., 210
Deese, M., 375
Deutsch, A., 4
Dickerson, W. L., 150
Dingman, H. F., 122, 123, 131, 132, 133,
    140, 141, 143, 153, 384
Dittman, L. L., 71, 386
Doll, E. E., 274, 276
Doman, G., 30, 43
Doughty, R., 220, 227, 304
Drucker, P. F., 146
Dugdale, R. L., 12

Dunn, L. M., 308, 310
Dybwad, G., 70, 79, 296, 303

Eagle, E., 300
Ebbinghaus, H., 373
Edgerton, R. B., 132, 139, 140, 141, 143
Edwards, M., 304
Eichorn, O. H., 30, 34
Ellis, N. R., 30, 36, 201
Elonen, A. S., 302
Eyman, R. K., 122, 125, 128, 130

Farber, B., 249
Ferryman, Z. C., 385
Ferster, C., 206, 208, 210, 211, 212, 227,
    228, 234
Filipizak, J., 232, 233
Fitzhugh, K. B., 383
Fitzhugh, L. C., 383
Freud, A., 165
Freud, S., 375
Fuller, P., 209
Fulton, R. T., 333, 346, 348, 353, 385

Galton, S. F., 11, 373
Gardner, J. M., 383
Gardner, W. I., 262, 377, 381
Girardeau, F., 201, 209, 304
Gibby, R. G., 379
Griffin, G. S., 333
Giles, D., 209
Gingland, D. R., 360, 363
Gladwin, T., 150
Glovsky, L., 302
Goddard, H. H., 10, 11, 12, 374
Goldberg, I., 280, 291
Goldfarb, W., 30, 34
Goldiamond, I., 214, 223
Goldschmidt, M., 376
Goodman, L., 385
Gorton, C., 202, 209
Gottsleben, R. H., 331, 333
Gottwald, H. L., 303
Gould, L. J., 177
Graves, W. S., 385
Green, M. J., 264
Greene, M., 279
Grissey, O. L., 167
Grould, K., 360
Guess, D., 302

Guggenbuhl, J. J., 5
Gunzburg, H. C., 379, 382
Guthrie, G. M., 382

Hackenbush, F., 374
Hall, J., 51, 373
Hamilton, J., 217, 218, 219, 220, 227, 304
Harlow, H. F., 30, 34
Harrison, J. H., 385
Haskel, R. H., 16
Hayden, F. J., 360
Heber, R., 118, 124, 255, 310
Heilman, A. E., 248
Henriksen, K., 220, 227, 304
Henry, J., 140, 157
Hersh, A., 253
Herzberg, F., 236
Hicks, C. B., 147
Hinojosa, V., 39, 40, 53
Hobbs, M. A., 277
Hobbs, M. T., 150
Hobbs, N., 385
Hollis, H., 202, 209
Holmes, J., 12
Holt, R. R., 375
Holz, W., 214, 215, 216, 217, 221
Horowitz, H., 67
Horsfield, E., 1
Horton, M. M., 340
House, B. J., 225
Howe, S. G., 4, 5, 6, 8, 9, 11
Hudson, M. G., 329
Humphrey, H. H., 78
Hundziak, M., 227
Hunt, J. G., 383
Hunter, R. M., 130, 277
Hurder, W. P., 37
Hutt, M. L., 379

Immel, R. K., 327
Irwin, J. V., 330
Itard, J. M., 2, 273, 327

Jackson, S., 301
James, W., 373
Jaslow, R., 264, 318
Jenkins, I., 376, 378
Jenne, W. G., 249
Jervis, J., 118
Johnson, A., 10

Johnson, D., 385
Johnson, O., 276, 281
Jones, R. W., 379
Jordan, J. E., 310
Jordine, J. E., 367
Jordon, T. E., 331
Jorsweick, E., 382

Kahne, M. C., 145
Kallikak, M., 374
Kanner, L., 374
Kantor, L. A., 275
Kaplan, A. R., 386
Kennedy, R. C., 384, 385
Kephart, N. C., 167
Kerlin, I. N., 10
Kerr, C., 144, 149
Kidder, J. D., 383
Kilburn, V. T., 361
Kim, P. J., 130
Kime, W. L., 264
King, R. D., 71, 88, 173, 197
Kinde, S., 331, 334
Kirk, S. A., 124, 276, 281, 308, 310, 331
Kish, G., 207, 216, 217
Klaber, M. M., 34, 38, 43, 53, 170, 177,
    178, 183, 193, 197, 198
Klackenberg, G., 164
Kloswowski, R. K., 209, 226
Knowles, K. G. J. C., 144
Kott, M. G., 264
Kraft, I., 3
Kretch, D., 145
Kweback, S., 128

Lake, D., 253
Lawson, R., 206
Lazersfeld, P., 130
Leach, R., 340, 342, 346, 352
Lent, J., 210, 220
Lerman, J. W., 333
Levene, S., 301
Levinson, B. J., 117
Liepmann, C., 365
Lilly, R., 304
Lilywhite, H. S., 331
Lindsley, O., 213
Lipton, R. C., 30, 34
Lohmann, W., 123
Lombardi, T. P., 353

Lord, F. M., 125
Lovaas, I., 217, 221
Lloyd, L., 340, 342, 346
Ludkte, R., 385
Luther, M., 2
Lyle, J. G., 165
Lyons, W. F., 328

MacAndrew, C., 141
McCandless, B. R., 29
McCarthy, J. J., 331
McCullough, O. C., 12
Maisner, E. A., 382
Malloy, J. S., 331
Malpass, L. F., 383
Maney, A., 277
Marge, M., 330
Margolin, J. B., 144
Mason, L. F., 386
Martin, C. H., 382
Matthews, J., 327
Mehlman, B., 382
Menefee, A. R., 317, 318
Menninger, K. A., 382
Mercer, J. R., 258
Mercer, J. M., 70, 133, 139
Miller, C. R., 130, 131
Mischel, W., 154
Moore, O. K., 30
Moos, R. H., 157, 223
Morel, 3
Morphet, M., 300
Morrison, D. F., 277
Morrissey, J. R., 257
Morse, W., 213
Mouton, J. S., 50, 51
Mueller, M. W., 334
Muench, H., 121, 122
Mundy, L., 382
Murray, H. A., 375

Nicosia, D., 211

O'Connor, G., 130
O'Connor, N., 382
O'Gorman, G., 143
O'Leary, V., 51
Ohrenstein, D. F., 253
Olsen, K. N., 267
Olsen, M. E., 267

Olshansky, S., 248, 264
Orser, R., 208, 209, 210, 211

Pace, R., 277
Parnicky, J. J., 258, 384
Patton, W. F., 150
Pearson, P. H., 88, 317, 318
Peck, R. F., 140, 143, 145, 146, 149, 384
Peins, M., 352
Pero, J. F., 384
Perrott, M., 234
Peters, R., 301
Peterson, R., 229
Philips, S. U., 141
Pinel, P., 3
Polzien, M., 302
Poole, R. G., 353
Popick, B., 257
Porter, R. M., 254
Powers, G. R., 333
Premack, D., 207, 213
Pritchard, D. G., 275, 302
Provence, S., 30, 34
Pursley, N., 304

Rabin, A. I., 165
Raynes, N. V., 173, 197
Reed, E. W., 13
Reed, S. C., 13
Reese, E., 203
Rheingold, H. L., 165
Richards, J., 6
Rigrodsky, S., 302, 333, 352
Robbins, R. C., 133
Roberts, J. A., 386
Robins, S., 37, 51
Robinson, H. B., 329, 379, 381, 382
Robinson, N. M., 329, 379, 381, 382
Rogers, D. P., 61, 70
Rolland, J., 340, 342, 346
Roethslisberger, F. J., 145
Roos, P., 30, 35, 36, 39, 40, 41, 53
Rorschach, H., 375
Roselle, E. N., 71
Rosen, M., 390
Rosenthal, N. H., 144
Rosenzweig, M. R., 30, 34
Rotberg, J., 305
Rotter, J. B., 380

Sanders, C., 208, 209, 210, 211, 225, 226, 227
Sarason, S. B., 150, 381
Savagh, G., 122, 131
Savage, M. J., 261
Savino, M. T., 384, 385
Schaefer, E. S., 188
Scheer, R. M., 255
Scheerenberger, R. C., 20, 37, 147, 363
Scheff, T. J., 145
Schein, E. H., 37, 51
Schiefelbusch, R. L., 329, 331, 335, 339, 349
Schlanger, B. B., 331, 333, 334, 339, 351
Schneider, B., 340
Schreiber, M., 268
Scott, W. D., 145, 147, 149
Sechrest, L., 382
Seguin, E., 2, 3, 4, 5, 7, 9, 11, 327
Seitz, S., 143
Schaefer, E. S., 188
Schaeffer, M. L., 333
Shafter, A. J., 123, 139, 301
Sharpe, W. M., 255
Shaw, M. W., 386
Shearer, W. M., 333
Sherman, J. A., 229
Shotwell, A. M., 30, 34, 153, 384
Shipe, D., 30, 34
Shubert, O. W., 348, 353, 385
Sidman, M., 210, 223, 224, 225, 226, 227, 228
Silberman, C. E., 152, 153
Silverstein, A., 376, 379, 380, 381, 384
Simon, T., 374
Sircin, J., 328
Skeels, H. M., 16, 29, 165, 166, 197
Skinner, B. F., 198, 206, 210
Skodak, M. A., 29
Smaltz, J., 211, 228, 365
Smith, H. L., 117
Smith, J. O., 329, 331
Smith, M., 385
Snyder, R., 382
Sorrels, I., 376
Spachman, C. L., 361
Spitz, R. A., 30, 34
Spotts, J. V., 303
Spradlin, J., 202, 209, 210, 304, 331, 348, 349

Spreen, O., 331, 334
Spriegel, W. R., 145
Spykman, N. J., 155
Stagner, R., 144, 149
Standifer, F. R., 268
Stanton, J., 300
Stedman, D. J., 30, 34
Steer, M. D., 352
Stein, D., 376
Stephens, H. A., 310
Stephens, L., 219, 220
Sternlicht, M., 378, 382
Stevens, H. A., 118, 124
Stoddard, L., 223, 224, 225, 226, 227, 228
Strauss, A. A., 167
Styles, S., 363
Suchman, R., 226
Sullivan, H. S., 145, 148
Sumner, F. G., 328
Swartz, J. D., 152, 159

Tague, C. M., 383
Talbot, M. E., 274, 277
Tarjan, G., 59, 61, 68, 70, 71, 88, 117, 119, 123, 129, 130, 153, 254, 278, 280, 384
Tate, B., 217, 218
Taylor, D., 217, 218
Taylor, H. G., 145
Terman, L. M., 373
Terrace, H., 223, 225
Terry, G. R., 146, 149
Thormahlen, P. W., 166, 167, 173, 178, 197, 198
Thorne, G., 37, 295, 297
Tizard, J., 64, 66, 69, 70, 71, 76, 83, 87, 93
Toigo, R., 249
Toombs, W. S., 365
Touchette, P., 223
Trabasso, T., 226

Ullman, L. P., 155

Vallon, J., 340
Van de Wall, W., 365
Vanden Henvel, C. M., 348
Van Riper, C., 333, 340

Wallin, J. E. W., 16

Washburne, C., 300
Watson, D. P., 366
Watson, L., 30, 36, 43, 206, 208, 209, 210, 211, 212, 218, 225, 227, 383, 385
Watson, R., 373
Weaver, S. J., 334
Webb, C. E., 331, 334
Weiss, A., 340
Weltman, R., 261
Wesissman, H., 376
West, R., 327
Whaley, D., 217
White, J., 217, 218
Whitney, L., 209
Wilbur, C. T., 7
Wilcox, G. T., 382
Wilensky, H. L., 144
Willard, H. S., 361
Williams, R. J., 81, 150
Windle, C., 119, 120, 123, 139, 301

Wishik, S., 318
Wolf, M., 213, 383
Wolfensberger, W., 192, 307, 316, 386, 387, 388, 389
Woody, R. H., 262, 382

Yonge, K. A., 382
Yarrow, L. J., 164
Younie, W. J., 280, 287, 288, 291, 304, 305, 306

Zarfas, D. E., 261
Zeaman, D., 225, 226
Ziegler, R. C., 384
Zigler, E., 34, 150, 167, 177, 197, 256, 378, 380
Zipf, G. K., 124
Zisk, T. K., 333
Zubin, J., 118
Zwarensteyn, S. B., 302

Subject Index

Acceptance of retarded child, 248
American Association on Mental
    Deficiency, 19, 21, 22, 31, 282,
    330–331
American Breeder's Association, 14, 15
American Speech and Hearing
    Association, 330, 336
Association of Medical Officers of
    American Institutions for Idiotic
    and Feebleminded Persons, 4
Attendants, 24, 25–26
    attitudes of, 189–190

Behavior
    accelerating, 208
    antisocial, 277
    decelerating, 213
    modification, 383
    shaping and maintaining, 204, 229
Boundaries in the institution
    temporal, 143–154
    spatial, 143, 154–158

Classification by statistical technique,
    131–132
Clinical psychology
    assessment, 379
    therapeutic function, 381
Community
    provision for the retarded, 15–16
    and the retarded, 132–133
    services, 60
    social agencies, 133–134

Computer
    use in institutions, 123
Connecticut Regional Center Program
    outpatient services, 167–169
    residential services, 170–172
    service list, 172
Current trends in residential care, 60

Dental work, 322
Deprivation, early environment, 30
Diagnosis and evaluation, medical,
    319–320

Education
    administrative view, 296
    effectiveness in institutions, 300
    evaluation, 285
    foreign country programs, 308
    future developments, 302
    objectives in institutions, 280–283
    of the public, 80
    residential, 283
    time allocation, 294
Effects of institutionalization, 164–167
Employees of institutions, 138
    absenteeism, 144–149
    employer relationship, 146–149,
        153–154
    work hours, 149–150
Equipment
    selection of, 96
Etiology, medical classification, 22–23
Eugenics Movement, 11–14, 19

Financing residential facilities
  federal grant programs, 30, 31
  planning, 69
  sources of funding, 391
Foster care, 36
  Grandparent Program, 39
  home supervision, 83
French Academy of Sciences, 273

Half-way House, 35
"Hawthorne" effect, 39
Hearing in the retarded, 333–334
Hospital improvement program, 39
Hospitals, 14
  records and research, 118–119
  "day or night" care, 83

Inservice training, 37, 384
Institutions, 9, 117
  administration, 196–199
  aims, 173
  architecture, 42
  behavior classification, 21–22
  boundaries, 143–158
  characteristics influencing educational
    programming, 291
  characteristics of residents, 21, 277–280
  current status, 19–26
  electro-chemical process, as, 121
  future goals, 78
  maintenance costs, 22, 24
  personnel, 24–25
  populations, 16–19, 277–280
  programs, 22–23, 78
  rated capacity, 20
  research in, 27
  short-term care, 19–20
  space, patient and employee, 154–158
  waiting lists and periods, 20–21
Intelligence tests, 10, 19
Inter-institutional research, 172–196
  attendant attitudes, 187–190
  attendant behavior, 183
  institutional routine, 185–187
  parents of retardates, 193–196
  professional staff, 190–193
  retardate interpersonal behavior,
    184–185
Jet-age syndrome, 147

Latent Class Model, 130–131
Language in the retarded, 334–335

Manpower development within the
    institution, 79
Markov chain, 125–129
Medical model, 316–317
Medical needs of retardates, 317–318
Medical Services
  components, 316
  counseling with parents, 320
  diagnostic and evaluation, 319–320
  laboratories, 323
  organization, 316–317
  preventive medicine, 320–322
  pharmacy, 323–324
  physical medicine, 324
  records, 324–325
  supportive programs, 322–323
Moonlighting, 152–153
Moral treatment, 3
Multivariate analyses, 130–132

National Association for Retarded
    Children, 30, 39, 276
Negroes in institutions, 21
Net change model, 119–120

Operant conditioning, 30, 202
  see also Behavior, modification

Parents of Retardates, 193–196
  counseling, 385
Patient care, 78
Pauper Idiot Law, 4
Personnel employment in education, 298
Personnel shortage in institutions,
    192–193
Planning
  architect, 67
  collection of data for, 64
  cross agency, 62
  description of construction project,
    88, 89
  preliminary steps, 64
  projected population of facility, 81
  residential facilities, 61
  specialized services, 90
  supportive systems, 103–104

Philosophy and goals of residential facility preliminary statement, 70
Physiological methods and education, 2–3, 7, 9, 273
Populations, *see* institutional populations
Possessions of patients, 142
Pre-admission services, 34
Premack hypothesis, 207
President's Panel on Mental Retardation, 19, 117
Prevention of mental retardation, 30
Professional staff in institutions, 38, 190–192
Programs in institutions
    evaluative, 124–129
    multivariate approach, 130–132
    socialization, 35
    speech and hearing, 340–349
    writing of, 73
Public Schools, the retarded in, 16

Quarter-way House, 35

Rehabilitation, 151
Reinforcement, 206
    of institutional personnel, 236
Release-Return Models, 119–121
Research
    in the institution, 39–40, 79, 95, 118, 387
Self-care scale, 179–180
Self-help training, 275–276
Sensory stimulation, 275, 276
    see also physiological method
Shaping and maintaining behavior
    retardates, 204
    institutional personnel, 229
Special classes, 16, 92
Speech in the retarded, 331–333
Speech and hearing programs, 340–349
    administrative location, 341–342
    case selection, 344–345
    effectiveness, 348–349
    facilities, 346–348
    personnel considerations, 345–346
    present and future, 349–354
    therapist's qualifications and responsibilities, 342–344

Speech and hearing objectives with mental retardation, 338–340
Speech and hearing therapist, 335–336
    qualifications, 342
    responsibilities, 342–344
    standards, 331
    training in mental retardation, 336–338
Social work
    admission process, 252
    discharge of patients, 258
    formulating institutional policies, 263
    implication of institutional setting casework practice, 261
    manpower problems, 267
    placement services, 257
    post-admission services, 253
    pre-admission services, 247
    role problems, 265
    services outside the institution, 250
    services to the community, 259
Southern Region Education Board Attendant Training Project, 37
Stimulus control, 222
    of institutional personnel, 239
Sub-professionals in Psychology, 385

Teaching Behavior Modification: Principles, 231, 235
Therapy
    adjunctive, 367
    industrial, 365
    music, 362
    occupational, 361
    recreational, 358
Trainable retarded, 9
    education of, 284–285
    programs for, 28
Training
    of patients, 79
    of staff, 37
Treatment of patients, 78

University affiliated centers, 40, 91

Volunteers in the institution, 38–40, 151, 367